NUCLEAR MEDICINE
A TEACHING FILE

Nuclear Medicine
A Teaching File

Frederick L. Datz, M.D.
Professor of Radiology
Director of Nuclear Medicine
The University of Utah School of Medicine
Salt Lake City, Utah

Gregory G. Patch, M.D.
Department of Radiology
The University of Utah School of Medicine
Salt Lake City, Utah

John M. Arias, M.D.
Department of Radiology
The University of Utah School of Medicine
Salt Lake City, Utah

Kathryn A. Morton, M.D.
Associate Professor of Medicine
The University of Utah School of Medicine
Chief of Nuclear Medicine
Veterans Administration Medical Center
Salt Lake City, Utah

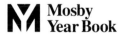 **Mosby Year Book**

St. Louis Baltimore Boston Chicago London Philadelphia Sydney Toronto

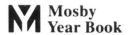
Mosby
Year Book

Dedicated to Publishing Excellence

Sponsoring Editor: Anne S. Patterson
Assistant Editor: Dana Battaglia
Assistant Managing Editor, Text and Reference: George Mary
    Gardner
Senior Production Assistant: Maria Nevinger
Proofroom Manager: Barbara Kelly

1 2 3 4 5 6 7 8 9 0 CL MV 96 95 94 93 92

Library of Congress Cataloging-in-Publication Data
Nuclear medicine : a teaching file / Frederick L. Datz . . . [et al.]
        p.   cm.
    Includes bibliographical references and index.
    ISBN 0-8016-6365-2
    1. Diagnostic imaging. 2. Nuclear medicine. I. Datz, Frederick
L.
    [DNLM: 1. Diagnostic Imaging. 2. Nuclear Medicine. WN 440
N9655]
RC78.7.D53N83 1992   91-46180
616.07'57—dc20   CIP
DNLM/DLC
for Library of Congress

To Terry and Katie—F.D.
*To Janene, Russell, Annie, Katie, and
Lizzie*—G.P.
*To Lenora, Manuel, and Blanca
Lilia*—J.A.

PREFACE

This book provides a review of all the major areas of nuclear medicine, including those that have recently entered the scene, such as SPECT brain scans. More than 200 cases are included.

The book is divided into eight chapters based on organ systems. Each chapter has case studies that cover all of the different types of imaging examinations used for that organ system. Each case consists of a set of images, a short history, and a query for a diagnosis. This is followed by the correct diagnosis, information about the imaging study (e.g., how IV dipyridamole thallium scans are performed), and a discussion of the disease process. The discussion is sufficiently detailed that the reader will have a firm grasp of how to tailor the examination to the symptoms or disease, criteria for the scan diagnosis, and other details about the disease helpful to an imager. The relationship of nuclear medicine studies to other imaging modalities in the particular disease process also is discussed. Because the appearance of different types of nuclear medicine studies varies so dramatically, and because some of the less commonly performed studies may not be familiar to some readers, we have provided normal cases, as well.

We hope you learn as much by reading this book as we did in writing it. Please feel free to contact us about suggestions for future editions.

FREDERICK L. DATZ, M.D.
GREGORY G. PATCH, M.D.
JOHN M. ARIAS, M.D.
KATHRYN A. MORTON, M.D.

CONTENTS

CHAPTER 1

Endocrine

CASE 1

History.—24-year-old woman complained of feeling tired all the time.

Labs.—Thyroid function test results were normal.

Scan.—^{123}I thyroid scan.

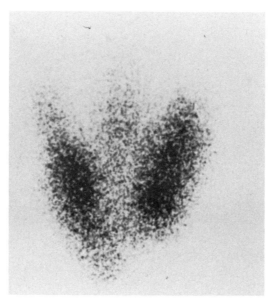

Anterior view of neck.

Findings.—Prominent midline projection of activity from isthmus.

Diagnosis.—Normal thyroid gland with prominent pyramidal lobe.

A pyramidal lobe is present in approximately 35% of patients. It usually arises from the isthmus or adjacent portion of the lobes, more commonly on the left.

In the embryo, the main anlage of thyroid cells develops as an endodermal downgrowth from the foramen cecum of the tongue. Cell remnants along this tract of lingual evagination often connect with the thyroid gland to produce the pyramidal lobe. In addition to being a normal variant, pyramidal lobe visualization is common in Graves' disease and Hashimoto's thyroiditis.

This scan also illustrates another common variant in thyroid anatomy: the left lobe is smaller than the right. The normal ratio of projected area of the lobes on anterior view is left/right = 0.8.

CASE 2

History.—Infant, 2½ weeks old, with low T_4 and elevated thyroid-stimulating hormone levels on newborn screening.

Scan.—The scan was obtained 20 minutes after IV administration of 1 mCi ^{99m}Tc pertechnetate.

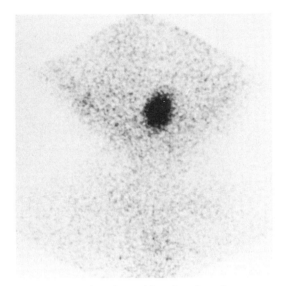

Anterior view of head and neck.

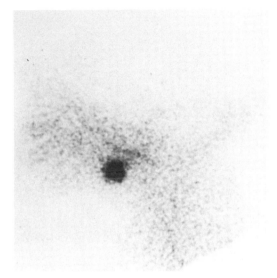

Left lateral view of head and neck.

Findings.—Functioning midline thyroid tissue located in the region of the posterior third of the tongue. Thyroid bed has no significant activity.

Diagnosis.—Lingual thyroid gland.

Neonatal hypothyroidism is detected on newborn screening in approximately 1 in 5,000 births. Evaluation of these infants usually includes a thyroid scan.

A lingual thyroid gland is caused by incomplete descent of the thyroid gland during the embryonic stage. A lingual thyroid gland usually is hypofunctional, and it is important that these children receive prompt full replacement doses of thyroxine (T_4) to assure normal intellectual development.

Lingual thyroid tissue also may manifest as a swelling or mass in the back of the tongue or upper part of the neck. Because this may be the patient's only functional thyroid tissue, it is important that a thyroid scan be performed to determine if thyroid tissue is present before a neck mass is excised; otherwise the patient could be left hypothyroid.

The thyroid gland develops as a median endodermal downgrowth from the foramen cecum of the tongue. The remnant attachment of the foramen cecum to the thyroid in the neck is the thyroglossal duct. This normally disappears by the seventh week of development. Unusual variants of thyroid development include lingual thyroid gland, thyroglossal duct cysts (which may be functional or nonfunctional), substernal extension of the thyroid gland, and congenital absence of one lobe. A pyramidal lobe, thyroid tissue along the thyroglossal duct region, is present in approximately 35% of patients and most frequently arises from the isthmus or adjacent portions of the lobes, more commonly the left. Thyroid tissue is also rarely located in teratogenic cysts in the ovary and is called struma ovarii.

^{99m}Tc pertechnetate scans in newborn infants are helpful in localizing functional thyroid tissue because background activity in the salivary glands and soft tissues of the neck and face help show the position of the gland. Iodine 123 can be used, but requires markers for localization of activity.

Another consideration in choosing a radiopharmaceutical for thyroid scanning is the radiation dose to the thyroid gland. The total radiation dose to the newborn's thyroid gland using ^{123}I or ^{131}I may be underestimated because of the higher uptake of radioiodine by the thyroid gland during the first 2 weeks of life.

CASE 3

History.— 58-year-old man with a 3-month history of an enlarging neck mass and dysphagia.

Labs.— Thyroid test results were normal.

Scan.— Imaging was performed 4 hours after ingestion of 300 μCi ^{123}I.

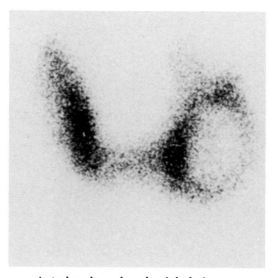

Anterior view of neck, pinhole image.

Findings.— A large "cold," or hypofunctioning, nodule in the left lobe of the thyroid gland is present.

Diagnosis.— Solitary cold thyroid nodule of the left lower pole.

The most common reason for performing a thyroid scan is to evaluate for a thyroid nodule. The scan not only detects nodules but also determines the risk for malignancy. A thyroid nodule that does not take up ^{123}I requires further evaluation because 10% to 20% of these are malignant. "Hot," or hyperfunctioning, nodules, on the other hand, usually are benign adenomas.

The thyroid scan sensitivity for detection of a cold nodule is related to its size:

6.6 mm	56%
1.2 cm	92%
>2 cm	100%

The risk for malignancy of a solitary cold thyroid nodule is increased in the following groups:

- Males or young females.
- Individuals older than 40 years of age.
- Those with a history of radiation exposure to the thyroid gland.

- Symptomatic patients (e.g., vocal cord paralysis, Horner's syndrome, dysphagia).
- Those in whom suppression with thyroid hormone fails to decrease the size of the nodule.

Fine needle aspiration is now widely used for evaluation of solitary cold nodules. This test is very sensitive and specific for thyroid cancer. The false negative rate is 6% to 10%, and the false positive rate is 0.6% to 2%.

Ultrasound also is helpful in evaluating solitary cold thyroid nodules by determining if the lesion is solid or cystic. Most thyroid carcinomas are solid and appear echogenic on ultrasound. If a lesion is cystic, a needle aspiration of the fluid can be curative. The specimen should be sent to cytology to exclude the possibility of malignancy.

Nonmalignant causes of a solitary cold nodule include adenoma, adenomatous hyperplasia, colloid cyst, hematoma, thyroiditis, fibrosis, or an extrinsic mass impinging on the thyroid gland.

CASE 4

History.— 43-year-old woman with a mass on the left side of her neck.

Scan.— ^{99m}Tc pertechnetate and ^{123}I thyroid scans.

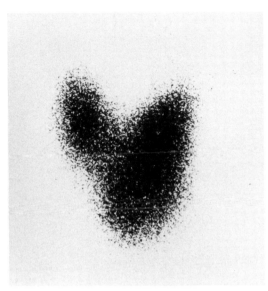 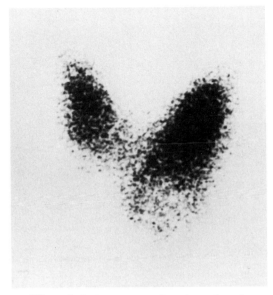

^{99m}Tc pinhole image, anterior view of neck. ^{123}I pinhole image, anterior view of neck.

Findings.— ^{99m}Tc pertechnetate: homogeneous uptake left lobe; ^{123}I: decreased uptake inferior pole on left.

Diagnosis.— Discordant nodule, thyroid carcinoma.

The use of ^{99m}Tc pertechnetate for imaging the thyroid gland requires some special precautions. ^{99m}Tc pertechnetate is trapped by the thyroid gland but not organified; ^{123}I, on the other hand, is both trapped and organified. Solitary nodules that are cold on ^{99m}Tc pertechnetate or radioiodine thyroid scan require further evaluation because 10% to 20% of these will be cancerous. In general, hot nodules on thyroid scan are benign and therefore do not require further evaluation with biopsy. One important exception is the discordant or disparate nodule, that is, a minority of nodules that appear hot or warm on ^{99m}Tc pertechnetate images but are found to be subsequently cold on radioiodine imaging. A number of these nodules have been shown to be carcinoma.

The phenomenon occurs because some well-differentiated thyroid carcinomas retain the ability to trap but not to organify. Therefore, on ^{99m}Tc pertechnetate scanning performed 20 minutes after injection, the thyroid nodule appears hot or warm. With radioiodine imaging performed at 24 hours, the same nodule appears cold because the iodine is not organified and therefore washes out over time. This same disparity can occasionally be found on radioiodine imaging with a nodule appearing warm on 4-hour images but cold on 24-hour images. Therefore, misdiagnosing a carcinoma as benign can be avoided by scheduling another set of images the following day for patients who have a warm or hot nodule on ^{123}I scan at 4 hours.

Other causes of a disparate or discordant thyroid nodule are adenomatous hyperplasia, follicular adenoma, and thyroiditis (subacute or chronic). Rare causes of a discordant nodule include colloid cyst, Hürthle cell adenoma, and thyroglossal duct cyst.

CASE 5

History.— 38-year-old man with history of radiation therapy to the region of the thymus as a child.

Scan.—^{123}I thyroid scan.

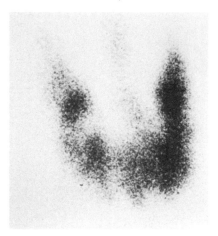

Anterior pinhole view of neck.

Findings.— Multiple cold nodules with prominent pyramidal lobe.

Diagnosis.— Multiple cold thyroid nodules, multiple thyroid carcinomas or adenomas most likely.

The findings of multiple cold nodules on a thyroid scan can be a difficult problem. Possible causes include:

- Multinodular goiter (Plummer's disease)
- Multicentric carcinoma
- Follicular adenoma
- Thyroiditis

A previous history of head and neck irradiation is important in this setting. In the past, external beam radiation was used to treat such benign conditions as tonsillar hypertrophy, cervical adenopathy, acne, and thymic enlargement. It was subsequently found that this radiation exposure increased these patients' risk for thyroid disorders in general and thyroid carcinoma specifically. Twenty percent of these patients developed some type of thyroid abnormality, with 5% to 7% developing thyroid cancer. This compares with a risk of 1 in 27,000 for nonirradiated individuals. Those found to be at highest risk were irradiated before 6 years of age. The average latency period for development of thyroid carcinoma is 20 years.

The incidence of thyroid cancer grows with increasing doses of thyroidal radiation up to 1,500 rad. With higher doses the thyroid is destroyed, and hypothyroidism, rather than cancer, results. Doses of less than 6.5 rad do not significantly increase risk above that of the normal population.

In a nonirradiated population, the finding of multiple nodules in the thyroid gland lessen the risk of cancer compared with a solitary cold nodule. The opposite is true if a patient has had prior head and neck irradiation. Thirty percent to 40% of patients with multiple thyroid nodules and a history of thyroid radiation will have thyroid cancer.

The types of thyroid malignancies found in patients with thyroidal irradiation are the same as those found in the general population. The majority are papillary and follicular carcinomas, which do not act any more aggressively than similar tumors in nonirradiated patients.

The thyroid scan is important in evaluating patients with a history of prior irradiation. The thyroid scan is more sensitive for identifying nodules than is a physical examination, and the frequency of malignancy in nodules found only with scanning is 20%.

The recommended follow-up of patients with a history of head and neck irradiation is as follows:

1. Perform careful palpation and baseline thyroid scan.
2. If the scan is normal, the patient should have a yearly follow-up examination with palpation (yearly thyroid scans are controversial).
3. If the scan is abnormal, the patient should probably undergo surgery because of the high likelihood of malignancy.
4. With diffuse enlargement without nodules on scan, suppress with thyroid hormone and reexamine in 6 months; if the scan shows a cold area, suppress with thyroid hormone and reexamine in 6 months; surgery is not indicated unless the nodule becomes palpable, because it is likely the patient has benign hypertrophy or Hashimoto's thyroiditis.

Suppression of the thyroid gland with thyroid hormone in patients with a history of previous head and neck irradiation may reduce the risk for thyroid cancer by decreasing thyroid-stimulating hormone (TSH) stimulation of the thyroid gland.

CASE 6

History.— 35-year-old woman with nervousness, palpitations, weakness, sweating, weight loss, neck fullness, and exophthalmos.

Labs.— T_3 and T_4 levels are elevated; TSH level is 0.

Scan.— After oral administration of 300 µCi of ^{123}I, thyroid uptake measurements were made at 4 and 24 hours. Multiple thyroid gland images were obtained at 4 hours.

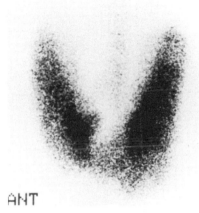

ANT

Anterior pinhole view of neck.

Findings.— The [123]I 4-hour uptake was 66% (normal range, 6%–16%); the 24-hour uptake was 80% (normal range, 10%–35%).
The scan shows diffuse homogeneous uptake in an enlarged thyroid gland with a prominent pyramidal lobe.

Diagnosis.— Graves' disease.

Graves' disease, or diffuse toxic goiter, is an autoimmune disease in which antibodies bind to thyroid-stimulating hormone (TSH) receptors of the thyroid cells, stimulating gland hypertrophy and increasing synthesis and secretion of thyroid hormone. It is a relatively common disorder, with a peak incidence in the third and fourth decades, but it may occur at any age. It is more common in women, with a female/male ratio of 5:1.

Manifestations of Graves' disease include general symptoms of hyperthyroidism and specific signs and symptoms of Graves' disease itself. Hyperthyroidism, if severe, is manifested by symptoms of nervousness, emotional lability, tremor, tachycardia, heat intolerance, weight loss, weakness, and diarrhea.

Increased mucopolysaccharide deposition causes the specific signs of Graves' disease, exophthalmos, pretibial myxedema, and acropathy (clubbing). Laboratory findings include elevated levels in thyroid function tests and increased radioiodine uptake. An elevated level of thyroid-stimulating immunoglobulin is specific for Graves' disease.

In Graves' disease, the thyroid scan shows diffuse homogeneous uptake with a prominent pyramidal lobe. Occasional cases show decreased uptake, suggesting cold nodules. This has been described in about 3% of cases and is often referred to as Marine-Lenhart syndrome. These patients require higher therapeutic doses of ^{131}I to ablate the thyroid gland than the usual case of Graves' disease.

Treatment options for Graves' disease include drug therapy, surgery, or radioiodine ablation. Drug treatment with blocking agents such as propylthiouracil cures only about 25% of patients. Those with the best chance of responding to drug treatment include younger patients, those with smaller glands and less severe disease, and those with recent onset of symptoms. Surgery cures 85% of patients; however, 15% relapse, and as many as 25% become hypothyroid in the first 10 years. Surgery is used infrequently at present.

Treatment with ^{131}I is effective, simple, and economical compared with surgery. Complications of therapy with ^{131}I include hypothyroidism, radiation thyroiditis, and, rarely, thyroid storm.

Thyroid storm can be avoided by interrupting antithyroid medication a few days before treatment and then resuming antithyroid therapy 3 to 4 days after treatment. β-Blockers need not be discontinued, because they have no effect on iodine concentration of the thyroid gland. A pregnancy test and careful history should be obtained on women of childbearing age to prevent radioiodine administration during pregnancy. Breast-feeding should be stopped before radioiodine therapy.

CASE 7

History.—50-year-old woman with heat intolerance and a left-sided neck mass.

Labs.—Elevated T_4, T_3, and T_3-RU levels and low TSH level.

Scan.—^{123}I thyroid scan.

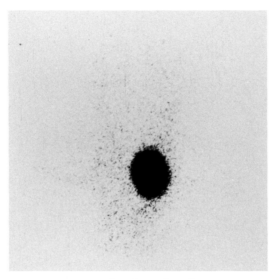

Anterior view of neck.

Findings.—Solitary focus of increased activity in the left side of the neck. The remainder of the thyroid gland is not visualized.

Diagnosis.—Toxic adenoma.

An autonomous nodule is an uncommon cause of hyperthyroidism. These nodules are hyperfunctioning adenomas. About one half are autonomous; the increased thyroid hormone they produce suppresses the remainder of the gland's function. In general, an adenoma must be 2.5 to 3.0 cm to produce enough hormone to cause hyperthyroidism.

An adenoma can be differentiated from a toxic adenoma by a suppression test. The patient is given triiodothyronine (T_3) for 1 week, and repeat imaging and thyroid uptakes are performed. If the activity is not significantly changed, the patient has an autonomous nodule. Thyroid-stimulating hormone (TSH) also can be given and the imaging repeated to prove the patient has normal but suppressed thyroid tissue.

Treatment of toxic adenoma is similar to multinodular goiter. Higher doses of ^{131}I are used than with Graves' disease. Because the remainder of the thyroid gland is suppressed, radioiodine treatment rarely causes hypothyroidism.

CASE 8

History.—30-year-old obese woman with hyperthyroidism.

Labs.—The T_4 level was elevated; the TSH level was low.

Scan.—After oral administration of 300 μCi of ^{123}I, thyroid uptake was measured at 4 and 24 hours. Thyroid scan was obtained 4 hours after ingestion.

Anterior pinhole image of neck.

Findings.—The 4- and 24-hour uptakes were 2.7% (normal, up to 16%), and 1.3% (normal, 10%–35%), respectively. The scan shows very little uptake of iodine by the thyroid gland.

Diagnosis.—Thyrotoxicosis factitia.

After further discussion with the patient, it was discovered she had been surreptitiously taking L-thyroxine sodium (Synthroid) to lose weight. Taking a patient's history before performing a thyroid scan is very important. Many substances will suppress the thyroid gland's uptake of radioiodine. These must be withheld for an appropriate interval before thyroid scanning. Medications that can decrease iodine uptake in the thyroid gland include thyroid medications (e.g., Synthroid, thyroglobuin [Proloid], and triiodothyronine sodium [Cytomel]); antithyroid medications (e.g., propylthiouracil, methimazole); medications containing iodine (e.g., providone-iodine [Betadine], antitussives, amebicides, iodinated radiographic contrast media, kelp); and penicillin, thiopental, sulfonamides, and antihistamines. The time when a scan can be performed after these substances are discontinued varies. The following provide some guidelines:

Medication	Waiting Time
Oil-based iodinated contrast	1–12 mo
Oral cholecystographic agents	1–6 mo
Intravenous (IV) contrast agents	1–2 mo
Thyroid replacement medications	1–3 mo
Antithyroid medications, antibiotics, antihistamines, thiopental sodium, antiparasitics	1–2 wk

A drug class that does not affect thyroid uptake is β-blockers. This allows a patient with hyperthyroidism to be treated with these medications during scanning and ^{131}I therapy.

One other notable cause of decreased iodine uptake by the thyroid gland is renal failure. Poor renal excretion of iodine results in an increased circulating iodine pool.

CASE 9

History.—47-year-old woman, clinically euthyroid, with an enlarging neck mass. Multiple thyroid nodules were present on palpation.

Labs.—Thyroid function test results were normal.

Scan.—After the oral administration of 300 μCi of ^{123}I, thyroid uptake was measured at 4 and 24 hours. Multiple images of the thyroid gland were also obtained 4 hours after ingestion.

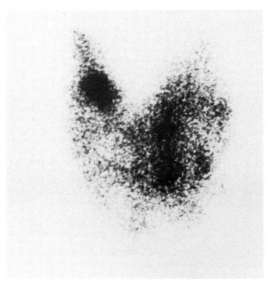

Anterior pinhole view of neck.

Findings.—The 4-hour uptake was 9.6% and the 24-hour uptake 22.0%; both results were normal. The scan shows multiple hot and cold nodules throughout the thyroid gland.

Diagnosis.—Multinodular goiter (Plummer's disease).

The development of multinodular goiter may be related to iodine deficiency. It also has a familial tendency. Multinodular goiter is more common in women than men, with a 3:1 distribution. It usually starts in adolescence and gradually progresses with advancing age. Hyperthyroidism usually does not develop until the fourth decade or later.

Results of the 4- and 24-hour uptakes are frequently normal, even if the patient is thyrotoxic. The thyroid scan shows multiple hot and cold nodules within the thyroid gland. These represent thyroid adenomas, some of which are hyperfunctioning and others of which are suppressed.

The natural history of this disease is progression to hyperthyroidism. This occurs when one of the hyperactive adenomas becomes autonomous; as the patient becomes thyrotoxic, the remaining thyroid gland is suppressed. The average duration of multinodular goiter before development of hyper-

thyroidism is 17 years. Sixty percent of patients more than 60 years of age with multinodular goiter are thyrotoxic.

Therapy for toxic multinodular goiter is similar to that for Graves' disease, with two exceptions: (1) multinodular goiter is more radioresistant than Graves' disease and is treated with higher doses; and (2) the development of hypothyroidism after therapy is much rarer in toxic multinodular goiter than in Graves' disease because the suppressed areas of the gland do not take up the radioiodine and therefore are not ablated. After eradication of the hyperfunctioning nodule, the previously suppressed tissue begins to function.

The association of multinodular goiter with thyroid cancer is somewhat unclear. Surgical specimens have been found to contain carcinoma in between 4% and 17% of cases. However, the number of clinical cases of carcinoma in multinodular goiter is much less.

CASE 10

History.— 40-year-old woman with painless enlargement of the neck.

Scan.—^{123}I scan.

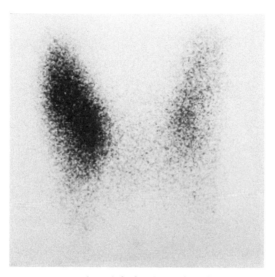

Anterior pinhole view of neck.

Findings.— Inhomogeneous with less uptake in left lobe than right.

Diagnosis.— Hashimoto's thyroiditis.

Hashimoto's thyroiditis is a common chronic disorder of the thyroid gland. Its etiology is autoimmune, and it frequently coexists with other autoimmune diseases such as pernicious anemia, Sjögren's syndrome, systemic lupus erythematosus, rheumatoid arthritis, Addison's disease, and Graves' disease. The autoimmune nature of the disease is reflected by high titers of antithyroglobulin and antimicrosomal antibodies and by lymphocytic infiltration of the thyroid.

The reported incidence of this disease is 3 to 6 per 10,000, but this likely underestimates the true incidence because of underdiagnosis. Hashimoto's thyroiditis usually affects middle-aged women. In the early stages, most patients are euthyroid and have painless enlargement of the neck. As the disease progresses, the thyroid gland becomes replaced by fibrosis and lymphocytic infiltrate, leaving the patient hypothyroid. Patients usually require chronic thyroid replacement therapy.

On palpation, the thyroid gland has a firm rubbery consistency; it is enlarged, and the pyramidal lobe may be prominent. Laboratory findings include normal to low T$_4$ levels and elevated levels of antithyroglobulin and antimicrosomal antibodies.

The thyroid scan findings vary considerably. The gland may appear normal, with a prominent pyramidal lobe. Patchy uptake, as well as overall poor thyroid visualization, are frequently seen. About 50% of patients have nodules. These may be hot or cold and solitary or multiple. The appearance can simulate a multinodular goiter (Plummer's disease).

Radioiodine uptake is variable. It is elevated early in the disease and falls to less than normal as the patient becomes hypothyroid. Because of an organification defect in Hashimoto's disease, the 2- or 4-hour uptake may be elevated in the face of a lower 24-hour uptake.

A ^{99m}Tc pertechnetate scan will often show better thyroid visualization than will an ^{123}I scan. Again, this is because of the ability of the thyroid gland to trap but not organify in Hashimoto's disease.

The organification defect can be demonstrated with a potassium perchlorate washout test. An oral dose of ^{131}I is given and a 2-hour uptake measured. The patient is then given an oral dose of potassium perchlorate, which competitively displaces iodide that has been trapped but not organified. Serial uptakes every 15 minutes are then performed for 90 minutes. Test results are abnormal if the uptake falls 15% below the 2-hour value.

Hashimoto's disease is associated with an increased risk of lymphoma. A biopsy should be performed on a dominant or enlarging cold mass on thyroid scan in these patients.

CASE 11

History.— 32-year-old woman with history of recent upper respiratory tract infection and subsequent development of painful enlargement of the thyroid gland, low-grade fever, and symptoms of hyperthyroidism.

Scan.—^{123}I scan and uptake.

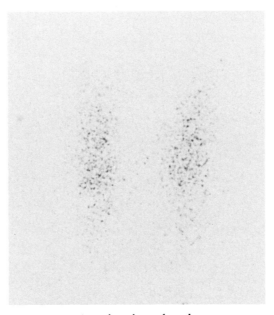

Anterior view of neck.

Findings.— 24-hour uptake = 0.9%. The thyroid gland showed little uptake even with prolonged imaging.

Diagnosis.—Subacute thyroiditis.

Painful enlargement of the thyroid gland may be caused by subacute (DeQuervain's) thyroiditis, acute suppurative thyroiditis, thyroid cancer (particularly anaplastic carcinoma), hemorrhage into a thyroid cyst or nodule, or rapid onset of Hashimoto's thyroiditis. The diagnosis can be narrowed by a careful history and physical examination and by laboratory tests.

Subacute thyroiditis and Hashimoto's thyroiditis sometimes have similar clinical manifestations. However, distinguishing between them is important because they have very different clinical courses.

Subacute thyroiditis is more common than Hashimoto's thyroiditis. The onset of subacute thyroiditis is gradual—over 1 to 2 weeks, with the disease fluctuating for an additional 3 to 6 weeks. Recurrences of diminishing intensity may extend over many months. The majority of patients recover without therapy and do not suffer any long-term ill effects. Ten percent of patients develop permanent hypothyroidism. Hashimoto's thyroiditis, on the other hand, causes long-term hypothyroidism, requiring chronic replacement therapy in the majority of patients.

Subacute thyroiditis is often associated with a history of a recent upper respiratory tract infection. This is commonly accompanied by fever, malaise, anorexia, and a sore throat. Results of laboratory tests show a mild leukocytosis, moderately elevated erythrocyte sedimentation rate, and mildly increased thyroid functions. Antithyroid antibodies are absent.

The thyroid scan findings of subacute thyroiditis are decreased 4- and 24-hour uptakes and poor or nonvisualization of the gland. In as many as 20% of patients, only one lobe is involved initially, showing decreased uptake. As this area resolves, the other lobe may become involved.

The decreased radioiodine uptake is usually in the presence of an elevated T$_4$ level. Other causes of an elevated T$_4$ level in the face of a low or normal ^{123}I or ^{131}I uptake include the use of thyroid medications (Synthroid), Hashimoto's thyroiditis, multinodular goiter, and struma ovarii.

Treatment is usually symptomatic, with analgesics for pain and a β-blocker for hyperthyroid symptoms.

CASE 12

History.— 24-year-old woman with increased nervousness, suspected of having Graves' disease. She denied any history of drug ingestion or recent intravenous contrast study. We were requested to do a 24-hour uptake in anticipation of ^{131}I therapy.

Labs.— T_4: 18.7 (μg/dL (high); antimicrosomal antibodies: negative; TSH: 0.03 μU/mL (low).

Scan.— Uptake was measured over the neck. 24 hours after the oral ingestion of 5 μCi of ^{131}I.

Findings.— The 24-hour uptake over the neck was 1%, verified with repeat measurement and calculations by a second technologist.

Diagnosis.— Elevated T_4 level and low ^{123}I uptake of unknown cause.

This is a perplexing situation where all clinical and laboratory evidence suggests Graves' disease and the patient has a low (or normal) radioiodine uptake. The patient was interviewed a second time and questioned about any possible ingestion of medication or iodine. The possibility of factitious thyroid hormone use was raised and denied. The referring physician had performed an initial evaluation for thyroiditis, which was negative. Yet this patient has clinical hyperthyroidism and is seen for possible thyroid ablation with ^{131}I.

Possible causes of elevated T_4 levels and low or normal ^{131}I uptake are:

- Exogenous iodine administration (e.g., IV iodinated contrast administration, medications, kelp)
- Thyroid medication
- Thyroiditis (subacute or chronic)

Uncommon and rare causes include:

- Thyrotoxicosis with rapid turnover rate
- Toxic adenoma
- Toxic nodular goiter
- Metastatic thyroid carcinoma
- Struma ovarii
- Trapping defect with thyrotoxicosis

An uptake dose at 2 to 4 hours will pick up cases of thyrotoxicosis with rapid turnover rate. If no cause for the low uptake can be found, we repeat the uptake in 1 month. Often the uptake will be elevated then. Presumably there is interference from a drug that the patient did not remember taking.

CASE 13

History.—56-year-old woman with follicular thyroid carcinoma who underwent total thyroidectomy 6 weeks earlier and now is seen for metastatic work-up.

Labs.—The TSH level is 76 μU/mL.

Scan.—A preoperative scan was performed with 300 μCi of ^{123}I. Postoperatively, the patient underwent an ^{131}I uptake, ^{99m}Tc pertechnetate scan, and 10 mCi of ^{131}I whole-body scan.

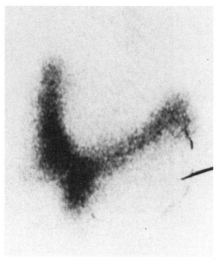

Anterior view of neck, ^{123}I scan.

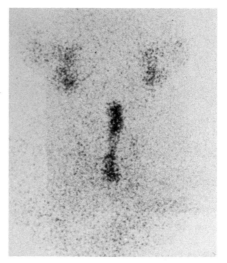

^{99m}Tc pertechnetate scan, anterior view of neck.

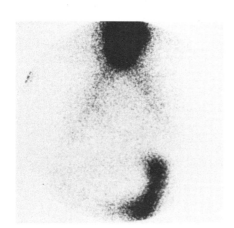

Anterior view of chest, ^{131}I scan.

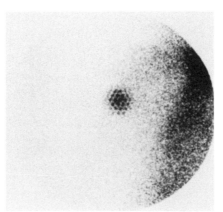

Right shoulder, ^{131}I scan.

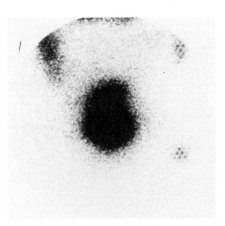

Anterior view of pelvis,^{131}I scan.

Findings.—Preoperative ^{123}I scan shows a large cold nodule in the left lower pole of the thyroid gland. Postoperative 24-hour ^{131}I uptake is 7%. ^{99m}Tc pertechnetate scan reveals a hypertrophied pyramidal lobe. ^{131}I whole-body imaging shows neck, right proximal humeral, and left femoral uptake.

Diagnosis.—Follicular thyroid carcinoma with bony metastases.

The majority of thyroid cancers are either papillary or follicular, with papillary being more common; often the tumor is a mixture of these two types. The age at diagnosis peaks in the second and third decades.

The presenting sign in 95% of cases is a palpable mass in the thyroid gland. The initial thyroid scan most often shows a cold nodule confirmed to be cancer by biopsy. The initial form of treatment should be a total thyroidectomy, followed by ^{131}I therapy of any remaining normal thyroid tissue and tumor. The patient should then be maintained on long-term suppression with high-dose thyroid hormone replacement to completely suppress TSH levels.

Complete surgical removal of the thyroid gland before ^{131}I therapy is necessary for cure (a significant percentage of thyroid cancers are bilateral) and to improve follow-up cancer surveillance. The rise in serum thyroid-stimulating hormone (TSH) after total thyroidectomy dramatically increases sensitivity of the whole-body ^{131}I scan for metastases.

With proper treatment, the prognosis for patients with thyroid carcinoma is very good. Patients with papillary carcinoma have a 10-year survival of 90% or better; with follicular carcinoma, this drops to 80%. However, for those with metastatic disease outside the neck, 10-year survival is as low as 25%. At presentation, the incidence of metastatic disease outside the neck is only about 1% for papillary and 4% for follicular carcinoma.

Factors that worsen prognosis include metastases outside the neck, follicular histology with vascular invasion, advanced patient age, male sex, and a primary lesion greater than 1.5 cm. Surprisingly, the presence or absence of local lymph node metastases in the neck does not affect prognosis.

Individuals who have received therapeutic external radiation to the head and neck in infancy or childhood have an increased risk of developing well-differentiated thyroid carcinoma. These radiation treatments were used to treat thymic enlargement, lymphatic hypertrophy, and acne. Radiation-induced thyroid cancers are not more aggressive than naturally occurring tumors. However, the risk of multicentric thyroid carcinoma is increased.

The metastatic work-up of well-differentiated thyroid cancer cannot begin until after all thyroid tissue is removed; otherwise, all the radioiodine administered will be taken up by the native thyroid gland.

After a total thyroidectomy, thyroid replacement is withheld for 6 weeks to allow the TSH level to rise. A TSH level greater than 30 to 50 μU/mL should be reached before the ^{131}I whole-body scan is done. Pregnancy must be excluded by history and testing of serum β-human chorionic gonadotropin (β-HCG) in women of reproductive age. In addition, women are warned not to become pregnant for 6 to 12 months after whole-body ^{131}I scanning or therapy.

A 24-hour ^{131}I uptake is obtained using 5 μCi of ^{131}I. Then, if the uptake is appropriate, a whole-body ^{131}I scan is performed using 10 mCi ^{131}I. If there is evidence of residual thyroid tissue in the neck or evidence of distant metastases, the patient is treated with 150 to 200 mCi of ^{131}I to eradicate any functioning thyroid tissue. A posttherapy whole-body scan increases the sensitivity for distant metastatic disease.

If the uptake is high, the surgeon may have left too much normal thyroid tissue in place. In these cases, a lower dose of 30 mCi may be given before any high-dose therapy.

The following is a summary of our approach to the workup and treatment of well-differentiated thyroid cancer:

1. Perform a total thyroidectomy.
2. Do not prescribe T$_4$ replacement for 6 weeks after surgery (or prescribe T$_3$ for the first 4 weeks).
3. Six weeks postoperatively, check TSH level; if it is more than 30 μU/mL, proceed with step 4; if it is less than 30 μU/mL, wait 1 week and redraw TSH level, or do low-dose uptake and scan to evaluate for possible incomplete thyroidectomy.
4. By history and serum β-HCG level, exclude the possibility of pregnancy in reproductive-age women.
5. Check chest x-ray film, complete blood cell counts and chemistry panel for any evidence of metastatic disease.
6. Administer a dose of 5 μCi of ^{131}I for 24-hour uptake.
7. Measure 24-hour ^{131}I uptake in the neck the next day. If uptake is low (<1%–7%), give 10 mCi ^{131}I whole-body scanning dose. If higher uptake, consider ^{99m}Tc pertechnetate scan to evaluate remaining thyroid gland, and consider ablation of remaining thyroid remnant with 30 mCi. Proceed with whole-body scan in 3 to 6 months.
8. Do an ^{131}I whole-body scan 72 hours later. If there is no detectable uptake, start Synthroid at doses of 0.3 mg/day or as high as tolerated. (This is to completely suppress TSH production by the pituitary gland.) Then skip to step 12.
9. If uptake is present in the neck with no distant metastases, admit the patient to the hospital for therapy with 150 mCi. If uptake is needed in the neck and lungs, use 175 mCi. If uptake is needed in the neck and bones, treat with 200 mCi.
10. Perform posttherapy whole-body scan 5 days later.
11. Start or restart Synthroid at doses of 0.3 mg/day (or as high as tolerated) after performing step 10.
12. Repeat steps 2 through 8 yearly until results are normal for 2 to 3 consecutive years; then repeat every 3 to 5 years.
13. In addition, follow progress with serum thyroglobulin levels every 6 to 12 months and yearly chest x-ray studies.

CASE 14

History.— 48-year-old woman with papillary thyroid carcinoma after thyroidectomy.

Scan.—^{201}Tl whole-body scan and ^{131}I whole-body scan.

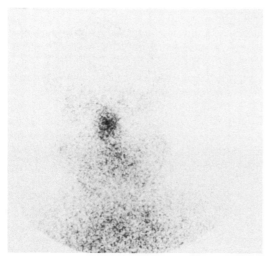

Anterior view of head and neck, ^{201}Tl scan.

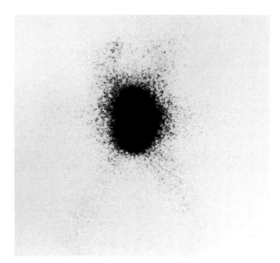

Anterior view of neck, ^{131}I scan.

Findings.—^{201}Tl: no definite neck uptake; ^{131}I: intense neck uptake.

Diagnosis.— Recurrent thyroid carcinoma.

The correct metastatic work-up of patients with well-differentiated thyroid carcinoma has been debated recently. The current standard is to image after total thyroidectomy 6 weeks later to allow the thyroid-stimulating hormone (TSH) level to rise above a minimum level of 30 μU/mL. At that time, a whole-body ^{131}I scan is performed to detect any residual thyroid tissue in the neck or any evidence of metastatic disease. If either is present, the patient is given a therapeutic dose of ^{131}I. A posttherapy whole-body scan with increased sensitivity for the detection of metastases is then performed.

An alternative to the ^{131}I whole-body scan is whole-body thallium 201 scanning. Thallium has been shown to concentrate in well-differentiated thyroid cancer. The mechanism is unclear. Thyroid cancer will usually manifest as a cold nodule on radioiodine scan. If the patient is subsequently injected with ^{201}Tl and images of the neck are obtained, the cold defect fills in. The combination of the two studies may be helpful in establishing the cause of a cold nodule. The pre-

ferred way to evaluate a cold nodule seen on thyroid scan, however, is percutaneous biopsy.

The principal advantage of whole-body ^{201}Tl imaging in patients with thyroid cancer is that they do not need to stop thyroid hormone before the study. This avoids a period of symptomatic hypothyroidism and avoids the necessary elevation in TSH levels, which theoretically can stimulate tumor growth.

The main disadvantage of the whole-body ^{201}Tl scan is its poor sensitivity for metastatic disease. The sensitivity of ^{201}Tl scanning was initially reported as being better than that of the whole-body iodine scan. Several subsequent investigators reported much poorer sensitivity. In our experience, whole-body ^{201}Tl imaging is about half as sensitive for metastatic disease as whole-body ^{131}I scans. Sensitivity for metastases may be better than for residual thyroid tissue.

^{201}Tl scanning can be a useful adjunct in selected patients, but it should not replace the ^{131}I scan.

CASE 15

History.— 30-year-old woman with papillary carcinoma. She had delivered a child 3 months earlier, and had recently ceased breast-feeding.

Scan.— 10 mCi of ^{131}I for whole-body scan.

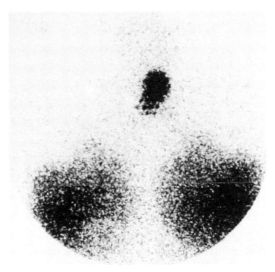

Anterior view of neck and chest.

Findings.— Focus of uptake in the neck and two foci in the chest area.

Diagnosis.— Recurrent tumor in the neck. Breast uptake because of recent breast-feeding.

^{131}I is concentrated in several tissues other than thyroid tissue. It is common to see activity in the salivary glands, stomach, colon, kidneys, and bladder. Liver activity is sometimes seen.

^{131}I will also concentrate in the breast tissue of female patients. The iodine is excreted into the breast milk. Therefore, it is imperative that patients cease breast-feeding before being given ^{131}I. The activity will be excreted for such a long time after administration that breast-feeding must be terminated rather than delayed as is done with Tc agents.

Even if the patient has ceased breast-feeding, some patients continue to lactate for a significant period of time. In these cases, blocking agents may be necessary. In this case, to prevent unnecessary radiation to the breast, high-dose therapy was delayed for several months to allow lactation to completely resolve.

Radioiodine is contraindicated during pregnancy; hyperthyroidism should be treated with antithyroid medication. Treatment after approximately the first trimester will result in fetal thyroid ablation. Treatment earlier than this will not affect the fetal thyroid gland because it does not function. However, the radiation effects on the fetus preclude its use in this period as well.

CASE 16

History.— 57-year-old woman with recurrent calcium oxalate renal calculi.

Labs.— Hypercalcemia, hypophosphatemia, and an elevated PTH level were found.

Scan.— Parathyroid scan using both a ^{201}Tl scan and a ^{99m}Tc pertechnetate scan. A subtraction image was also done.

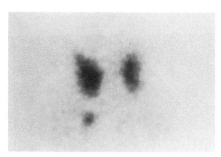 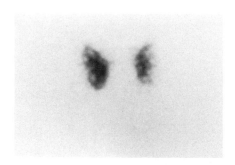 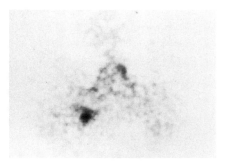

^{201}Tl anterior pinhole view of neck.　　　^{99m}Tc pertechnetate anterior pinhole view of neck.　　　Subtraction image.

Findings.— Focus of ^{201}Tl activity inferior to right lobe of thyroid gland.

Diagnosis.— Parathyroid adenoma causing primary hyperparathyroidism.

Hyperparathyroidism is caused by increased circulating parathyroid hormone (PTH) levels. Abnormal calcium and phosphate metabolism occur, with clinical signs most often related to elevated calcium levels. The disorder occurs in about 1 in 700 patients, with a 70% female predominance. The average age at onset is 56 years; it is very rare in children.

The most common cause of hyperparathyroidism (90%) is a single benign parathyroid adenoma. The remaining 10% of cases are caused by secondary hyperplasia (due to renal failure), primary hyperplasia, and rarely parathyroid carcinoma.

Hyperparathyroidism can be part of a hereditary syndrome that includes multiple endocrine abnormalities. Multiple endocrine neoplasia type I (MEN I) includes tumors or hyperplasia of the parathyroid glands, pituitary gland, adrenal cortex, thyroid gland, and pancreatic islet cells. MEN II consists of pheochromocytoma, medullary thyroid carcinoma, and, in 50% of cases, parathyroid hyperplasia.

Signs and symptoms of hyperparathyroidism classically involve the kidney and skeletal system. Renal involvement occurs in 60% to 70% of patients and is manifested by either recurrent nephrolithiasis or nephrocalcinosis. Generalized osteopenia, osteitis fibrosa cystica, and phalangeal tuft resorption with subperiosteal resorption are the main skeletal manifestations. Other associated findings include neuromuscular weakness, psychiatric disorders, duodenal ulcers, chondrocalcinosis, and pseudogout.

Parathyroid imaging is performed using two isotopes, ^{201}Tl and ^{99m}Tc pertechnetate. ^{201}Tl is taken up by parathyroid and thyroid tissue. ^{99m}Tc pertechnetate is concentrated only in the thyroid gland and is subtracted from the ^{201}Tl view. Any remaining activity represents parathyroid tissue.

Specifically, an initial wide field of view image and then pinhole views of the neck are obtained after ^{201}Tl injection. This is followed by ^{99m}Tc pertechnetate injection, with additional pinhole images of the neck obtained without moving the patient. A computer subtraction is then performed.

Most parathyroid adenomas are evident by visual inspection of both images without computer subtraction; however, a minority will be seen only on the computer subtraction image.

Normal parathyroid glands and about one half of hyperplastic glands are not detected using this technique. The scan has an overall sensitivity of 80% to 90% for pathologic conditions, with sensitivity for a given adenoma dependent on its size. The scan's sensitivity is 70% to 80% for parathyroid adenomas that are 500 to 1,500 mg; in larger adenomas, the sensitivity approaches 100%. Smaller tumors are infrequently imaged. Because hyperplastic glands (excluding renal failure patients) are smaller than adenomas, they are more likely to be missed.

It is important to remember that parathyroid imaging is not used to diagnose hyperparathyroidism; the diagnosis is made by clinical and laboratory findings. Imaging is performed to localize parathyroid adenomas before surgical exploration. Preoperative localization reduces surgical time, especially if the gland is ectopic. When the information from the scan is used, 90% to 95% of patients are cured with one operation.

CASE 17

History.—55-year-old man with hyperparathyroidism referred for preoperative localization of a probable parathyroid adenoma. A palpable mass was present in the right side of his neck.

Scan.—^{201}Tl-^{99m}Tc parathyroid scan.

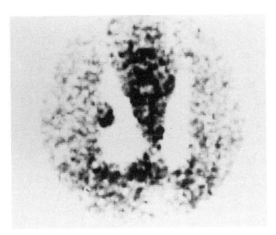

Anterior subtraction image of neck.

Findings.—Focal area of activity in the mid–right lobe remaining on the subtraction image.

Diagnosis.—Thyroid nodule simulating a parathyroid adenoma.

^{201}Tl has an affinity for a variety of neoplasms in addition to parathyroid adenomas. The cause of uptake is unknown but may be related to increased blood flow or to increased potassium content in tumors (^{201}Tl is a potassium analogue). This can produce false positive parathyroid scans.

The most common false positive cause is a thyroid tumor, benign or malignant. Thyroid nodules are common in the age range that parathyroid adenomas occur (average age, 56 years). In fact, 40% of individuals more than 50 years of age will have a thyroid nodule. Careful palpation of the neck before scanning is important to determine if the patient has a thyroid nodule. Unless parathyroid adenomas are quite large, they are usually not palpable.

Other causes of false positive parathyroid scans are:

- Chronic thyroiditis
- Hodgkin's lymphoma
- Lymph node involvement from sarcoidosis, metastases, etc.
- Normal pyramidal lobe
- Subtraction artifacts

CASE 18

History.—36-year-old woman with persistent hypertension and elevated catecholamine levels.

Scan.—^{131}I MIBG and ^{99m}Tc DTPA renal scan. The renal scan was subtracted from the MIBG image.

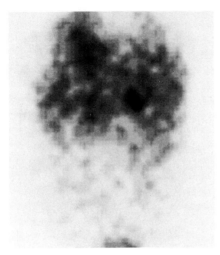

Posterior MIBG image of abdomen.

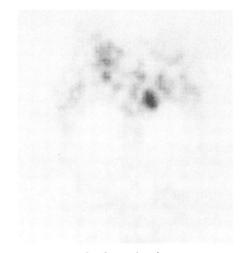

Renal subtraction image.

Findings.—MIBG: ill-defined area of increased uptake in right side of abdomen; subtraction image: focus of uptake in right adrenal gland.

Diagnosis.— Pheochromocytoma.

Pheochromocytoma is an uncommon neuroectodermal tumor arising from chromaffin cells of the sympathetic adrenal system. They produce excessive quantities of catecholamines, which are released continuously or episodically. Pheochromocytomas occur in 0.01% to 0.001% of the adult population and 0.1% of hypertensive patients. The tumor is an important correctable cause of hypertension, which if left untreated is commonly fatal. Autopsy series indicate more than one third of pheochromocytomas go undiagnosed, and most probably contributed to the death of the patient.

Pheochromocytoma is the "tumor of tens":

- 10% occur in children.
- 10% are extra-adrenal.
- 10% are malignant.
- 10% occur occur familialy (MEN IIA and IIB)
- 10% are bilateral.
- Most are <10 cm in diameter.

Clinical features of pheochromocytoma are most often related to hypertension. Sixty percent of patients have sustained hypertension, with only 40% having episodic hypertension. The paroxysmal hypertensive crises can be accompanied by anxiety attacks or even seizurelike symptoms. With time, the frequency of attacks increases. The onset of the paroxysmal attacks is sudden, with headache, palpitations, apprehension, sweating, and a sense of impending doom.

The diagnosis can be suspected in the proper clinical setting, and is established by measurement of elevated catecholamine levels or catecholamine metabolites in a 24-hour urine collection.

The role of imaging in pheochromocytoma is not for diagnosis but for localization before surgical resection. X-ray computed tomography (CT) is the primary technique for localization. Radionuclide imaging with metaiodobenzylguanidine (MIBG) is reserved for confirmation of equivocal CT findings and for identification of suspected extraadrenal sites.

MIBG is similar to norepinephrine in structure and localizes in sympathetic tissue. It is normally labeled with ^{131}I or ^{123}I. It is administered intravenously after saturated solution of potassium iodide (SSKI) to block thyroidal uptake. Imaging is done 24, 48, and 72 hours after injection. A renal scan is also performed with this study to both localize the kidneys and evaluate the bladder region. A computer subtraction can be helpful in localizing pheochromocytomas in these locations.

Normal activity can be seen in the liver, spleen, salivary glands, heart, and urinary bladder. A minority of normal persons also have activity visible in the adrenal glands and large bowel.

An abnormal study shows increased activity in the region of the adrenal gland or anywhere from the base of the skull to the bladder. The sensitivity of this study for pheochromocytoma is 85% to 90%.

CHAPTER 2

Skeletal

CASE 19

History.— 59-year-old man with newly diagnosed prostate cancer. Bone scan was performed to evaluate for osseous metastases.

Scan.—^{99m}Tc MDP bone scan.

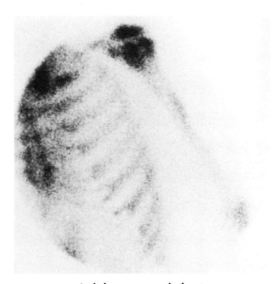

Left humerus and chest.

Findings.—Linear increased uptake in proximal third of humerus.

Diagnosis.—Normal bone scan (deltoid tuberosity uptake).

^{99m}Tc phosphate bone agents are phosphate residues with either inorganic (P-O-P) or organic (P-C-P) bonds. The inorganic phosphates, which were the original bone agents, are used infrequently today. However, ^{99m}Tc pyrophosphate (which contains two phosphate residues) is superior to other currently used bone agents at localizing necrotic tissue and is used in diagnosing myocardial infarction.

The organic diphosphonates offer numerous advantages over their inorganic counterparts, including no susceptibility to enzymatic hydrolysis in vivo, increased renal excretion because of less plasma protein binding, and negligible binding to red blood cells. The major diphosphonates are ^{99m}Tc hydroxyethylene diphosphonate (HEDP) and ^{99m}Tc methylene diphosphonate (MDP).

The primary mechanism of phosphate uptake by bone is chemisorption, which occurs via chemical bonding at kink and dislocation sites on the surface of hydroxyapatite crystals. Tin and ^{99m}Tc are hydrolyzed and bind to bone either separately or together as hydrated tin oxide and technetium dioxide. Large surface areas, such as growth centers and metabolically active bone lesions, allow enhanced chemisorption and thus show more activity. Binding to the organic matrix and to enzyme and enzyme receptor sites may also play a role in localization.

The three primary determinants of phosphate uptake are skeletal metabolic activity, blood flow, and sympathetic tone. Metabolic bony turnover is the most important. It is related to both blood flow and surface area and accounts for the increased uptake seen at growth centers, osteoblastic lesions, and other metabolically active regions. As blood flow increases, bony uptake also increases, although not linearly. A threefold to fourfold increase in blood flow will increase bony uptake 30% to 40%. Sympathetic tone is also important, although less so than metabolic activity. Because sympathetic tone is responsible for capillary tone, loss of sympathetic innervation results in vascular dilatation, locally increased flow, and recruitment. This causes the increased activity seen after stroke or hemiplegia. Hyperemia secondary to sympathetic dysfunction can also be seen in osteomyelitis, fractures, and tumor.

The most important feature of a normal bone scan is symmetry. In an adult, the bones are well seen with minimal soft tissue activity. Both of the kidneys should be visualized with mild uptake. The bladder is usually seen and the ureters and renal pelves are sometimes identified as well. If imaging has been delayed more than 4 hours, the kidneys may not be visualized, and soft tissue activity may be virtually absent, giving the false appearance of a "superscan." Because renal excretion of the ^{99m}Tc phosphates is the key to keeping background activity low, patients with poor renal function often show extensive soft tissue activity and may require more delayed images.

The normal scan may show numerous areas of increased activity. These include the acromioclavicular joints, sternoclavicular joints, scapular tips, costochondral junctions, sternum, parasagittal skull, cervical and lumbar spine (secondary to lordosis), and the sacroiliac joints. Other normal variants include uptake at the deltoid tuberosity of the proximal humerus at the insertion site of the deltoid muscle. This is seen in 7% of patients and may be asymmetric. Vertical linear activity in the posterior ribs is also seen in 7% of scans and is secondary to the insertion of the iliocostalis portion of the erector spinae muscles. Increased uptake in the patellae, the "hot" patella sign, has been shown to be degenerative disease in virtually all cases. This sign carries an extremely low probability of representing metastatic disease, even in patients with known skeletal metastases. Finally, lower cervical spine activity, which may be secondary to lordosis, thyroid cartilage uptake, or free ^{99m}Tc pertechnetate in the thyroid gland, is often seen.

Numerous technical factors and patient variations may produce asymmetry and simulate lesions. Patient rotation is the most common cause of asymmetry. Also, breast prostheses may produce asymmetric appearance of the chest. Simulated lesions can be seen secondary to urinary collecting system activity (especially in the renal calyces), contamination of clothing by radioactive urine, and recent dental procedures or dental disease. "Cold" defects may be present secondary to belt buckles, earrings, necklaces, or other metal objects. Cold lesions may also be simulated by retained barium in the gastrointestinal (GI) tract after a recent x-ray series.

Radiopharmaceutical problems may occur. Free TcO_4 from breakdown of tag will localize to the thyroid gland and GI tract. Colloid formation will show activity in the reticuloendothelial system and may show biliary excretion. Finally, aluminum contamination during preparation of the radiopharmaceutical results in pulmonary activity.

CASE 20

History.—57-year-old woman with a 1-year history of persistent left shoulder pain unresponsive to therapy. She denies trauma.

Scan.—⁹⁹ᵐTc MDP bone scan.

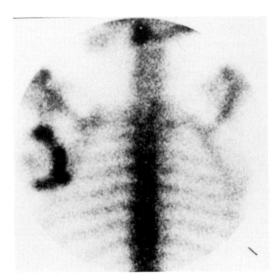

Posterior view of upper back.

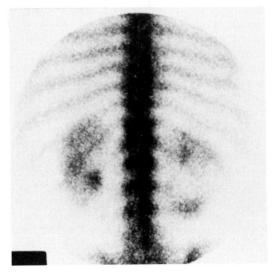

Posterior view of lower back.

Findings.— Increased uptake in the inferior left scapula. No other osseous abnormalities are present. There is a cold defect in the right kidney.

Diagnosis.— Metastatic disease to the left scapula from a primary renal cell carcinoma.

The solitary focal bone scan lesion is a nonspecific finding, although specificity in spinal lesions can be improved using high-resolution parallel-hole and pinhole collimators. It can be a significant problem in pretherapy scans because the therapeutic approach is dependent on the presence or absence of osseous metastases.

Osseous metastatic disease manifests as a solitary focus in 10% to 15% of cancer patients. When metastatic disease is present, approximately 80% of metastases will be located in the axial skeleton, 10% in the skull, and 10% in the long bones. Within the axial skeleton, the distribution of metastatic disease is 39% in the vertebrae, 28% in the ribs and sternum, and 12% in the pelvis. Long bone metastases tend to occur in the proximal portion of the bone.

A solitary bone scan lesion in a patient with no known malignancy carries a low probability of being malignant. In patients with known extraskeletal primary malignancies, the overall probability of a solitary lesion representing metastasis is approximately 15%. Location of the lesion affects the likelihood of metastatic disease, with a vertebral or pelvic lesion being more likely to represent metastatic disease than a lesion in a rib or extremity. The probability of a solitary lesion being metastatic is 80% in the vertebral column, 60% to 65% in the pelvis, 10% to 17% in the ribs, and approximately 20% in the skull.

In children, solitary lesions represent metastatic disease in 39% of patients. Solitary metastatic lesions in children do not have a predilection for the axial skeleton.

The solitary lesion secondary to benign disease is frequently apparent on plain films, making confirmation of its benign nature possible. This is unlike the metastatic lesion, which is often undetectable by conventional radiography. In the skull, most benign lesions occur in the regions of the sutures and are thought to represent small cartilaginous rests. Nonmalignant causes of solitary rib lesions include benign traumatic fractures (40%), radiation therapy (27%), and idiopathic (24%). Uptake near joints is usually degenerative joint disease. The combination of a scintigraphically apparent and radiographically hidden lesion commonly implies metastatic disease, although this is less true in the skull and ribs.

Location and characteristics of the lesion are often useful in distinguishing benign from malignant disease. In the vertebral column, a single lesion that is intense, inhomogeneous, and primarily in the region of a pedicle is likely to be a metastasis. Conversely, uptake across an entire end plate probably is a compression fracture. Activity spanning a disk space is suggestive of infection. Magnification and pinhole views can be helpful in distinguishing these lesions.

Features of malignancy in a rib lesion are linearity and inhomogeneity. A small circular lesion is more likely benign, such as a rib fracture. Lesions in unusual locations are more likely to be secondary to malignancy than to benign disease. For example, a single lesion in the scapula is probably metastatic because this is a very atypical location for benign disease.

In this patient the solitary osseous abnormality is seen in the left scapula. Close examination of the remainder of the scan, however, reveals a large photopenic area in the midinferior portion of the right kidney. Renal ultrasound showed a 10-cm mass in the right kidney, found to be a renal cell carcinoma at surgery.

CASE 21

History.—75-year-old man with a 2-year history of prostate cancer, admitted because of lower GI bleeding. The scan was obtained to assess the status of his prostate cancer.

Scan.—^{99m}Tc MDP bone scan.

Skull and cervical spine.

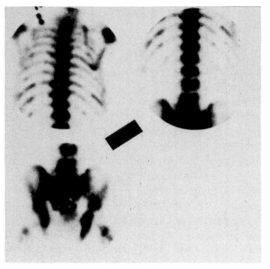

Posterior view of thoracic spine, lumbosacral spine, and pelvis.

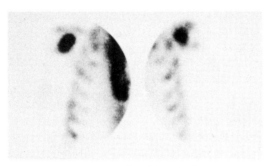

Anterior view of shoulders and chest.

Findings.—Markedly increased uptake of ^{99m}Tc MDP in the axial skeleton, especially the vertebral column, ribs, pelvis, and shoulder girdles. The calvarium and extremities are poorly visualized, showing little uptake compared with the axial skeleton. Almost no soft tissue activity is present. The kidneys are not seen.

Diagnosis.—This is a superscan, or "beautiful bone scan," representing widespread metastatic disease from prostate cancer.

In a superscan, diffusely increased uptake throughout the skeleton is seen with a lack of kidney activity and near-total absence of soft tissue activity. Early bone uptake can be seen on images taken in the first 10 minutes after injection.

Metastatic disease is a frequent cause of superscans, with prostate carcinoma the most common tumor type. Other causes include breast, lung, and bladder cancer and lymphoma.

Metabolic bone disease can also cause a superscan. Hyperparathyroidism, osteomalacia, Paget's disease, and fibrous dysplasia are nontumorous causes of superscans.

Superscans that result from metabolic bone disease can be distinguished from metastatic disease by examining the activity in the calvarium and extremities. Metabolic bone disease tends to involve the calvarium and long bones, whereas metastatic disease tends to spare them. Another feature that distinguishes metastatic from metabolic superscan is symmetry. If even slight asymmetry is present, the scan is more likely secondary to metastatic disease.

Although widespread metastases and metabolic bone disease must always be considered, the most common cause of a superscan is factitious. If there is a delay of 4 or more hours before imaging, renal excretion causes the kidney activity to disappear, soft tissue activity to decrease, and skeletal activity to appear increased.

CASE 22

History.—53-year-old man with newly diagnosed lung cancer. The patient gave a 2-month history of lumbar spine pain. He denied any history of trauma.

Scan.—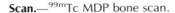^{99m}Tc MDP bone scan.

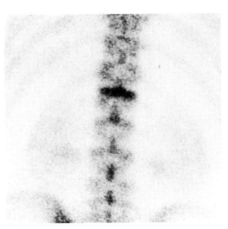

Posterior view of lumbar spine.

Findings.—Increased uptake in L-1 involving the superior end plate. The remainder of the vertebral column and skeleton is normal. The kidneys show a mild degree of uptake.

Diagnosis.— Compression fracture of L-1 vertebral body.

Distinguishing between benign compression fractures and metastases is a frequent clinical problem. Although compression fractures and metastases are more common in most patient populations, infection can also manifest in a similar manner.

Compression fractures can occur secondary to repeated trauma or stress in normal bone or in bone morphologically weakened by metabolic bone disease. They commonly occur in the thoracic and lumbar spine areas where metastases and infection are also common.

Compression fractures usually involve either the superior or inferior vertebral end plate; occasionally both are involved. Superior end plate fractures are the most common, and isolated inferior end plate fractures are less common.

In addition to delayed images at 2 to 4 hours, pinhole collimator views of the vertebral body in question can also be helpful. The pinhole images are obtained for 400,000 to 500,000 counts at a distance of 5 to 10 cm from the patient. These enlarged images increase the spatial resolution of the scan, better characterizing the findings. This improves specificity compared to routine views.

Compression fracture, metastases, and infection all show nonspecific increased uptake on parallel-hole collimator images. On pinhole collimator views, each has a more specific pattern. Compression fractures characteristically show boardlike involvement of the entire length and thickness of the involved vertebral end plate. The demarcation between the involved and uninvolved portion of the vertebral body is sharp in three fourths of cases. Interestingly, the boardlike nature of the uptake cannot be recognized in more than 75% of cases without special views. Disk space narrowing is not a feature of compression fracture and is more suggestive of infection. Burst fractures of a vertebral body, unlike compression frac-

tures, show diffuse uptake throughout the vertebral body and may be difficult to differentiate from metastases.

The majority of metastases (87%) show increased activity in a vertebral body, which may be either focal or diffuse. Involvement of the pedicles also favors metastatic disease. Approximately 13% show short areas of uptake along an end plate. Metastatic disease does not show disk space narrowing.

Infection in the vertebral column shows two patterns of uptake, depending on whether the infection is tuberculous or pyogenic. Tuberculous involvement of the spine (Pott's disease) shows homogeneous involvement of the vertebrae in three fourths of cases, much like metastases. However, disk space narrowing is usually present as well, unlike metastases or fractures.

Pyogenic vertebral infection shows uptake localized to the end zone of opposing vertebral bodies, with an intervening cold disk space producing a sandwichlike appearance early; disk space obliteration occurs later in the course of the disease.

The infecting organism most commonly localizes in the end zone vascular arcades. Disk space invasion follows end zone involvement. Thus the cold disk space is seen early in the course of pyogenic infection and the disk space obliteration later if left untreated.

In summary, pinhole collimation is the key element in the evaluation of compression fracture vs. metastases vs. infection. The nature of vertebral body uptake, as well as the presence or absence of disk space involvement, helps differentiate the causes. In this case, we see end plate uptake and no disk space narrowing, indicating a benign compression fracture.

CASE 23

History.— 27-year-old man with testicular carcinoma.

Scan.—^{99m}Tc MDP bone scan.

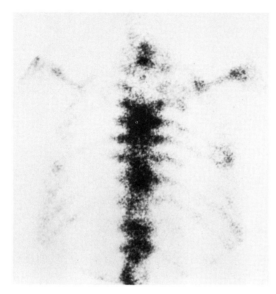

Posterior view of thoracic spine.

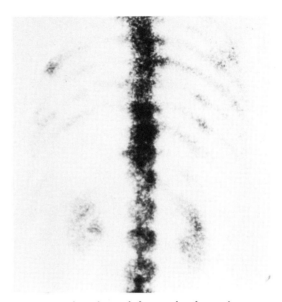

Posterior view of thoracolumbar spine.

Findings.— Hot and cold defects in spine and ribs.

Diagnosis.— Metastatic disease.

The uptake of phosphate bone agents is determined by bony metabolic activity, blood flow, and sympathetic tone. Of these, metabolic activity is the most important. Increased metabolic activity accounts for the uptake seen at epiphyseal growth centers and in osteoblastic lesions.

Increases in regional blood flow produce a diffusion-limited increase in bone uptake. A threefold to fourfold increase in flow will produce a 30% to 40% increase in uptake.

Loss of sympathetic tone leads to an inability to close capillaries. The resultant increase in blood flow causes increased tracer accumulation, as seen in patients with stroke or hemiplegia.

There are several mechanisms for producing cold defects on bone scan. Bone that is either avascular or subject to low flow shows little or no uptake. This is the mechanism by which bone infarcts and certain stages of avascular necrosis appear as cold lesions. This also sometimes occurs early in the course of osteomyelitis, especially in children. Subperiosteal pus and inflammation elevates the periosteum dissecting small vessels. Pus in the bone marrow increases pressure, compromising endosteal flow as well. The result is a cold defect. Tumors can cause a cold defect by compromising blood flow or replacing so much normal bone that no significant uptake occurs.

Artifacts are a common cause of cold areas on bone scan. Cold lesions in the abdomen can be produced by residual barium. Jewelry (e.g., earrings, medallions, rings), clothing (e.g., buttons, belt buckles), and coins in pockets are frequent causes of cold defects.

The relationship between the radionuclide scan findings and radiographically "lytic" and "blastic" lesions is often misunderstood. The majority of radiographically lytic, or lucent, lesions will show increased uptake on bone scan, often as intense as blastic lesions. This is because of increased reactive bone metabolism and repair at the periphery of the lesion. Purely lytic lesions, causing little to no osseous reaction, however, can be missed on scintigraphy. This is the case in multiple myeloma and also in some highly anaplastic, rapidly growing tumors.

Metabolically vigorous lesions show intense uptake of the radiotracer; however, metabolically indolent lesions may show little or no uptake of radiotracer while still being blastic on plain film because of the different nature of the two modalities. The radiograph images morphology, as reflected by bone density. The bone density at any given time is the net sum of all previous metabolic activity and not necessarily a reflection of current metabolic activity. In contrast, the radionuclide scan is dependent on bone physiology, with active bone metabolism the primary determinant of uptake. A radiographically blastic lesion that reflects low metabolic rate can produce a false negative radionuclide scan. This occurs in the late phases of Paget's disease, for example.

CASE 24

History.— 60-year-old man with new-onset back pain. Rule out compression fracture vs. metastases.

Scan.—^{99m}Tc MDP bone scan.

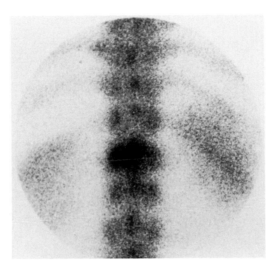

Posterior high-resolution view of thoracolumbar junction.

Findings.—Asymmetric uptake in L-1.

Diagnosis.—Metastatic disease of the lumbar spine.

The tumors most likely to metastasize to bone include renal cell carcinoma, breast cancer, lung cancer, lymphoma, thyroid cancer (follicular and papillary), prostate cancer, and neuroblastoma.

Bone scanning is much more sensitive than plain radiography for the detection of metastatic disease. Normal plain films are seen in 30% to 50% of patients with abnormal bone scans, because the demineralization of at least 30% to 50% of bone is required for plain film detection. However, approximately 5% of patients with normal bone scans will have abnormal radiographs. This is secondary to low metabolic activity and is usually associated with multiple myeloma, thyroid cancer, purely lytic lesions, and some anaplastic tumors.

Bone scan is more sensitive for metastases than are alkaline and acid phosphatase, calcium, and clinical symptoms. In one series of patients with prostate cancer only 45% had symptoms at the time of discovery of metastases, whereas 12% of patients without metastases complained of pain.

Most (90%) metastases are multiple. The axial skeleton is the site for 80% of metastases, with approximately 39% in the vertebrae, 28% in the ribs and sternum, and 12% in the pelvis. The skull and long bones are each involved about 10% of the time. In the long bones, metastases are more often located proximally than distally.

The significance of solitary bone scan lesions depends on whether the patient has a known malignancy and on their location. A solitary lesion in a patient with no known malignancy carries less than 1% chance of representing metastases. In a patient with a known primary neoplasm, however, a solitary lesion carries an overall probability of 15% to 80% of representing metastatic disease, depending on the location of the lesion.

A rib lesion in a patient with a known extraskeletal malignancy carries an approximately 10% to 17% chance of being metastatic. Rib lesions not representing metastases are usually secondary to benign traumatic fractures (40%), radiation therapy (27%), and idiopathic (24%). Skull lesions carry a 15% to 20% chance of being malignant. Activity near suture lines is less likely to be tumor.

Vertebral uptake (which is not degenerative) has a very high probability of representing metastases. Because degenerative disease is so common, the distinction between metastases and degenerative disease is important. Approximately 11% of bone metastases occur in areas of degenerative disease, however.

CASE 25

History.—70-year-old man with bronchogenic carcinoma who complains of pain in the knees and ankles.

Scan.—^{99m}Tc MDP bone scan.

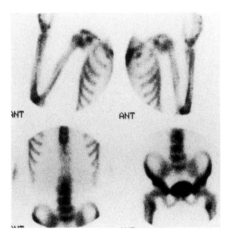

2-hour delayed anterior views of both arms, abdomen, and pelvis.

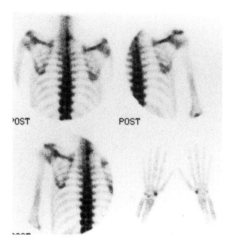

Posterior view of spine, both arms, and hands.

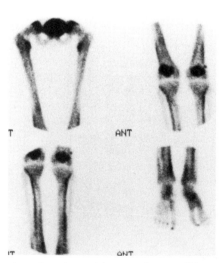

Anterior view of femurs, knees, tibias, and feet.

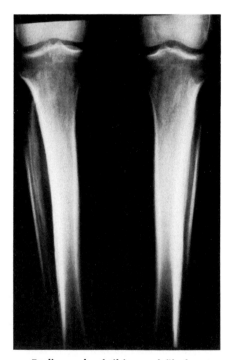

Radiograph of tibias and fibulas.

Findings.—Increased uptake in both distal upper extremities, with marked periarticular uptake in the hands is seen. There is increased uptake in the distal lower extremities also, especially in the tibias and fibulas. The remainder of the bone scan is unremarkable.

Diagnosis.—Hypertrophic pulmonary osteoarthropathy or secondary hypertrophic osteoarthropathy.

There are two types of hypertrophic osteoarthropathy (HOA): the less common primary form, also called pachydermoperiostitis, and the more common secondary form, associated with a variety of disease processes, usually intrathoracic. Clinically, HOA is a form of periostitis and typically manifests as joint pain.

Primary HOA is familial and is more common in males than females. Onset is in adolescence, and its course is usually self-limited, with spontaneous arrest of the process in young adulthood. The spectrum of findings range from simple periostitis to the complete picture, which includes clubbed digits resulting in pawlike hands and thickening of skin.

Secondary HOA occurs secondary to a number of conditions, usually intrathoracic. It is most commonly associated with bronchogenic carcinoma; other intrathoracic causes include other types of pulmonary malignancy, benign lung diseases, chronic suppurative lung disease, and cyanotic heart disease. Occasionally HOA occurs secondary to abdominal diseases, including malignancy, hepatic and biliary cirrhosis, and inflammatory bowel disease. How these diseases induce periostitis is not known. There is no specific therapy for HOA, but treatment of the underlying disease generally produces clinical remission, with rapid resolution of radionuclide scan findings and slower radiographic resolution.

Both plain radiography and radionuclide scanning are useful for the evaluation of HOA. On radiographs the joints are normal, but the affected long bones show thick periosteal reaction. The classic findings on standard radionuclide bone scan are increased uptake in the distal extremities, both upper and lower. HOA usually is a bilateral process but can be asymmetric.

CASE 26

History.—60-year-old man with lung cancer.

Scan.—^{99m}Tc MDP bone scan.

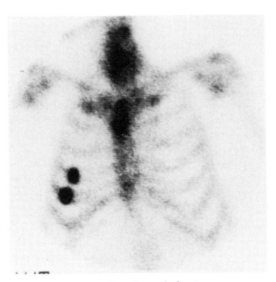

Anterior view of chest.

Findings.—Two foci of uptake in ribs.

Diagnosis.—Rib trauma, no metastases.

Isolated rib uptake on bone scan is frequently encountered in nuclear medicine. Is the activity the result of trauma or metastatic disease?

The normal bone scan shows homogeneous uptake throughout the ribs. The costal cartilages may or may not be visible. When visible, they produce a Christmas tree appearance.

The location and characteristics of rib uptake are the two most useful features in interpreting increased rib uptake. Rib uptake caused by trauma is frequently located anteriorly near the costochondral junction. At this site, it is usually focal and may involve several costochondral junctions in a row. Rib trauma can also be seen posteriorly or laterally, either as a result of direct trauma or transmitted force (e.g., steering wheel impact). In these situations, uptake is again focal and will usually involve serial adjacent ribs. Because of the mechanisms of rib trauma, it is highly unusual to have trauma cause either focal or multiple areas of increased uptake isolated to a single rib.

Ribs are a common site of metastases. Tumors most likely to metastasize to bone include prostate, breast, lung, thyroid, renal cell, lymphoma, and neuroblastoma. Of all bone metastases, 80% are located in the axial skeleton. The overall distribution of metastases within the axial skeleton are 39% vertebrae, 28% ribs and sternum, and 12% pelvis.

A solitary rib lesion in patients with a known extraskeletal malignancy carries only a 10% to 17% chance of representing metastatic disease. The location of metastatic rib uptake is more variable than in trauma. The characteristics of metastatic rib uptake also differ. Metastatic lesions are more likely to involve a solitary rib, which is distinctly uncommon in trauma. The uptake may be linear over a significant length of the rib and may give the rib a beaded appearance. This is in sharp contrast to trauma-induced uptake, which is usually focal. Diffuse involvement of the ribs by metastatic disease may show a heterogeneous beaded pattern of uptake.

Rib films are sometimes helpful; however, a significant number of patients with normal rib films (no fracture) and solitary uptake are still proved not to have metastatic disease.

CASE 27

History.—60-year-old man with prostate carcinoma who had recently undergone orchiectomy. The PSA level had fallen, and the patient was feeling better.

Scan.—^{99m}Tc MDP bone scan done 1 week before orchiectomy. Repeat scan 5 weeks after orchiectomy.

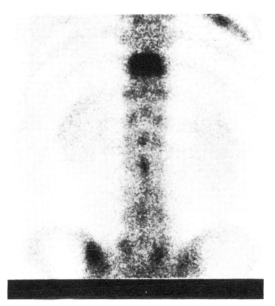

Posterior view of thoracic spine 1 week before orchiectomy.

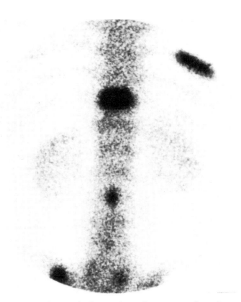

Posterior view of thoracic spine 5 weeks after orchiectomy.

Findings.—Initial scan: uptake in lower thoracic vertebra and right rib; posttherapy scan: increased uptake in all lesions.

Diagnosis.—Flare phenomenon.

The bone scan is commonly used to follow treatment response in patients with malignancies metastatic to the skeleton. Such tumors include carcinoma of the prostate, lung, breast, and kidney.

When following treatment response, signs of progression of metastatic disease are an increase in the number, extent, or intensity of activity of bone lesions. Improvement is shown by the opposite findings. Stable bone scans show no significant change in findings. Stability of bone scan findings does not necessarily indicate an unfavorable treatment response. Patients with stable bone scan findings have survival rates similar to patients showing improved bone scans.

Increased activity in metastatic lesions on bone scan in a patient clinically responding to therapy is called the "flare phenomenon." It has been described in a variety of tumors,

most commonly in breast and prostate carcinoma in response to hormonal manipulation. It is also seen after other types of chemotherapy and radiation treatment.

Two factors are thought to be involved: (1) increased blood flow caused by the inflammatory response of healing may lead to increased deposition of the radionuclide; and (2) as bone heals, the increased turnover of hydroxyapatite in the newly deposited bone may also increase uptake of the bone agent. The clinician is faced with a management problem when the bone scan and clinical picture seem to present conflicting data. The flare phenomenon is uncommon. Follow-up bone scan at 3 months is helpful if the cause of the scan findings is uncertain. If the activity has resolved, flare phenomenon was the cause.

CASE 28

History.—57-year-old man with lung cancer has pain in back and wrist. He is currently undergoing chemotherapy.

Scan.—^{99m}Tc MDP bone scan.

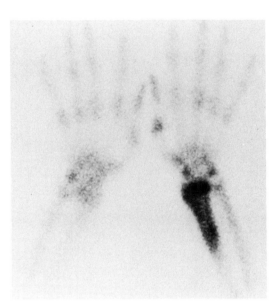

Hands.

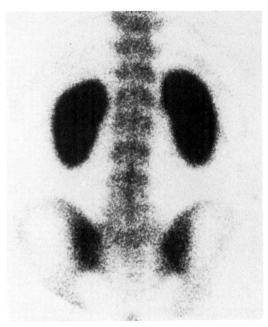

Posterior view of abdomen.

Findings.—Uptake in distal radius. Diffusely increased uptake in both kidneys.

Diagnosis.—Osseous metastases. Diffusely increased kidney uptake secondary to chemotherapy.

Soft tissue uptake of ^{99m}Tc organophosphates may be seen in any organ system. Normal areas of soft tissue uptake include the breast, renal parenchyma and calyces, and calcified cartilage (costal, thyroid, cricoid). Technical causes of soft tissue activity include uptake at the injection site, instrument contamination with isotope, urine contamination, recent ^{99m}Tc sulfur colloid scan, free ^{99m}Tc secondary to radiopharmaceutical breakdown, and radiopharmaceutical colloid formation.

Inflammation or cellular injury is probably responsible in uptake from cellulitis, burn injury, and muscle trauma. In-

farcts (myocardial, cerebral, splenic), muscle necrosis, benign and malignant soft tissue tumors, and metastases are other common causes of soft tissue uptake of bone agents.

In this patient, there is diffuse increased renal activity. The cause is chemotherapy, which resulted in renal parenchymal injury. Other causes of diffuse increased kidney uptake of bone agents include urinary tract obstruction, metastatic calcification, pyelonephritis, acute tubular necrosis, postradiation therapy, the use of radiographic contrast, iron overload, and hemoglobinopathies.

CASE 29

History.—60-year-old man with possible prostate carcinoma on biopsy.

Scan.—^{99m}Tc MDP bone scan.

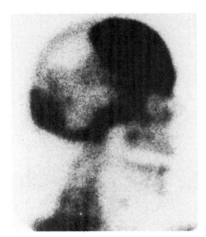

View of skull.

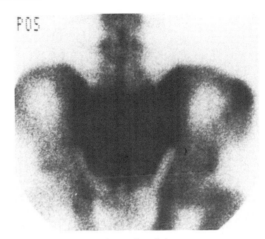

View of pelvis.

Findings.—Increased uptake in skull and pelvis.

Diagnosis.—Paget's disease.

Paget's disease is a metabolic bone disease in which abnormal increased remodeling of bone involving both osteoblastic and osteoclastic activity occurs, resulting in bone that has thickened, disorganized, and fragile trabeculae. It is one of the most common chronic skeletal diseases, affecting 3% of the population older than age 40 years. It affects males more commonly than females, and is rare before age 40. Although its cause is unknown, it may be of viral etiology.

Patients are often asymptomatic. When symptoms are present, skeletal pain is the most frequent complaint. Other signs and symptoms include bowing of the long bones, pathologic fracture, and degenerative joint disease. Although the bone is weakened, affected bone does enlarge, especially the cranium. Occasionally deafness occurs secondary to either cranial nerve compression or ossicle involvement. Spinal cord signs may also be seen with platybasia or other types of compression. Rarely, high-output congestive heart failure occurs secondary to increased blood flow to the metabolically hyperactive bone.

Laboratory findings include increased serum alkaline phosphatase level and elevated serum and urinary hydroxyproline levels. These values reflect osseous formation and resorption, respectively, and vary greatly with the severity of disease.

Radiographically there are three sequential stages of Paget's disease: (1) the lytic phase, (2) the mixed lytic and blastic phase, and (3) the sclerotic phase. Initially, geographic destruction of bone with well-defined borders is seen. The mixed phase shows cortical accretion and bony enlargement. The bone continues to increase in both density and size in the sclerotic phase and ultimately may become quiescent as osteoblastic activity ceases.

The bone scan is abnormal in the lytic and mixed phases of Paget's disease because both blood flow and metabolic activity are increased. The uptake often involves the entire bone or large portions of the bone. In osteoporosis circumscripta, a cold lesion with increased activity at the edge is seen in the skull. As osteoblastic activity ceases in the sclerotic phase, the bone scan may return to normal.

Sixty percent of lesions are seen on both radiographs and bone scan. Approximately 27% of lesions are seen on bone scan only, and 13% are visible only on plain films. Early lesions that have high metabolic activity and blood flow but little change in bone density are more likely to be seen on the bone scan. Late lesions that reflect long-standing changes in bone size and density but may be metabolically quiescent are more likely to be seen only on radiographs.

Paget's disease most commonly involves the pelvis (80% of patients). The spine is involved in 75%; the lumbar and thoracic vertebrae are affected more commonly than the cervical spine. Cranial involvement occurs in 65% of cases and usually begins in either the frontal or occipital bones. Tubular bones are affected in 35% of patients, most commonly the femur, tibia, and humerus.

Paget's disease can be misinterpreted on bone scan as metastatic disease, especially in patients with prostate cancer. Diffuse involvement of the pelvis and an entire long bone should raise the suspicion of Paget's disease. Plain films should be obtained in these patients to exclude Paget's disease.

Complications from Paget's disease include pathologic fracture, osteoarthritis, osteoporosis, benign giant cell tumors, and malignant degeneration. Although malignant degeneration to sarcoma may occur (osteosarcoma more commonly than fibrosarcoma), it is rare, being found in less than 1% of patients. In patients with widespread disease, the chance of malignant degeneration may increase to 5% to 10%.

CASE 30

History.—18-year-old man with a 9-month history of crippling right hand pain, especially with temperature changes. His hand is exquisitely sensitive to touch. He reports having had a car door slam on his hand approximately 1 year ago.

Scan.—^{99m}Tc MDP bone scan.

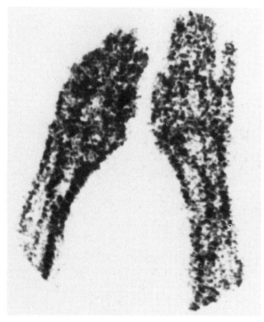

Flow study of hands.

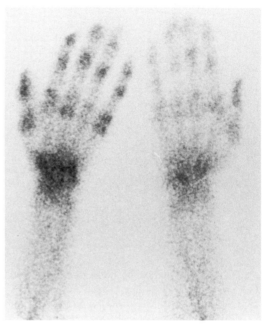

Delayed hand view.

Findings.— Angiographic and blood pool images over both distal upper extremities show hyperemia and increased blood pool to the right hand and forearm. Delayed images at 2 hours also show increased uptake in the right arm. Increased periarticular uptake that extends proximally is seen on the delayed images.

Diagnosis.— Reflex sympathetic dystrophy.

Reflex sympathetic dystrophy syndrome (RSDS), causalgia, Sudeck's atrophy, and shoulder-hand syndrome all refer to the same entity: a syndrome characterized by pain, tenderness, vasomotor instability, swelling, and dystrophic skin changes, usually of the upper extremity. There is often a preceding history of trauma or injury, although it can also be seen with neurologic disease, after surgery, and with a variety of other entities.

Trauma is the precipitant in 30% of cases of RSDS. Types of trauma that have been shown to precipitate RSDS include fracture, crush injury, contusion, sprain, laceration, and thermal injury. Neurologic disease has been implicated in 20% of cases. Neurologic causes include cerebrovascular accident, head injury, spinal cord injury, and peripheral nerve entrapment or injury. In the case of peripheral nerve entrapment, ulnar, median, and brachial plexus entrapment are most common. RSDS has been seen postoperatively after carpal tunnel decompression, ganglion excision, Dupuytren's contracture repair, hip or knee surgery, and cardiac or intrathoracic surgery. A number of other reported precipitants of RSDS include myocardial infarction, infection, neoplasm, metabolic bone disease, herpes zoster, and cervical osteoarthritis.

Three clinical states have been described. The first stage lasts up to 6 months and is characterized by either abrupt or gradual onset of a painful, stiff shoulder, and diffuse intensely burning pain, swelling, and stiffness of the hand and fingers. The pain may be exacerbated by exposure to cold. The hand will be diffusely tender, swollen, and dusky and may appear red, pale, or mottled.

In stage 2, usually lasting 3 to 6 months, the shoulder pain may improve, but stiffness and diffuse burning pain remain in the shoulder, wrist, and hand. There is often periarticular tenderness at the wrist and metacarpophalangeal joints, as well as wasting of the subcutaneous tissues and intrinsic muscles of the hand. Flexion deformities of the fingers may be seen, and hand-grip weakness may become pronounced. The hand is cool and pale, gray, or cyanotic, possibly with thickened palmar fascia and loss of hair. The nails appear dystrophic, cracked, or brittle.

Stage 3 may last several months or become chronic. Pain may spread proximally, and there is either marked or total limitation in motion of the shoulder and small joints of the hand, with pronounced wasting of the intrinsic muscles of the hand and subcutaneous tissues. Contractures are frequently present. Skin is atrophic with a smooth, glossy, or glazed appearance. The distal extremity is cool and pale.

RSDS may follow a benign and self-limited course, or it may become chronic and irreversible. Prognosis is improved when RSDS is recognized early in its course and therapy promptly instituted. Complete recovery is less likely when diagnosis occurs in stage 2 or later. The nature and severity of the precipitant does not influence the severity of the syndrome.

Therapy of RSDS is controversial; however, sympathetic blockade (local, regional, or by surgical sympathectomy), and corticosteroid administration are currently the two most widely accepted modes of treatment.

Radiographic and nuclear studies are the two main techniques to confirm RSDS. The most common plain film finding is osteopenia, seen in about 70% of cases. It is usually not present until 6 weeks after onset of symptoms. Erosions of the subchondral or periarticular bone in the small bones of the hands and feet or in the wrist and ankles may also be seen.

CASE 31

History.—Elderly woman with low back pain.

Scan.—^{99m}Tc MDP bone scan.

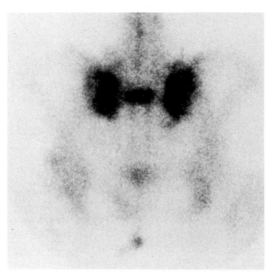

Posterior view of pelvis.

Findings.—Linear increased uptake bilaterally in region of sacral alae. Transverse area of uptake in midsacrum.

Diagnosis.—Sacral insufficiency fracture.

Stress fractures are of two types: (1) fatigue fractures, which occur when repeated abnormal stress is placed on normal bone (e.g., in runners); and (2) insufficiency fractures, which occur when normal stress is placed on abnormal bone. Insufficiency fractures are commonly seen with metabolic bone disease, such as osteoporosis, osteomalacia, Paget's disease, fibrous dysplasia, and after radiation.

Sacral insufficiency fractures are secondary to normal stress on abnormal bone. As with other insufficiency fractures, they are often difficult to diagnose by plain radiography because of underlying bone disease. When visible on radiographs, they appear as a dense vertical line parallel to the sacroiliac joint.

The bone scan is more sensitive for sacral insufficiency fractures than is the plain film. They appear as bilateral linear areas of increased uptake in the region of the sacral alae. Sacral insufficiency fractures usually appear different from sacral fractures associated with trauma, which may be trans-verse (direct trauma) or vertical with interruption of sacral foramina and neural arches (complex pelvic trauma).

Osteoporosis is the most common metabolic bone disease. It is associated with reduction in bone mass, cortical thinning, fragmentation, and loss of medullary trabeculation. The radionuclide bone scan is often normal in osteoporosis, although in severe cases, decreased uptake, especially in the spine, may be seen because of reduced osteoblastic activity.

Disuse osteoporosis is associated with increased blood flow, increased bone formation, and an even greater increase in bone resorption. Because of the increased flow and osteoblast activity, increased uptake is frequently seen.

Focal abnormalities on bone scan are also seen in regional migratory osteoporosis. This disease generally affects middle-aged men. They develop severe joint pain, often in the hip. Bone scans show increased blood flow on angiographic images and increased periarticular uptake at the involved joint. The areas of uptake migrate on serial scans.

CASE 32

History.— 30-year-old renal transplant patient with right hip pain.

Scan.—^{99m}Tc MDP bone scan.

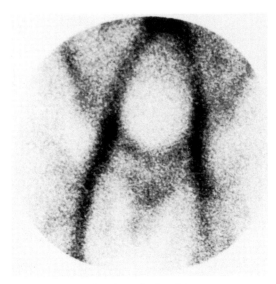

Blood pool of pelvis.

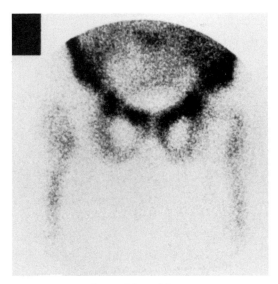

2-hour delayed image.

Findings.— Cold defect in right femoral head.

Diagnosis.— Avascular necrosis of the right hip.

Avascular necrosis (AVN) of the hip is a disease of both adults and children. It is defined as necrosis of bone at the epiphysis. The pathologic causes of AVN are trauma with vascular damage, vascular compression, or intraluminal obstruction. Common sites of AVN include the femoral head, lunate, scaphoid, and body of the talus.

Causes for vascular compromise leading to necrosis include trauma (delayed reduction of dislocation or subcapital fracture); corticosteroids (increased pressure secondary to increased adipocyte size); ethanol abuse (increased marrow pressure from fat emboli); sickle cell disease (vascular occlusion in sickle crisis); Gaucher's disease (sinusoids packed with glucosylceramide-laden cells); caisson disease (nitrogen embolization following rapid decompression); radiation (direct radiotoxic effects to vascular supply); pancreatitis (fat necrosis); and systemic lupus erythematosus (additive effects of vasculitis and corticosteroid therapy).

Legg-Calvé-Perthes (LCP) disease is a specific subset of AVN; it is AVN of the hip in children, primarily young boys 4 to 8 years old.

Multiple imaging modalities are used to evaluate possible AVN. Plain radiographs, scintigraphy, and magnetic resonance imaging are helpful. Plain radiographs are normal early in the course of the disease; the earliest plain film changes may not be seen for 6 months. The first radiographic change is sclerosis, followed by a linear subchondral fracture (crescent sign), flattening of the head, and bony deformity. Secondary degenerative changes may occur later. The cartilage is normal on plain films because it receives its blood supply from the synovium.

Radionuclide scintigraphic findings vary in AVN, depending on the stage of the disease. Immediately after fracture, bone scans may be normal for the first 48 hours, then show decreased uptake for a varying period of time. As the bone's reparative processes are activated, the bone scan will show progressively increasing activity. Acetabular uptake is seen when degenerative complications of AVN develop later in the disease. Single-photon emission computed tomography improves sensitivity for AVN.

Bone marrow imaging can be used in AVN as a predictor of bone viability. At our institution we use ^{99m}Tc sulfur colloid. Both hips are imaged for comparison purposes. Normal, symmetric radiocolloid uptake implies an intact vascular supply. Asymmetric absence of radiocolloid uptake indicates vascular impairment and nonviable bone.

The presence or absence of marrow uptake in normal individuals varies with age. In 11- to 19-year-old persons, 100% will show femoral head uptake. In the 70- to 79-year age range, only 39% have uptake; thus the marrow scan has limited utility in older patients.

CASE 33

History.— 14-year-old youth with hip pain, worse at night.

Scan.—^{99m}Tc MDP bone scan.

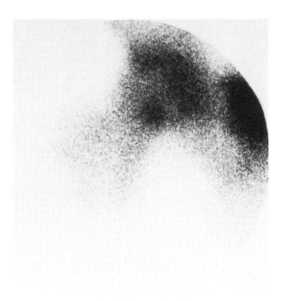

Anterior view of right hip.

Findings.— Increased uptake in right hip with more focally intense area in neck.

Diagnosis.— Osteoid osteoma.

Osteoid osteomas are benign primary bone tumors usually occurring in the second or third decades. They are most commonly cortically based in the tubular bones; however, they can be intramedullary (and intracapsular, e.g., in the proximal medial femoral neck), or, least commonly, subperiosteal (talus).

The spine is a common site for cortically based osteoid osteomas. These are located in the posterior elements and spare the vertebral body. Clinical findings include the classic triad of aching pain that is worse at night, relieved by both aspirin and exercise. In the spine, osteoid osteomas may cause a painful scoliosis, with the apex at the lesion concave on the side of the lesion, and no rotatory component.

Bone scan sensitivity for the diagnosis of osteoid osteoma is excellent. A normal scan virtually rules out the diagnosis. On bone scan, increased flow and blood pool activity is almost always present, and intense, focally increased uptake is seen on delayed imaging. Delayed images may also show the classic "double-density" sign, a focal area of intensely increased uptake surrounded by a more diffuse area of less intense activity. The focal area of activity is thought to represent the nidus, and it may be centrally or eccentrically located within the whole lesion.

Injection of ^{99m}Tc MDP just before surgery is sometimes done so that the surgical specimen can be examined to be certain the nidus has been removed. The bone scan may also be useful in the postoperative follow-up of osteoid osteoma. Recurrent or persistent pain associated with persistently increased bone scan activity suggests incomplete surgical resection.

CASE 34

History.— 22-year-old man with right knee pain.

Scan.— ^{99m}Tc MDP bone scan.

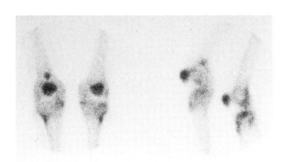

Anterior and lateral views of the knees.

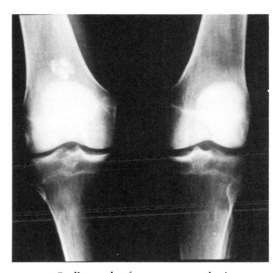

Radiograph of same area as in A.

Findings.— There is a focus of increased uptake in the right distal
femur. Plain radiograph correlation shows a corresponding focus
of increased density.

Diagnosis.— Enchondroma.

Benign primary bone tumors can show MDP uptake. An osteoid osteoma, classically accompanied by the clinical triad of aching pain, worse at night, relieved by aspirin and exercise, is readily seen on bone scintigraphy. Osteoid osteoma shows increased blood pool activity and usually intense uptake on delayed imaging. The so-called double-density sign, representing a central, intensely hot nidus surrounded by a ring of less intense, more diffusely increased uptake, is the classic scintigraphic finding for osteoid osteoma.

Bone islands may show minimally increased uptake. Visualization of bone islands is more likely with lesions 3 cm or more, superficial lesions, and rapidly growing lesions. Like bone islands, bone cysts may show normal or minimal uptake. More intense uptake in a bone cyst is usually seen with fracture through the cyst. Fibrous cortical defects (nonossifying fibroma) also may show normal or minimal bone scan uptake.

Multiple other benign bony lesions can show increased uptake; these include fibrous dysplasia, eosinophilic granuloma, Brown's tumor of hyperparathyroidism, aneurysmal bone cyst, chondroblastoma, enchondroma, and bone infarct.

Enchondromas are benign tumors composed of lobules of hyaline cartilage that develop in the medullary cavity. They occur most commonly in the hand, especially the metacarpals and proximal and midphalanges. Other common sites include the bones of the feet, humerus, femur, tibia, and ribs. They appear in the third and fourth decades of life; men and women are equally affected.

Enchondromas are usually asymptomatic, especially those involving the hand. The onset of pain raises the question of malignant transformation, an infrequent occurrence. Malignant degeneration is more common in enchondromas that involve the tubular bones.

When multiple enchondromas occur, it is called Ollier's disease.

History.—Athletic 48-year-old man with a 6-month history of persistent left proximal femur pain at a site of previous fracture.

Scan.—^{99m}Tc bone scan.

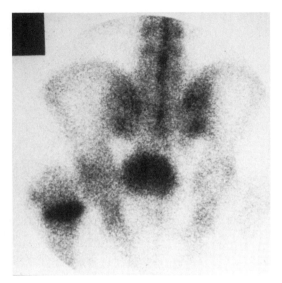

Posterior view of pelvis.

Findings.—Delayed bone scan images over the pelvis show an area of intensely increased uptake in the intertrochanteric region of the left femur.

Diagnosis.—Nonunion of a left intertrochanteric fracture.

Traumatic bone fractures usually become scintigraphically positive within 24 hours. Bone scan sensitivity for acute fracture is 80% at 24 hours, 95% at 72 hours, and 98% at 1 week. The results in older patients may take longer to become abnormal and longer to return to normal. Scintigraphic resolution of fractures requires at least 5 to 7 months. By 1 year, approximately two thirds will have returned to normal. Ninety percent will return to normal by 2 years. Approximately 10% of fractures will remain abnormal for 3 or more years. This is seen more commonly in fractures of long bones with callus formation and increased bony mass. In general, acute fractures show intense uptake, whereas old fractures show either normal or mildly increased uptake.

Increased bone scan uptake is also seen after orthopedic surgery. The bone scan will usually return to near-normal within 6 to 9 months after placement of a prosthetic joint.

Bone scanning has been used to evaluate treatment of frac-

ture nonunion. In patients with nonunited fractures who may be treated with percutaneous, low-grade, direct-current stimulation, bone scanning appears useful in predicting response to electrical stimulation. When intense uptake is seen at the fracture site, patient response to electrical stimulation is excellent. Patients with fibrous nonunion will show a linear area of decreased uptake at the fracture site, with increased uptake on both sides of the fracture. These patients respond poorly to electrical stimulation.

This patient shows intense uptake at the fracture site in the intertrochanteric region of the left femur. This uptake is much more intense than would be expected from an old healed fracture, especially in an otherwise healthy middle-aged man. This is consistent with a nonunion of the fracture. Differential diagnosis for increased uptake includes tumor and infection, because increased uptake is a nonspecific sign of increased osteoblastic activity.

CASE 36

History.—27-year-old diabetic man with Wiskott-Aldrich syndrome who had a 2-week history of right ankle pain, erythema, and draining ulcer.

Scan.—Four-phase ^{99m}Tc MDP bone scan.

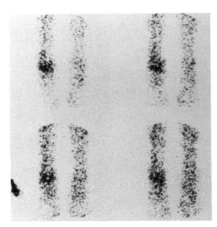

Anterior flow study of lower legs.

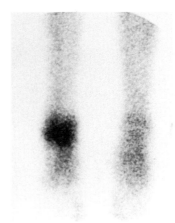

Blood pool.

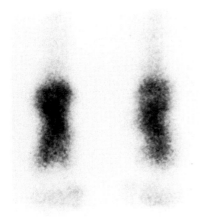

2-hour delayed image.

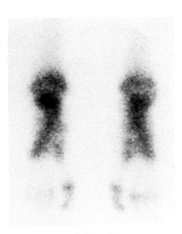

6-hour delayed image.

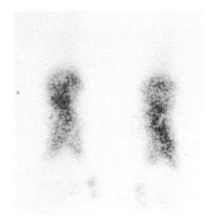

24-hour delayed image.

Findings.—The angiographic and blood pool phases show hyperemia to the right ankle. The delayed images show progressive washout of tracer from the bones of the affected ankle so that both ankles appear symmetric by 24 hours.

Diagnosis.—Cellulitis of the right ankle.

A common clinical problem is whether a known soft tissue infection has extended into bone. The bone scan can distinguish between cellulitis and osteomyelitis. Many institutions use a three-phase bone scan to determine the presence of osteomyelitis. The three phases are angiogram, blood pool, and 2-hour delayed image. At our institution we use a four-phase bone scan, which improves the specificity of the three-phase scan. The fourth phase is a 24-hour image. This gives a sensitivity and specificity of 76% to 91%.

Angiographic and blood pool phases will show hyperemia and increased blood pool activity in both cellulitis and osteomyelitis, reflecting hypervascularity to the tissues. The third and fourth phases show progressively increasing bony uptake in osteomyelitis with a higher bone/soft tissue ratio over time because of the increased osteoblast activity that occurs as a response to infection. In cellulitis there is progressive washout of activity from the soft tissues so that the bone/soft tissue ratio falls over time. However, delayed images sometimes show mild diffusely increased uptake in the affected extremity and may show mild focal activity as well.

Ulcerations, cellulitis, osteomyelitis, and neurotrophic osteoarthropathy are features of the diabetic foot. Ischemia and sympathetic denervation make the foot highly susceptible to trauma. Because of the osteoarthropathic changes of the diabetic foot, the four-phase bone scan may show mild diffuse and focal increased uptake in all four phases, even in the absence of osteomyelitis. Degenerative sites sometimes show false positive increasing uptake as well.

CASE 37

History.—68-year-old woman with a history of diabetes and an ulcer on the right great toe and second toe. Bone scan was performed to evaluate for possible osteomyelitis.

Scan.—Four-phase ^{99m}Tc MDP bone scan.

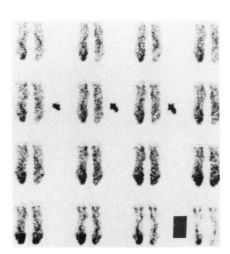

Flow study of feet.

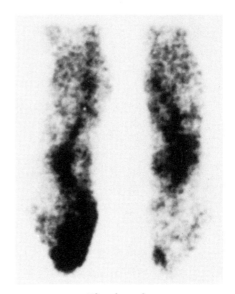

Blood pools.

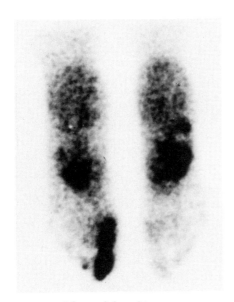

2-hour delayed image.

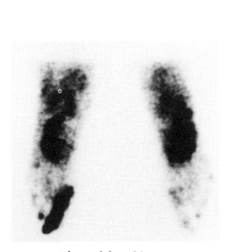

6-hour delayed image.

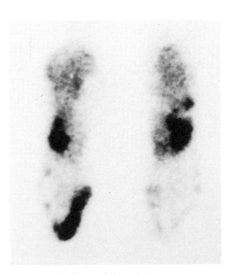

24-hour delayed image.

Findings.—On the angiographic images, asymmetric flow is seen with hyperemia to the medial right foot. Blood pool images show increased uptake in this region as well. Delayed images at 2 hours show increased activity of the first and second toes, with progressively increasing bony uptake, especially in the second toe, and decreasing soft tissue uptake over 24 hours.

Diagnosis.—Osteomyelitis.

The four-phase bone scan is used to differentiate soft tissue inflammation from osteomyelitis. The four phases are angiogram, blood pool, 4-hour delayed image, and 24-hour image. After the routine 4-hour delayed image, views of the area of concern are obtained for 100,000 counts. At 24 hours, these same views are obtained again for 100,000 counts. The 100,000-count views at 4 and 24 hours are used to compare the intensity of bone uptake at these intervals. Osteomyelitis should show increasing uptake over this interval, being most intense at 24 hours, whereas soft tissue infections will decrease in intensity over time.

In children, osteomyelitis is caused by the hematogenous spread of an acute infection. Osteomyelitis occurs in the metaphyseal-epiphyseal region, where the growing epiphyseal ends have the greatest blood flow. The vessels here end in vascular arcades that slow local flow. Spread to adjacent joints usually does not occur except in infants, where the growth plate does not serve as an effective barrier. Pus may spread, however, along the periosteum or through the marrow cavity, with eventual cortical penetration via the haversian system. Occasionally, increased pressure or periosteal stripping by purulent exudate may produce local ischemia and a cold defect on bone scan.

In adults, the pathogenesis is different. Approximately half of adults will give a history of a superficial *Staphylococcus* infection; in these cases, infection tends to occur by contiguous spread. The most common locations for osteomyelitis are about the knee, the ankle, and the shoulder. Plain films are usually normal the first 10 to 14 days, and blood cultures are positive in only 50% of cases. When spread is hematogenous in adults, osteomyelitis usually occurs in the vertebral column. This is commonly seen in intravenous drug abusers.

Both the sensitivity and specificity of the four-phase bone scan for osteomyelitis are approximately 76% to 91%. Sensitivity is decreased for neonates and elderly patients and possibly also in the face of antibiotic therapy. The bone scan is usually abnormal within the first 24 hours of symptoms. The classic bone scan findings for osteomyelitis are increased flow, increased blood pool, and increased uptake on delayed images, with an increase in the bone/soft tissue ratio of activity over time. Soft tissue infections such as cellulitis also show increased angiographic and blood pool activity but will show washout of activity over time. The fourth phase of the scan improves specificity for osteomyelitis approximately 8% to 10% over a three-phase scan.

As mentioned previously, osteomyelitis occasionally produces a cold lesion on bone scan. This occurs more commonly in children early in the course of the disease. It is thought to be secondary to increased pressure compromising blood flow, periosteal stripping by pus, and interruption of blood supply by thrombosis and sludging. These patients are at increased risk for sequestrum formation. The lesion will usually subsequently become hot, passing through a phase of normal uptake.

Gallium 67 citrate and indium 111 oxine are other radiopharmaceuticals useful in the evaluation for osteomyelitis, especially in the cases of equivocal bone scan findings.

CASE 38

History.—60-year-old man with a painful right hip prosthesis 6 months after implantation.

Scan.—^{99m}Tc MDP bone scan.

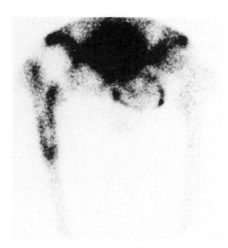

Anterior view of pelvis.

Findings.—Diffuse increased uptake involving the femoral and acetabular components of right hip prosthesis.

Diagnosis.—Infected prosthesis.

Radionuclide bone scanning using ^{99m}Tc MDP is frequently used to diagnose prosthetic joint complications. Painful prostheses can be caused by loosening, infection, heterotopic ossification, inflammatory bursitis, breakage of fixation wires, fracture, and dislocation of the prosthesis. Although the bone scan is more sensitive than plain radiographs for detecting complications, plain radiographs should be obtained first, because if they are abnormal, the work-up can stop.

The bone scan can be useful in two ways. First, a normal bone scan (and plain films) makes significant pathologic conditions as the cause of pain extremely unlikely. Second, the pattern of uptake can suggest a specific diagnosis such as loosening or infection.

Bone scan evaluation of prostheses should include angiographic, blood pool, and 3- to 4-hour delayed imaging. A normal, mature prosthesis should show no evidence of increased blood flow or blood pool activity. Delayed images show a photopenic defect corresponding to the prosthesis. Diffuse or focal areas of increased uptake may be seen, depending on the age of the prosthesis. Activity around the prosthesis, including at the tip, may be seen for 9 to 12 months postoperatively in normal individuals and has occasionally been reported as late as 36 months after surgery. Increased activity in the region of the greater or lesser trochanter is normal, regardless of prosthesis age. It is helpful to use the contralateral hip as a control if it does not also have a prosthesis.

Loosening of the prosthesis usually produces focal abnormalities on delayed imaging. In prosthetic hips, the femoral component tends to loosen early and the acetabular component late. In knee prostheses, it is the tibial component that fails more often, frequently without radiographic changes. With loosening, angiographic and blood pool images are normal. Delayed images show increased uptake around the prosthesis, which, in the case of total hip arthroplasties, is usually focal at the tip of the femoral component. Although diffuse uptake around the prosthesis can be seen with loosening, it is more characteristic of infection.

Infection of a prosthesis will produce abnormal bone scan findings in all three imaging phases. Angiographic and blood pool images show hyperemia and increased blood pool activity. Delayed images show increased uptake diffusely around the prosthesis. As earlier, this pattern is sometimes seen with loosening. Because infection causes loosening, it is not surprising that characteristics of both can be present.

Two other prosthetic complications that can be detected on bone scan are heterotopic ossification and inflammatory bursitis. Both of these cause increased uptake outside the normal confines of bone. The activity of heterotopic ossification usually parallels the prosthetic femoral neck. Inflammatory bursitis produces increased angiographic, blood pool, and delayed images in the expected location of the bursae.

CASE 39

History.— 19-year-old female college student majoring in dance who was also an avid jogger. The study was obtained to evaluate lower extremity pain.

Scan.—^{99m}Tc MDP bone scan.

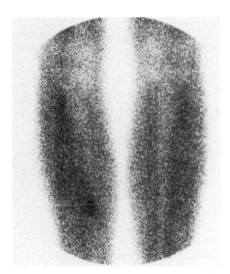

Blood pools of lower extremities.

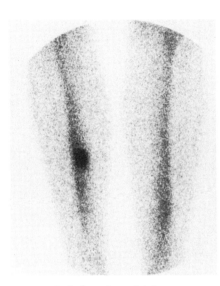

Anterior view of 2-hour delayed images.

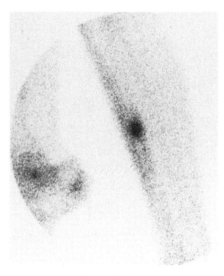

Lateral view.

Findings.— There is focal hyperemia to the right lower extremity on the blood pool images. In the posteromedial aspect of the tibia, there is focal uptake on delayed images involving less than one fifth of the bone's length.

Diagnosis.—Stress fracture of the tibia.

The bone scan is much more sensitive than plain films in the detection of stress injuries. There are two types of stress fractures: fatigue and insufficiency. Fatigue fractures are secondary to abnormal stress on normal bone, as in runners and other athletes. Insufficiency fractures occur in abnormal bone, as in osteoporosis.

If the fatigue fracture is acute (< 1 month), angiographic and blood pool images show increased uptake. In both acute and nonacute stress fractures, delayed images show increased uptake.

A common location of stress fractures is the posteromedial tibia at the junction of the middle and distal thirds of the shaft. The activity is focal, involving less than one fifth the length of the tibia. It often is fusiform shaped longitudinally, usually involving the posterior tibial cortex, and should extend across more than half the width of the bone. Other sites for stress fracture include the metatarsals, tarsals, and, occa-

sionally, the proximal femur and pelvis. Insufficiency fractures occur in abnormal bone.

Shin splints are the main consideration in the differential diagnosis of stress fractures. They occur in the same patient population (young, healthy, active people). Shin splints occur in the same location as tibial stress fractures, in the distal third of the tibia at the posteromedial cortex. The mechanism of injury and scan findings, however, are different. Shin splints are thought to be secondary to abnormal stress of the soleus muscle at its tibial origin. The angiographic and blood pool images are normal. Delayed images show longitudinal, linear uptake on the posteromedial tibial cortex involving at least one third of the length of the bone, often longer. This is in contrast to stress fractures, which involve less than one fifth of the bone. Because stress is the cause of both types of injuries, it is not uncommon to see both shin splints and stress fractures in the same patient.

CASE 40

History.— 7-year-old boy with left hip pain.

Scan.—^{99m}Tc MDP scan with pinhole images.

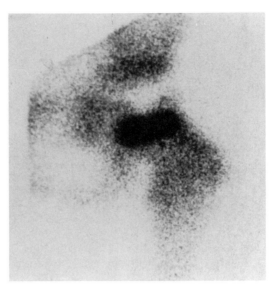

Anterior pinhole view of left hip.

Findings.— Decreased epiphyseal activity in left femoral head.

Diagnosis.— Legg-Calvé-Perthes disease.

Legg-Calvé-Perthes disease is necrosis of the capital femoral epiphysis, which affects primarily children ages 4 to 8 years old. It is thought to be secondary to compromise of the vascular supply to the femoral epiphysis. Males are affected more than females, and it is usually unilateral, although 10% of cases are bilateral. After loss of vascular supply, there is necrosis of the femoral capital epiphysis, which may be followed by revascularization and bone healing.

The bone scan is useful in both the diagnosis and management of Legg-Calvé-Perthes disease. It has a sensitivity of 98% and specificity of 95% compared with 92% sensitivity and 78% specificity with conventional radiography. Bone scan findings precede radiographic changes by several months.

The findings on bone scan depend on the stage of disease. Early decreased activity in the femoral capital epiphysis with increased uptake in the acetabulum is seen, caused by loss of vascularity to the femoral head epiphysis and associated synovitis.

The femoral head receives its blood supply from a single capsular branch of the medial circumflex artery, which is vulnerable to compromise. Decreased activity is seen on bone scan when elevated joint pressure is sufficient to impair vascular supply. Thus in severe or long-standing joint effusions, femoral head infarction may occur.

As revascularization and bone healing occurs in Legg-Calvé-Perthes disease increased uptake is seen in the femoral head. This finding indicates a better prognosis. Demonstration of bone healing is useful in predicting viability of the femoral head. Pinhole images are best.

CASE 41

History.—63-year-old man with chronic renal failure and lumbar pain.

Scan.—^{99m}Tc MDP bone scan.

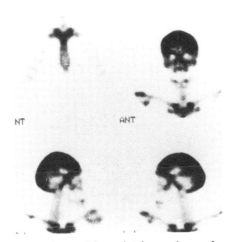

Anterior and lateral 2-hour views of head and chest.

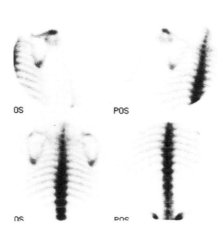

Posterior view of shoulders and back.

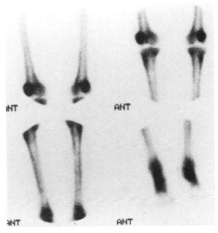

Anterior view of femurs, knees, tibias, and feet.

Findings.— There is marked skeletal uptake of ^{99m}Tc MDP diffusely and symmetrically with little or no soft tissue activity. The increased uptake involves the calvarium and extremities equally, as well as the axial skeleton. The kidneys are not visualized.

Diagnosis.— Secondary hyperparathyroidism.

There are three types of hyperparathyroidism: primary, secondary, and tertiary. Although all are characterized by elevated serum calcium and parathyroid hormone levels, their bone scan appearance varies.

Primary hyperparathyroidism is caused by hyperplasia or tumor of the parathyroid glands, which results in excessive production of parathyroid hormone. When tumor is present, it is almost always a benign parathyroid adenoma, although rarely, parathyroid carcinoma can cause hyperparathyroidism. Serologic features of primary hyperparathyroidism include increased levels of serum parathyroid hormone, calcium, and alkaline phosphatase, with a decreased serum phosphate level.

Approximately 50% to 80% of patients with primary hyperparathyroidism will have normal bone scans. Those scans that are abnormal show uptake in the same areas that characteristically demonstrate demineralization, erosion, or both. These areas include the calvarium, mandible, acromioclavicular joint, sternum, lateral humeral epicondyles, and hands. Calvarial involvement tends to be peripheral. When present,

brown tumors may show accumulation of the radiotracer or may appear as cold defects. Soft tissue calcification may also cause radioisotope accumulation. This may be seen in the lungs, stomach, kidneys, heart, and joints.

Secondary hyperparathyroidism is an acquired condition usually associated with chronic renal failure. In this condition, excessive destruction of renal parenchyma results in the inability to hydroxylate 25-hydroxycholecalciferol to its 1,25-dihydroxy form. This results in vitamin D deficiency, which causes a compensatory rise in parathyroid hormone levels.

Unlike the primary form, secondary hyperparathyroidism usually demonstrates an abnormal bone scan. If symmetric uptake is present, a superscan occurs. Excellent skeletal detail, absent renal activity, and calvarial and extremity uptake equal to axial skeleton activity are seen. Often secondary hyperparathyroidism results in asymmetric uptake. Focal abnormalities will be seen at the same sites as primary hyperparathyroidism. In addition, increased uptake in the metacarpals, proximal and distal phalanges, and costochondral regions may be seen. Soft tissue calcifications may also occur.

CASE 42

History.— 24-year-old woman with hypercalcemia.

Scan.— ^{99m}Tc MDP.

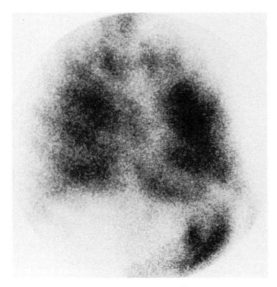

Anterior view of chest on bone scan.

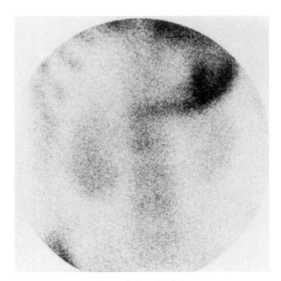

Anterior abdominal image.

Findings.— Chest and left upper quadrant activity is present.

Diagnosis.— Hyperparathyroidism.

In the lung, soft tissue uptake of bone agents occurs secondary to both benign and malignant disease. Malignant causes of pulmonary MDP uptake include metastatic calcification, bronchogenic carcinoma, metastases from osteosarcoma, and malignant pleural effusions. Benign etiologies of pulmonary activity include radiation therapy, fibrothorax, sarcoidosis, interstitial pulmonary calcification, berylliosis, and lung nodules in patients receiving chronic hemodialysis. Pulmonary uptake also has been described in hyperparathyroid patients with hypercalcemia and renal failure, and is thought to be secondary to tissue deposition of hydroxyapatite.

Hyperparathyroidism is associated with soft tissue calcification in other organs, including the stomach (as in this patient), kidneys, and adrenal glands.

History.— 58-year-old man with prostate cancer. Rule
out metastases.

Scan.—^{99m}Tc MDP bone scan.

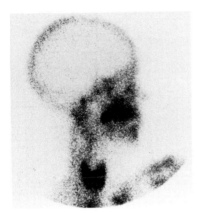

Lateral view of skull and cervical spine.

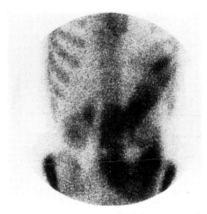

Anterior view of abdomen.

Findings.—There is no focal osseous uptake of MDP. However, ^{99m}Tc is seen in the thyroid gland, oral pharynx, and GI tract.

Diagnosis.—Soft tissue uptake of free ^{99m}Tc.

^{99m}Tc is eluted from a molybdenum 99 generator in its Tc +7 oxidation state as the ^{99m}Tc pertechnetate ion ^{99m}TcO$_4^-$. In this state, Tc will not tag the phosphate bone agents. Stannous chloride is used to reduce ^{99m}Tc pertechnetate to the Tc +4 oxidation state for bonding. In the +4 state, a ^{99m}Tc Sn-phosphate complex forms that localizes in bone.

Before use, all bone radiopharmaceuticals should be checked by chromatography for labeling efficiency. A 90% to 95% or more labeling efficiency is required for use. It is important that oxygen not be introduced into the mixing vial during the preparation of the radiopharmaceutical because oxidation of ^{99m}Tc reduces tagging efficiency. It is also important to use kits within 4 hours after their preparation because the tag breaks down with time.

Soft tissue uptake of ^{99m}Tc can be secondary to a poor tag with the formation of free ^{99m}Tc pertechnetate, hydrolyzed-reduced ^{99m}Tc, or pathologic processes that take up adequately tagged ^{99m}Tc MDP in soft tissues.

Bone radiopharmaceutical quality control is done with thin-layer chromatography. Chromatography separates a chemical mixture into its components based on their solubility (or polarity). Two chromatograms are necessary to fully evaluate ^{99m}Tc MDP. The first uses saline solution as the solvent to determine the proportion of hydrolyzed ^{99m}Tc and ^{99m}Tc Sn colloid (^{99m}Tc in a reduced state but not bound to diphosphonate). Radiochemical impurities hydrolyzed ^{99m}Tc and ^{99m}Tc Sn colloid remain at the origin, whereas ^{99m}Tc MDP and free ^{99m}Tc move with the solvent front. The second separation uses acetone or acetone and methanol as solvent. Free ^{99m}Tc moves with the solvent front, whereas ^{99m}Tc MDP and reduced ^{99m}Tc stay at the origin. The percentage radioactivity at the origin of the saline chromatogram is added to the percentage of activity at the solvent front of the acetone separation to obtain the total percent of radiochemical impurities. Less than 5% to 10% impurities is acceptable (although not ideal).

Free ^{99m}Tc pertechnetate is taken up and excreted by the thyroid gland, gastric mucosa, and the gastrointestinal tract. Bone scan activity in these areas is almost always secondary to free ^{99m}Tc pertechnetate and not a pathologic process.

Appropriately labeled ^{99m}Tc MDP can also be seen in soft tissues because of pathologic processes. Generalized soft tissue uptake can be secondary to renal failure and chronic iron overload (this may also be seen with poor radiopharmaceutical preparation). More focal uptake of phosphate bone agents in soft tissues is seen in malignant tumors and fluid collections (i.e., effusions and ascites). Ovarian cancer (usually mucinous), colon cancer, neuroblastoma, and hepatic metastases are also likely to accumulate bone agents.

Soft tissue calcifications may take up the bone agent. These include dystrophic and metastatic calcifications at injection sites and surgical scars or from hyperparathyroidism and tumoral calcinosis. Inflammation and tissue infarction as in myositis, polymositis, and stroke patients, can show bone agent uptake.

Breast uptake may be seen in estrogenically active individuals, both male and female, as in pubertal and lactating women, chronic liver disease, and prostate cancer patients on hormonal therapy. Breast uptake may also be seen with corticosteroid therapy. Soft tissue activity has been described in amyloid deposits, hematomas, and radiation therapy portals. Finally, one of the most common causes of soft tissue uptake is extravasation at the injection site. Although this is usually a straightforward situation, injection through "unusual" ports, such as chemotherapy catheters, may mimic lesions.

The kidneys normally are faintly visualized on bone scan. However, enhanced renal uptake may be seen with chemotherapy. Also, urine contamination of skin or clothing and renal or ureteral obstruction will show extrarenal activity.

CASE 44

History.—72-year-old man with lung cancer being evaluated for possible osseous metastases.

Scan.—^{99m}Tc MDP bone scan.

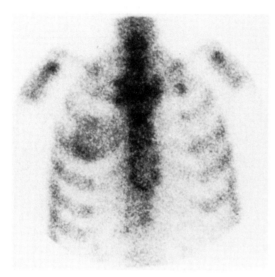

Anterior view of chest.

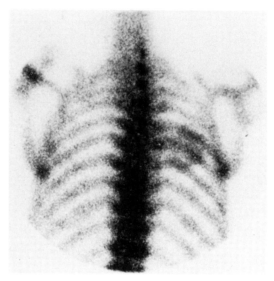

Posterior view of chest.

Findings.—The bones appear unremarkable. There is soft tissue uptake in the right thorax.

Diagnosis.—Soft tissue uptake of ^{99m}Tc MDP in primary bronchogenic carcinoma.

^{99m}Tc MDP is the most commonly used organophosphate bone agent. It has a high avidity for bone and is rapidly excreted by the kidney, resulting in a high target/background ratio.

Adequate patient hydration is essential for a high target/background ratio and optimal image quality. Patients with poor hydration or poor renal function have diminished target/background ratios with diffuse soft tissue activity.

Organophosphate uptake may be seen in many soft tissue lesions. Both heterotopic ossification and soft tissue calcification are visible on bone scanning and may also be seen radiographically. However, radiographically noncalcified soft tissue lesions are sometimes readily seen on bone scanning as well. The mechanism of localization of bone radiopharmaceuticals in nongrossly calcified soft tissues may be related to the influx of calcium from the extracellular space (microscopic calcification). In muscle injury, calcium enters the cell through the damaged sarcolemma, which has abnormal permeability. This is the mechanism responsible for uptake of organophosphates in acute myocardial infarction. Other possible mechanisms for soft tissue uptake include binding to immature collagen and phosphatase enzymes.

Soft tissue uptake of bone agent has been described in many conditions, including infection, primary tumor (benign or malignant), metastases, radiopharmaceutical breakdown, trauma, and injection sites. This patient shows uptake of MDP in his primary lung tumor.

CASE 45

History.—60-year-old man with bone pain, history of prostate carcinoma.

Scan.—^{99m}Tc MDP bone scan.

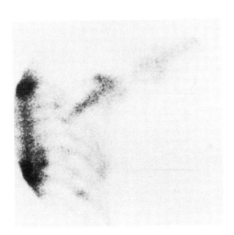

Posterior view of right shoulder.

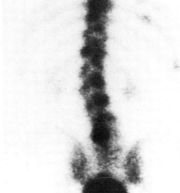

Posterior thoracolumbar spine.

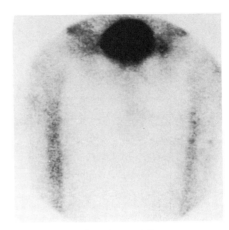

Anterior view of femurs.

Findings.—Increased uptake of ^{99m}Tc MDP in muscle of arms and legs.

Diagnosis.—Soft tissue uptake of ^{99m}Tc MDP secondary to intramuscular injections of narcotics, metastatic prostate carcinoma.

Soft tissue uptake of bone agents has been described at sites of injection of iron dextran for anemia and other drug injections, in surgical incisions, at sites of infiltrated calcium gluconate solution, with soft tissue inflammation, abscess, radiation therapy, fat necrosis, precordial electrical stimulation, after sympathectomy, in muscle trauma, and after radiographic contrast.

This patient shows uptake in the extremities. This was a common site for the patient to self-administer intramuscular narcotics.

CASE 46

History.— 32-year-old man with generalized, tonic-clonic ethanol withdrawal seizures 2 days before this study, followed by muscular edema and rising CPK levels.

Scan.—^{99m}Tc MDP bone scan.

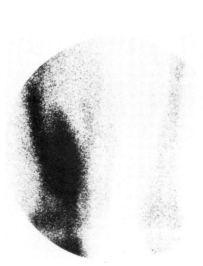

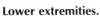

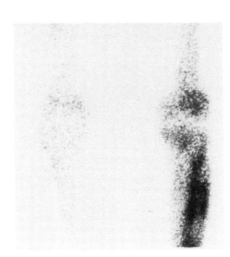

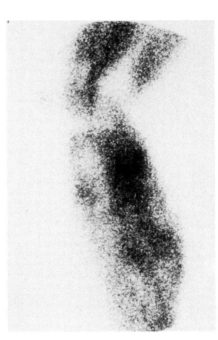

| Lower extremities. | Knees. | Lateral view of right calf. |

Findings.— Increased skeletal muscle uptake in the right lower extremity.

Diagnosis.— Rhabdomyolysis.

Rhabdomyolysis involves acute skeletal muscle injury. It is caused by a variety of disorders, including trauma, overexertion (seizures, long-distance runners), pressure necrosis (unconsciousness with an extremity under the body), heatstroke, and frostbite. The necrotic tissues release myoglobin into the blood, which can lead to acute tubular necrosis.

The uptake of bone agents into skeletal muscle is similar to what occurs in the heart with myocardial necrosis. Injury leads to an abnormal influx of calcium. The calcium binds the bone agent in various states, including hydroxyapatite crystals.

CASE 47

History.— 22-year-old motorcyclist who suffered a closed head injury in a motor vehicle accident 2 months earlier developed new hip pain.

Scan.—^{99m}Tc MDP bone scan.

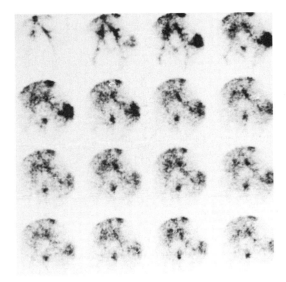

Posterior flow study of pelvis.

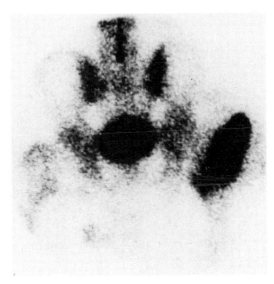

2-hour delayed image.

Findings.— Angiographic images show hyperemia to the soft tissues of the right hip. Delay images show intense uptake of ^{99m}Tc MDP in the same region.

Diagnosis.—HO of the right hip, which is skeletally immature.

Heterotopic ossification (HO), or posttraumatic periostitis, is a form of myositis ossificans associated with neurologic injury. Approximately 25% of patients with spinal cord injury develop HO, and 33% to 49% of patients with paraplegia are affected in the paralyzed area, most commonly the hips.

HO becomes clinically evident 4 to 10 weeks after injury. It can manifest as acute inflammation, which, in these posttrauma or postburn patients, may mimic deep venous thrombosis or infection. If left untreated, it will progress for 6 to 18 months and lead to joint ankylosis.

HO is classified as either immature or mature, based on osseous maturity. The radionuclide bone scan using ^{99m}Tc MDP is useful for both diagnosing HO and determining maturity. Early in the course of HO, the bone scan is more sensitive than plain radiography.

Typical findings of immature HO are increased uptake in the soft tissues on the angiographic, blood pool, and delayed phases of the scan. Immature HO also shows absence of uptake when marrow imaging agents such as ^{99m}Tc sulfur colloid are used.

HO patients are followed with serial ^{99m}Tc MDP bone scans to determine when maturation occurs. As HO matures, the angiographic and blood pool phase activity will normalize, and activity on delayed images will decrease and then plateau. Marrow uptake will be seen on ^{99m}Tc sulfur colloid scans, indicating marrow formation.

The treatment of HO is based on its maturity. During the immature stage of HO, pharmacologic therapy is used. Surgical resection of heterotopic bone is performed only on mature HO because this reduces the recurrence rate.

CASE 48

History.— 25-year-old man with a history of malignancy.

Scan.—^{99m}Tc MDP bone scan.

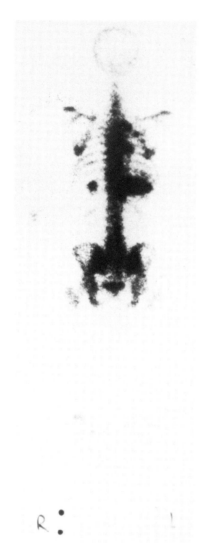

Whole-body image, posterior view.

Findings.—Increased uptake is seen in multiple ribs, scapula, and spine. One area of uptake on left is between the ribs.

Diagnosis.—Osteosarcoma metastatic to the pleura.

Soft tissue uptake of organophosphate bone agents can be seen with a variety of both benign and malignant conditions. The mechanism of uptake is related to soft tissue calcification, heterotopic ossification, or abnormally permeable sarcolemma, allowing abnormal influx of intracellular calcium.

There are numerous etiologies for soft tissue organophosphate uptake. Malignant causes of soft tissue bone agent uptake include primary neural tumors (cerebral tumors, schwannoma, neurolemmoma, neuroblastoma), brain metastases, endocrine tumors (calcified, well-differentiated thyroid carcinoma, medullary carcinoma), primary or metastatic breast cancer, lung tumors (bronchogenic carcinoma, malignant pleural effusion), GI tumors (cholangiocarcinoma, mucinous gastric adenocarcinoma, melanoma, colorectal cancer), renal or genitourinary malignancy (primary renal tumors, lymphosarcoma, ovarian carcinoma, seminoma), musculoskeletal (osteosarcoma, rhabdomyosarcoma, synovioma), and splenic malignancies (lymphoma, reticulum cell sarcoma, lymphosarcoma). Metastatic mucinous ovarian and colorectal carcinomas are especially prone to soft tissue uptake. With ovarian carcinoma, peritoneal metastases will show diffuse abdominal uptake. Mucinous colorectal carcinoma usually shows focal or diffuse liver uptake in liver metastases.

This patient has soft tissue uptake in the chest due to metastasis from osteosarcoma. Close scrutiny shows the activity is between ribs rather than the usual osseous location. Osteosarcoma frequently metastasizes to the pleura and can cause pneumothorax. Soft tissue uptake in metastases from osteosarcoma has also been described in the liver, skin, and subcutaneous tissues.

CASE 49

History.—54-year-old woman with biopsy-proved adenocarcinoma of unknown primary. We were asked to evaluate for metastatic disease.

Scan.—⁹⁹ᵐTc MDP bone scan and renal ultrasound.

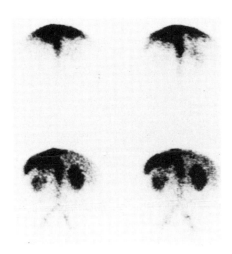

Flow study of kidneys.

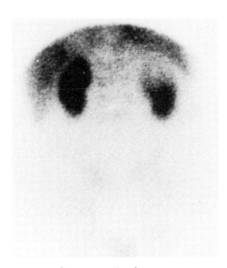

Images at 2 minutes.

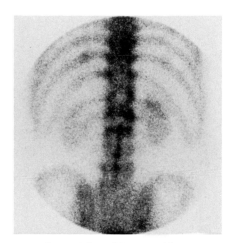

2-hour delayed image of lower lumbar spine.

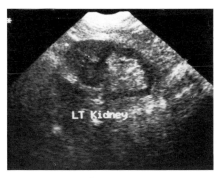

Renal ultrasound.

Findings.—Angiographic images over the kidneys show decreased flow to the upper pole of the left kidney. Blood pool images show a large photopenic area in the same region. Delayed images over the lumbar spine show a focal rib uptake on the left with diffuse thoracic spine activity. Ultrasound shows echogenic upper pole mass.

Diagnosis.—Renal cell carcinoma with osseous metastases.

At our institution angiographic and blood pool images over the kidneys are performed routinely. This is done for three reasons. Because MDP is excreted by the kidneys, it allows renal blood flow and function to be evaluated. Vascular structures such as the abdominal aorta and iliac arteries can also be evaluated; aneurysms will pool tracer on the flow study. Finally, early bone uptake on blood pool images can indicate a superscan.

Renal cell carcinomas are typically described as hypervas-

cular. However, a surprising number do not show increased flow on radionuclide flow studies. In this patient, ultrasound revealed a 10-cm renal mass, found at surgery to be renal cell carcinoma.

CHAPTER 3

Cardiovascular

CASE 50

History.—53-year-old nonsmoking man with epigastric discomfort. He has a previous history of peptic ulcer disease. Risk factors for coronary artery disease included positive family history and mildly elevated cholesterol levels.

Scan.—An exercise SPECT ^{201}Tl scan was performed. The patient reached maximal stress.

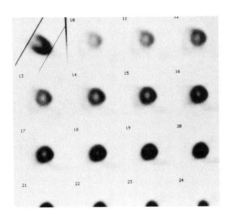
Stress short-axis view.

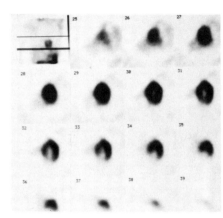
Stress horizontal long-axis view.

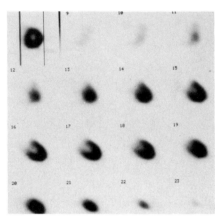
Stress vertical long-axis view.

Findings.—Short-axis stress views show an area of decreased uptake in the septum at the base of the heart; otherwise, there is homogeneous uptake of ^{201}Tl throughout the left ventricle, producing a full doughnut appearance. Horizontal and vertical long-axis views are normal; redistribution images in all three projections (not shown) were unchanged.

Diagnosis.—Normal stress ^{201}Tl scan.

Thallium 201 is a cyclotron-produced isotope that decays by electron capture, emitting mercury K−characteristic x-rays of 68 to 83 keV. It is a group IIIA metal with biologic properties similar to potassium. Like potassium, it is distributed primarily intracellularly. Transport across the cell membrane is dependent on the sodium-potassium pump.

Myocardial concentration of ^{201}Tl is dependent on two main factors: (1) myocardial blood flow and (2) myocardial extraction fraction. Because normally 85% of coronary artery ^{201}Tl is extracted by the myocardium in one pass, blood flow to the myocardium becomes the primary determinant of initial myocardial Tl concentration and the basis of the ^{201}Tl scan for ischemic disease.

Over time, the cardiac and noncardiac ^{201}Tl distribution (skeletal muscle, gastrointestinal tract, and kidneys) distribution changes. The three pools of ^{201}Tl (myocardium−blood pool−extracardiac tissues) continuously exchange in equilib-

rium. This is redistribution. Areas of stress-induced ischemia may show an initial perfusion defect that disappears on delayed images because of redistribution of ^{201}Tl. Nonreversible defects are associated with myocardial scars.

Normal ^{201}Tl scans show decreased uptake in the region of the basal septum, which represents valve plane or membranous septum. There are other areas of normal variation or artifact that can simulate defects in normal myocardium. Apical thinning on both stress and redistribution images mimics apical scar. Anterolateral defects are often seen in women and are secondary to breast attenuation. Inferior wall defects on stress images only may represent "cardiac creep," or increased superoinferior myocardial motion, because the diaphragmatic excursion increases with exercise. Likewise, fixed inferior defects may be seen secondary to diaphragmatic attenuation. These are more common in males.

CASE 51

History.—61-year-old woman with atypical chest pain.

Scan.—Stress ^{201}Tl SPECT scan.

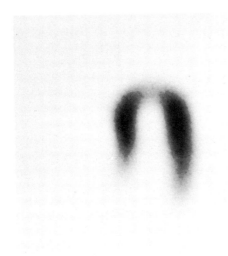

Horizontal long-axis stress slice.

Horizontal long-axis redistribution slice.

Findings.—This patient's ^{201}Tl scan shows a defect in the apex, seen on both stress and redistribution views.

Diagnosis.—Normal apical thinning.

Usually a fixed defect on ^{201}Tl scan that does not redistribute is a myocardial infarction (MI). This is not always the case, however.

A nonreversible ^{201}Tl defect can result from a variety of causes other than a previous MI. For example, the inferior wall and apex frequently show a fixed ^{201}Tl defect, which represents artifact and normal anatomic variant.

In the inferior wall, nonreversible defects can be caused by diaphragmatic attenuation such as when the patient's stomach is distended. On planar imaging, the patient can be placed in a left lateral decubitus position to lower the left side of the diaphragm, reducing attenuation. With single-photon emission computed tomography (SPECT), the patient can be imaged in the prone position, although special equipment is necessary to reduce both the camera's distance from the patient and attenuation from the table.

A related problem known as "heart creep" can cause inferior wall defects on stress images, which appear to redistrib-

ute on delayed images. It is thought that the increased diaphragmatic excursion during stress from deep breathing, possibly associated with gastric distention from air swallowing, raises the relative position of the diaphragm on stress images. This causes diaphragmatic attenuation of the inferior wall. At redistribution, the patient breathes normally, which places the diaphragm in a lower position. The degree of diaphragmatic attenuation is therefore reduced, producing a more normal appearance. Defects caused by heart creep may occur in up to 29% of cases.

Nonreversible apical defects caused by normal anatomic thinning are also commonly seen. Differentiation between normal apical thinning and apical infarct is a difficult problem. Complete absence of activity involving a substantial portion of the apex is more suggestive of infarct. Also, apical infarcts sometimes have associated aneurysms. Apical aneurysms have diverging walls on ^{201}Tl scan.

CASE 52

History.—70-year-old man with a 50-pack-year history of smoking.

Scan.—Resting ^{201}Tl SPECT image.

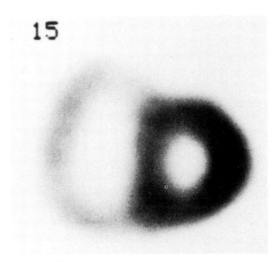

Short-axis reconstruction view.

Findings.—Right ventricular uptake.

Diagnosis.—Cor pulmonale.

The significance of right ventricular ^{201}Tl uptake depends on whether the images are stress, redistribution, or rest. Right ventricular uptake on stress ^{201}Tl images is normal. Right ventricular uptake is frequently seen on redistribution images as well, and again is usually normal. Resting ^{201}Tl images, however, show ^{201}Tl activity in the right ventricle only infrequently (15% of normal individuals).

There are numerous causes of abnormal right ventricular uptake of ^{201}Tl on resting studies; they are usually the result of right ventricular overload (volume or pressure). Causes of right ventricular overload include atrial septal defect, tetralogy of Fallot, corrected transposition of the great vessels, ventricular septal defect with Eisenmenger's complex, congestive cardiomyopathy, hypertrophic cardiomyopathy, valvular disease (aortic insufficiency, aortic and mitral stenosis, and pulmonic stenosis), cor pulmonale, pulmonary hypertension (primary or secondary to left ventricular dysfunction), cystic fibrosis, and sarcoidosis.

CASE 53

History.— 54-year-old man with atypical chest pain and epigastric discomfort. He had a remote history of peptic ulcer disease. CAD risk factors included strong family history, hypercholesterolemia, and a sedentary lifestyle. He was a nonsmoker.

Scan.—Stress ^{201}Tl SPECT scan.

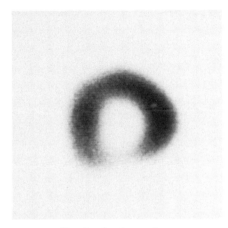

Short-axis stress view.

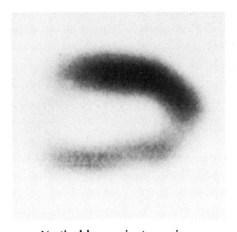

Vertical long-axis stress view.

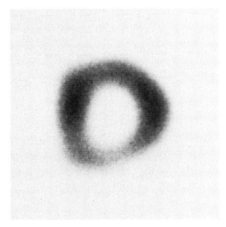

Short-axis redistribution view.

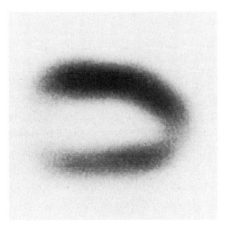

Vertical long-axis redistribution view.

Findings.— On the stress short-axis images, a defect is present in the inferior wall that shows reperfusion on the redistribution images. No other defects are seen.

Diagnosis.— Single-vessel ischemia supplying the inferior wall.

Ischemic heart disease is the most common reason for obtaining exercise ^{201}Tl scans. The sensitivity and specificity of planar ^{201}Tl scans approaches 85%. For single-photon-emission computed tomography (SPECT) Tl scans, the sensitivity improves to 90% or more, although there may be a decrease in specificity.

Sensitivity for detection of coronary artery disease (CAD) increases with the number of diseased vessels. Sensitivity is 73% for single-vessel disease, 87% for two-vessel disease, and 97% for triple-vessel disease.

Exercise ^{201}Tl scans often underestimate the extent of disease. Exercise is stopped when the patient becomes symptomatic; this occurs when the myocardium supplied by the most critical lesion becomes ischemic. Myocardium supplied by less critically diseased vessels are not stressed and may appear normal. Dipyridamole studies do not have this limitation.

Planar ^{201}Tl scanning is best at detecting left anterior descending artery (LAD) disease (sensitivity 74%) and right CAD (sensitivity 69%). It is poor at detecting circumflex artery disease, with reported sensitivities as low as 38%. SPECT studies significantly improve sensitivity for circumflex disease, although the highest sensitivity is still in the LAD and RCA distribution.

If both fixed and reversible defects are used as the criteria for coronary artery disease, the sensitivity increases to 100% for LAD lesions, 80% for right coronary artery (RCA) lesions, and 65% for circumflex lesions. These figures are based on ^{201}Tl studies in which maximal exercise is obtained. The sensitivity will decrease when exercise is submaximal.

Exercise ^{201}Tl scanning is helpful in patients in whom the exercise tolerance test (ETT) is nondiagnostic. This includes patients with an abnormal electrocardiogram on ETT with either nonanginal chest pain or absence of chest pain, patients with exercise-induced chest pain but no ECG changes, patients with abnormal baseline ECG (arrhythmia, left-bundle branch block, left ventricular hypertrophy), and patients taking medications that alter the ECG tracing, such as digoxin. Exercise ^{201}Tl scanning has been shown to be more sensitive than routine ETT in patients who have submaximal stress and in patients with atypical chest pain.

Bayesian analysis indicates ^{201}Tl scans are best for patient populations with an approximately 50% pretest probability of having CAD. In patients with a high likelihood for disease, an abnormal scan merely confirms already strong clinical suspicion, whereas a normal scan is likely a false negative. Conversely, in patients with a low likelihood of CAD, a normal scan again merely confirms clinical suspicion, whereas an abnormal scan is likely a false positive.

Because ^{201}Tl scanning is physiologically based, it is also helpful in the evaluation of the functional significance of known anatomic lesions. Usually lesions with less than 50% to 75% narrowing are not physiologically significant unless they are of sufficient length or eccentricity to be flow limiting or are in series with other stenoses. Borderline lesions can be evaluated with stress ^{201}Tl imaging. Assessment of the functional significance of collateral coronary arteries can also be done with ^{201}Tl scanning.

CASE 54

History.— 54-year-old man with severe rheumatoid arthritis experiencing angina-like symptoms. He has diabetes, controlled with oral hypoglycemics. He had a 30-pack-year smoking history and chronic obstructive pulmonary disease. A β-blocker had been prescribed for hypertension.

Scan.— An IV dipyridamole ^{201}Tl scan was performed.

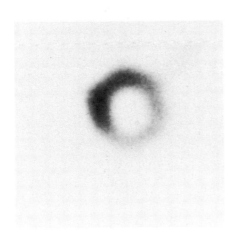

Short-axis stress image.

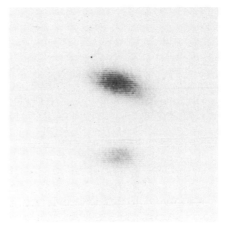

Vertical stress long-axis view.

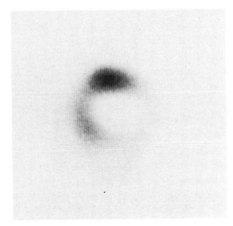

Short-axis redistribution view.

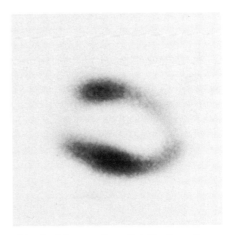

Vertical long-axis redistribution view.

Findings.—Stress: decreased activity in apicolateral wall; redistribution: filling-in of apicolateral wall.

Diagnosis.—Inferior, posterior, and apical ischemia.

The exercise ^{201}Tl scan is dependent on achievement of maximal stress during exercise for good sensitivity and specificity; however, in our institution, one third of all patients do not achieve maximal stress. Their ^{201}Tl scans represent submaximal exercise and have significantly decreased sensitivity for coronary artery disease, perhaps by as much as 50%.

The dipyridamole ^{201}Tl scan is useful in patients who cannot exercise adequately or who do not show the normal physiologic response to exercise as assessed by heart rate and blood pressure. This includes patients with arthritis, amputation, severe peripheral vascular disease, stroke, and diabetes. It is also useful in patients using β-blockers who cannot increase their heart rate adequately with exercise. Patients with dysrhythmias may tolerate dipyridamole stress testing better than exercise stress testing.

Two patient populations in whom the dipyridamole ^{201}Tl scan is the best predictor of prognosis are those with preoperative peripheral vascular disease patients or post-uncomplicated myocardial infarct (MI) before discharge. Specifically, the dipyridamole scan is superior to the submaximal exercise ^{201}Tl scan in the patient, with predischarge, post-uncomplicated MI.

Dipyridamole is a potent vasodilator. It acts by inhibiting the enzyme adenosine deaminase, which allows the accumulation of adenosine, a vasodilator. Normal coronary vessels respond to dipyridamole by dilating and increasing blood flow to the myocardium.

Diseased vessels narrowed by atherosclerotic plaque are already maximally dilated in an effort to preserve blood flow to the myocardium. These vessels will not show a response to dipyridamole. Because the flow through normal vessels increases and the flow through narrowed vessels does not, ^{201}Tl delivery to normal myocardium increases disproportionately. This causes a contrast between myocardium supplied by normal vessels and that supplied by narrowed vessels. Dipyridamole may also increase myocardial oxygen consumption.

Theophylline is a direct antagonist of dipyridamole; the only absolute contraindication to a dipyridamole ^{201}Tl scan is a patient taking a theophylline-related drug. In this case, the scan can be performed 24 to 48 hours after the discontinuation of the drug.

Dipyridamole may be given orally or intravenously; the oral dose is 300 mg, and the IV dose is 142 μg/kg/min infused over 4 minutes. Heart rate, blood pressure, and 12-lead ECG are monitored throughout the study.

In nondiabetic patients who have normal gastric emptying and take the drug orally, ^{201}Tl is injected 45 minutes after ingestion; imaging begins at 60 minutes. Diabetic patients are more likely to have delayed gastric emptying, so absorption is allowed to proceed longer. These protocols are based on differences in time to achieve peak serum levels of dipyridamole, which is 20 to 60 minutes for normal patients and as much as 120 minutes for diabetic patients. Serum levels from oral and IV administration are comparable.

With IV administration of dipyridamole, ^{201}Tl is injected at the peak time of effect, approximately 6.5 minutes after the beginning of infusion; imaging begins 5 to 6 minutes later.

If symptomatic, the patient may be rapidly reversed at any point during the examination. Patients in our department are frequently reversed with aminophylline given intravenously after the acquisition of their "stress" images before leaving the department. The acquisitions, both stress and redistribution, are performed identically to an exercise ^{201}Tl scan.

Count statistics for dipyridamole ^{201}Tl scans are higher than for exercise ^{201}Tl scans because of the potency of the vasodilator effects of the dipyridamole, which increase coronary blood flow greater than exercise. With maximal exercise, about 4.4% of the injected ^{201}Tl dose localizes to myocardium; about 3.5% localizes with a resting study. In contrast, 8% to 10% of the injected ^{201}Tl dose localizes using dipyridamole, a significant increase over rest and exercise ^{201}Tl studies. Sensitivity and specificity of dipyridamole ^{201}Tl scans for CAD are comparable with exercise ^{201}Tl scans.

CASE 55

History.—72-year-old woman with angina.

Scan.—Stress ^{201}Tl SPECT scan.

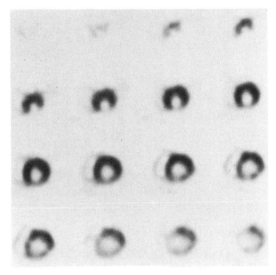

Transaxial stress images.

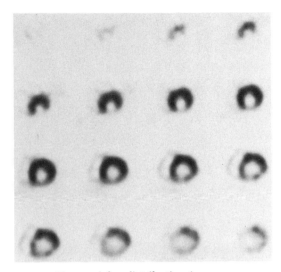

Transaxial redistribution images.

Findings.—Inhomogeneous, globally diminished uptake at stress, which is more homogeneous at redistribution.

Diagnosis.—Balanced triple-vessel ischemia.

Stress ^{201}Tl imaging is most commonly performed for the evaluation of ischemic heart disease. With planar imaging, the sensitivity for coronary artery disease is approximately 75% using reversible defects only and 80% to 85% using both reversible and fixed defects. Specificity is 95% for reversible defects and 85% to 90% using both reversible and nonreversible defects. With single-photon emission computed tomography (SPECT), sensitivity increases to 90% or more, whereas specificity is somewhat lower than with planar imaging.

For single-vessel disease, sensitivity varies depending on the individual vessel involved. Sensitivity with planar imaging is 74% for left anterior descending artery (LAD) lesions, 69% for right coronary artery (RCA) disease, and only 38% for narrowing of the circumflex artery. SPECT improves these figures, especially for the circumflex artery. If a fixed defect is present, the sensitivity for single-vessel disease increases to near 100% for LAD disease, 80% for RCA disease, and 65% for circumflex disease.

The sensitivity of ^{201}Tl scanning increases as the number of diseased vessels increases. Overall sensitivity is 73% for single-vessel disease, 87% for two involved vessels, and 97% for three-vessel disease.

A common concern is that triple-vessel disease may be equally balanced such that the scan will not have focal lesions. Theoretically, this leads to a diffuse decrease in uptake that could be missed. However, this is a rare occurrence. Quantitative programs that determine the degree of uptake and the rate of washout and compare these to a normal file will detect cases of balanced disease.

With single-vessel disease, the presence of a reversible ^{201}Tl abnormality in the distribution of a coronary artery with borderline narrowing is strong evidence the lesion is hemodynamically significant. The absence of a stress-induced abnormality in myocardium supplied by a borderline lesion is only moderately reliable for excluding hemodynamically significant disease. When multivessel disease and a second known significant lesion are present, the absence of stress-induced abnormality in a borderline lesion is not helpful in determining the hemodynamic significance of the borderline lesion. Sensitivity of stress ^{201}Tl studies is limited by the most critical lesions, making evaluation of coexistent, less critical lesions difficult. In these cases, dipyridamole ^{201}Tl scanning is superior.

CASE 56

History.—57-year-old man, 2 weeks after inferior MI. He received IV thrombolytic therapy with tissue plasminogen activator during the acute phase of infarct. Predischarge submaximal exercise ^{201}Tl scan was ordered to identify potential myocardium at risk.

Scan.—70% maximal exercise SPECT ^{201}Tl scan.

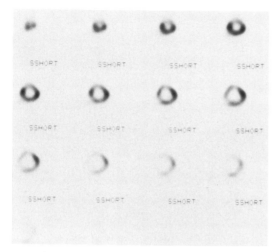

Short-axis stress SPECT reconstruction.

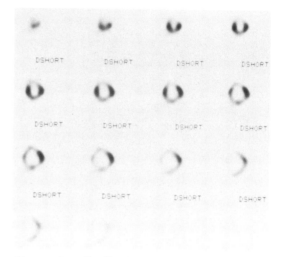

Short-axis redistribution SPECT reconstruction.

Findings.—Stress images show normal uptake in all walls of the left ventricle. Short-axis and vertical long-axis redistribution images show a prominent defect in the inferior wall not present on stress images.

Diagnosis.—Reverse redistribution.

^{201}Tl myocardial scanning is a sensitive technique for detecting ischemic disease. Perfusion defects that appear on exercise images and fill in on redistribution images are strong evidence for ischemic heart disease. However, on occasion defects are seen on redistribution images that were not present on stress images. Also, defects initially seen on stress views may appear even more prominent on redistribution images. This phenomenon has been termed "reverse redistribution," and its significance remains a point of debate.

Reverse redistribution has been described in normal, ischemic, and infarcted myocardium. It has been seen in a wide variety of patient populations including normal individuals, myocardial infarct (MI) patients with revascularization (either surgically or via thrombolytic drugs), and in patients with previous MI. Depending on the population, there has been a markedly different prognostic value for reverse distribution.

The incidence of reverse redistribution is 4% to 20%. One study looking at almost 800 consecutive ^{201}Tl scans showed a low positive predictive value (PPV) of 65% for any coronary artery disease (CAD), with an even lower PPV of 5% for sig-

nificant CAD. In other studies of reverse redistribution, the incidence of significant coronary disease has been higher. To date, all studies examining reverse redistribution have looked at planar exercise ^{201}Tl scans. Reverse redistribution is now known to be seen in single-photon emission computed tomography (SPECT) scans, as well as in dipyridamole ^{201}Tl scans.

A large variety of mechanisms have been proposed to explain the occurrence of reverse redistribution. Rapid washout of Tl in areas of reverse redistribution has been described in both patients who have undergone revascularization of ischemic myocardium and normal patients. Delayed wash-in of ^{201}Tl to ischemic myocardium may make an adjacent scar show reverse redistribution. Technical factors have been suggested as a cause of reverse redistribution. Background subtraction has been shown to cause reverse redistribution in certain patients. Because there is no universally accepted mechanism for reverse redistribution, its clinical significance and prognostic value remain unclear.

CASE 57

History.— 64-year-old man with symptoms of CAD.

Scan.— Stress planar ^{201}Tl scan.

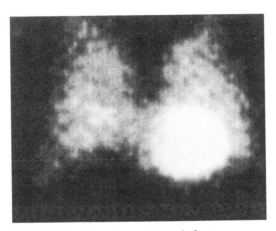

Anterior planar view of chest.

Findings.— Increased pulmonary uptake of ^{201}Tl is seen.

Diagnosis.— Pulmonary uptake of ^{201}Tl with CAD.

^{201}Tl is a group IIIA metal with biologic properties similar to potassium. Like potassium, the distribution of Tl ions after IV administration is primarily intracellular, and its transport across the cell membrane is dependent on the sodium-potassium pump. ^{201}Tl is cyclotron produced and decays by electron capture to mercury 201, which emits characteristic x-rays of 69 to 83 keV. Less abundant γ-rays are also emitted at 135 and 167 keV. The physical half-life of ^{201}Tl is 73 hours.

Two main determinants of initial regional concentration of ^{201}Tl are regional blood flow and myocardial extraction fraction of ^{201}Tl. Regional blood flow is the main determinant of ^{201}Tl concentration, and myocardial uptake is proportional to blood flow. Normally the myocardium extracts 85% of ^{201}Tl presented to it in a single pass. Myocardial extraction of ^{201}Tl is not affected by acidosis, β-blockers, insulin, or digitalis, but it is decreased by extremely high coronary flow rates, as seen with exercise, vasodilators, and hypoxia. Initial myocardial Tl uptake is rapid and peaks at about 10 minutes.

Because approximately 5% of cardiac output flows through the coronary arteries and 85% of ^{201}Tl presented to viable myocardium is extracted, about 4% of the total dose localizes to the myocardium.

Before ^{201}Tl reaches the systemic circulation, about 5% to 15% of the injected dose is extracted by the lungs. The amount of pulmonary uptake is proportional to the pulmonary circulation time. If the pulmonary circulation time is prolonged, pulmonary ^{201}Tl uptake is increased. Therefore, patients with left ventricular failure of any cause (ischemic, viral, valvular, congenital, or ideopathic) will have increased pulmonary uptake and, consequently, have lower heart/lung uptake ratios. Uncommon and rare causes for increased pulmonary uptake of ^{201}Tl are adult respiratory distress syndrome, hypertension, supine exercise, and injection in the supine position.

The remaining approximately 90% of ^{201}Tl is distributed into other organ systems. The systemic organs with the highest Tl uptake include skeletal muscle, the gastrointestinal tract, and the kidneys, which receive the largest radiation dose (1.2 rad/mCi).

Evaluating for increased pulmonary uptake of ^{201}Tl can be useful in two ways: (1) increased pulmonary uptake is a marker of coronary artery disease (CAD); (2) increased pulmonary uptake may indicate more extensive (i.e., multivessel) disease.

To evaluate pulmonary uptake, a 300,000-count planar image is done several minutes after exercise. Regions of interest are defined for the left lung and the myocardium with the highest activity. Ratios of mean counts/pixel (or point) greater than 0.3 to 0.5 are considered abnormal.

CASE 58

History.—49-year-old diabetic candidate for renal transplant. No known coronary disease.

Scan.—Stress SPECT ^{201}Tl scan.

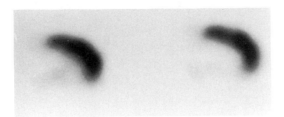

**Vertical long-axis reconstruction views. Stress
(left) and redistribution (right).**

Findings.—Fixed defect in inferoposterior wall.

Diagnosis.—Myocardial infarction of the inferoposterior wall.

Stress ^{201}Tl scanning for suspected ischemic heart disease is one of the most common procedures in nuclear medicine today. The heart can be stressed by exercising on a treadmill or injecting a pharmacologic agent such as dipyridamole. Immediate poststress and delayed images are acquired for SPECT single-photon emission computed tomography (SPECT) reconstruction. Reversible ^{201}Tl defects indicate myocardial ischemia, whereas fixed ^{201}Tl defects are due to myocardial infarction (MI).

The sensitivity of ^{201}Tl scanning for coronary artery disease (CAD) varies depending on the type of imaging performed and the diagnostic criteria used. With planar imaging, ^{201}Tl sensitivity is 75% and specificity 95% using reversible defects as the criteria for coronary disease. When both reversible and fixed defects are used as the diagnostic criteria, sensitivity becomes 80% to 85% and specificity 85% to 90%.

^{201}Tl scanning can be used to diagnose acute MI. The sensitivity of Tl for acute MI depends on the timing of the scan. A resting study obtained within the first 6 hours after infarction has a sensitivity approaching 100%. The high sensitivity is the result of peri-infarction ischemia contributing to the size of the defect. After 24 hours, sensitivity decreases to 75%. Sensitivity also varies with location and type of infarct. Sensitivity is 100% for anterior wall infarction and 85% for inferior wall infarction. For transmural infarction, sensitivity is 85% to 100%, whereas only 50% of nontransmural infarctions are discovered. Some studies have indicated stress-redistribution studies are more sensitive for remote infarction than resting studies alone.

Once an MI has occurred, it will usually remain visible on ^{201}Tl scan. Therefore, acute MI may be indistinguishable from past MI unless a previous Tl scan is available for comparison.

The sensitivity of ^{201}Tl scan for old MI is about 70%. The size of the infarct, scar retraction, and obscuration of infarct by overlying normal myocardium all contribute to the lower sensitivity of ^{201}Tl for old MIs.

A defect on a resting ^{201}Tl study is not specific for infarction. Patients with unstable angina can show resting defects. In this case, delayed imaging may be helpful because redistribution may occur.

CASE 59

History.—68-year-old man with a history of MI 4 years earlier. The patient was about to undergo a total hip replacement.

Scan.—Dipyridamole ^{201}Tl scan with SPECT imaging.

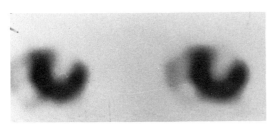

Short-axis reconstruction view in midventricle.

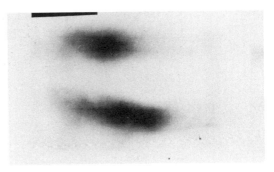

Vertical long-axis view.

Findings.—Stress and redistribution images show a large, nonreversible defect in the anterior wall, which also involves the apex. Furthermore, vertical long-axis views show the anterior and inferior walls of the left ventricle appear to diverge as they approach the apex.

Diagnosis.—Infarct involving the anteroapical walls of the left ventricle with apical aneurysm.

Large anterior wall infarcts will appear as nonreversible defects, best seen on the short-axis and vertical long-axis views. Extensive apical involvement such as seen here would make an LAD lesion the likely cause of the infarct. Often areas of reversible defects are seen adjacent to the infarct, representing peri-infarct ischemia in viable myocardium.

In patients with severe left ventricular dysfunction, the ventricle may appear larger during the stress than the redistribution views. This likely represents left ventricular decompensation and acute dilatation during stress. Diffuse subendocardial ischemia is another possible explanation.

This scan shows divergence of the septum and lateral walls as they approach the apex, seen best on long-axis views. This finding has been described in patients with ventricular aneurysm. When present, it usually occurs in patients with large anteroapical infarcts. The wide mouth of the aneurysm and apical location indicate a true aneurysm (all three coverings present) rather than a false aneurysm (epicardial covering only).

CASE 60

History.—34-year-old previously healthy man with newly diagnosed Hodgkin's lymphoma being considered for chemotherapy.

Scan.—Resting radionuclide ventriculogram (RNV).

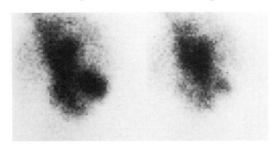

End-diastole *(left)* **and end-systole** *(right)* **in
45-degree LAO projection.**

Findings.—No wall motion abnormalities are present. The left ventricle contracts smoothly and symmetrically throughout. The right ventricle is also seen and has normal wall motion as well. The LVEF is 55%.

Diagnosis.—Normal resting RNV.

The radionuclide ventriculogram (RNV) is the most accurate and reliable noninvasive method of determining left ventricular ejection fraction (LEVF). It is also useful in assessing segmental wall motion.

Red blood cells labeled with technetium 99m are the most commonly used label for gated blood pool studies, having largely replaced ^{99m}Tc human serum albumin (HSA). There are currently three RBC labeling techniques: in vitro, in vivo, and a modified in vivo technique. All three involve the use of cold stannous pyrophosphate as a complexing agent between the globin portion of the hemoglobin molecule and ^{99m}Tc administered as ^{99m}Tc pertechnetate. The labeling efficiencies for the three techniques are 80% to 90% for in vivo labeling, up to 98% for modified in vivo labeling, and 98% or more for in vitro labeling using the Brookhaven National Laboratories technique. The standard dose is 20 to 30 mCi of ^{99m}Tc pertechnetate.

Using the ECG to physiologically synchronize, or "gate," and using the R wave as the electrical reference point for end-diastole, the cardiac cycle can be divided into 12 to 64 frames. Sixteen frames are used for routine scans.

The data can be acquired in either frame or list mode. In frame mode, the most commonly used technique, data from each cycle are added to counts already stored in each frame. The data are "buffered" so that before new counts are added to the already stored data, unwanted counts from nonrepresentative beats can be rejected by measuring the RR interval. Only beats with RR intervals varying less than 20% from sinus rhythm are saved. Once a sufficient information density is obtained, an "average" beat is created.

List mode is less commonly used but is helpful in patients with dysrhythmias, especially atrial fibrillation. Here each scintillation event is assigned x and y coordinates, time markers, and R-wave markers. The data are stored in a serial manner. List mode acquisition requires a significant amount of computer storage.

First-pass studies can be used to measure ejection fraction. These are frequently done to assess function of the right ventricle. Images are obtained in the right anterior oblique (RAO) projection, either gated or ungated, as the ^{99m}Tc RBCs make their first pass through the right ventricle after rapid bolus injection.

Visual analysis of the scan is aided by both temporally and spatially smoothing the images. This involves averaging pixels with other pixels that are adjacent in time and space, respectively. The frame with the highest number of counts is end-diastole, and the frame with the lowest number of counts is end-systole. The ejection fraction is calculated using the formula EF = (ED − ES)/ED (where EF = ejection fraction, ED = end-diastole, and ES = end-systole). Background activity should first be subtracted from ED and ES counts.

The normal LVEF is 50% to 65%. The normal right ventricular ejection fraction (RVEF) obtained by RNV is somewhat higher, because of technique. Physiologically the LVEF is higher than the RVEF, because the right ventricle has a larger end-diastolic volume and stroke volume must be the same for both sides of the heart.

Ventricular separation is critical for determining an accurate ejection fraction. Reasons for falsely elevated ejection fraction include poor atrial or ventricular separation, drawing a region of interest at end-systole that cuts off a portion of the left ventricle, and falsely high background determination. Reasons for a falsely low ejection fraction include falsely low background determination leading to insufficient background subtraction, end-diastolic areas of interest that exclude a portion of the left ventricle, and end-systolic areas of interest that, in addition to left ventricular activity, include atrial counts.

CASE 61

History.— 60-year-old man with borderline cardiomegaly on chest x-ray film.

Scan.—^{99m}Tc labeled red cell radionuclide ventriculogram.

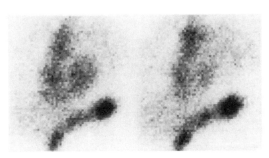

End-diastole *(left)* **and end-systole** *(right)* **in 45-degree LAO projection.**

Findings.—Normal ventriculogram. EF = 55%. Increased activity in stomach.

Diagnosis.—Normal ventriculogram with poor tag.

Gated cardiac blood pool imaging is performed using either ^{99m}Tc human serum albumin (HSA) or RBCs labeled with ^{99m}Tc. Both isotopes reach equilibrium in the blood pool and remain in the intravascular compartment over a long time. ^{99m}Tc HSA has been largely replaced by ^{99m}Tc RBCs because HSA leaks from the intravascular compartment, leading to significantly lower target/background ratios.

There are three techniques for RBC labeling with ^{99m}Tc: completely in vitro, in vivo, or modified in vivo technique (so-called in vivitro method). In all three techniques, a critical element for high labeling efficiency is the reduction of ^{99m}Tc pertechnetate with cold stannous pyrophosphate.

The most commonly used technique today is the modified in vivo method. Labeling efficiency of 98% is possible, with little free pertechnetate in the gastrointestinal tract. The labeling is performed in a closed system (butterfly needle, extension tube, three-way stopcock) attached to the patient's vein. First, cold stannous pyrophosphate is administered intravenously. Fifteen minutes later, after the line is flushed with heparinized saline solution, 5 to 10 mL of blood is withdrawn into a syringe containing 15 to 30 mCi of ^{99m}Tc pertechnetate and a small amount of anticoagulant. The syringe is agitated gently for about 10 minutes, after which the RBCs are reinjected via the indwelling butterfly catheter.

The in vivo labeling technique yields labeling efficiencies of 80% to 90%. First, cold stannous pyrophosphate is injected intravenously. Fifteen minutes later, 15 to 30 mCi of ^{99m}Tc pertechnetate is administered; labeling occurs in the intravascular compartment. The ^{99m}Tc binds to the globin portion of the hemoglobin molecule. It is important to mix the cold stannous pyrophosphate just before injection to reduce the chance of chemical oxidation of the stannous ion if free air is introduced into the vial.

At our institution, in vitro labeling is performed using the Brookhaven National Laboratories kit. Approximately 4 to 5 mL of the patient's blood is withdrawn into a heparinized syringe and then transferred to a kit Vacutainer containing a lyophilized stannous citrate mixture containing 2 μg of Sn^{2+}. The blood is incubated for 5 minutes. One milliliter of 4.4% ethylenediamine tetraacetic acid (EDTA) is added and mixed, and the tube is centrifuged upside down at 1,300 g for 15 minutes; 1.25 mL of the packed RBCs is then added into a vial containing 1 to 3 mL of ^{99m}Tc pertechnetate and mixed gently for 10 minutes. The RBCs are then reinjected. Labeling efficiency with the Brookhaven kit is approximately 98%.

Standard adult doses for multiple gated acquisition imaging are 20 to 30 mCi of ^{99m}Tc pertechnetate. The minimal pediatric dose is 2 to 3 mCi. Pediatric dose may also be calculated using 200 μCi/kg.

Meticulous attention to detail is necessary with all labeling techniques to prevent poor labeling. A number of medications may also reduce labeling efficiency, including certain antimicrobials, anticonvulsants, antihypertensives, cardiac glycosides, tranquilizers, heparin, and anti-inflammatory agents. Diseases and drugs associated with anti-RBC antibody formation reduce labeling efficiency. Manifestations of reduced labeling efficiency include free pertechnetate in the GI tract, thyroid gland uptake, and increased background activity. Ejection fraction calculations may be inaccurate in patients with poor labeling.

CASE 62

History.—60-year-old renal failure patient with shortness of breath.

Scan.—Resting RNV.

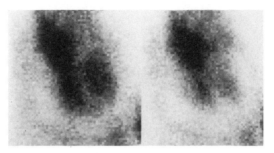

End-diastole *(left)* **and end-systole** *(right)* **in
45-degree LAO projection.**

Findings.—Line of decreased activity around the heart.

Diagnosis.—Pericardial effusion.

On the normal radionuclide ventriculogram (RNV), the liver, spleen, and lungs are visualized, as well as the heart and great vessels, reflecting labeled red blood cells in these organs. Because the labeled RBCs are in the cavity of the ventricles, the walls of the ventricles are seen as black lines (on black and white displays). Papillary muscles in the left ventricle may produce defects superolaterally on the 45-degree left anterior oblique view and at the inferoapical junction on the left lateral view.

An area of decreased activity representing ventricular wall and pericardial fat normally separates the heart from pulmonary and hepatic parenchyma. With ventricular wall hypertrophy, such as secondary to hypertension, the line around the left ventricular chamber will be thickened.

If the line that separates the heart from lung and liver is extremely thickened, the possibility of a pericardial effusion should be considered. Pericardial effusions may also show an abnormal cardiac silhouette, especially on the anterior projection.

Left ventricular hypertrophy can have an appearance similar to pericardial effusion. With effusion, the septum is not affected, the thickening involves the right border of the cardiac outline, and the line extends to the pericardial reflection above the top of the left ventricle.

The RNV is not a sensitive technique for diagnosing pericardial effusion; a significant amount of fluid must accumulate before it can be detected. An echocardiogram is much more sensitive for small pericardial effusions.

Pleural effusions can increase the separation between heart and lung, simulating pericardial effusion. A halo of decreased activity can also be seen as a result of pericardial or mediastinal hemorrhage in postthoracotomy patients.

Sequential images after injection of ^{99m}Tc pyrophosphate (PYP) have been used to differentiate pericardial transudate from exudate. In transudate, the normal halo of decreased activity disappears 1 hour after injection. With exudates, the halo is still discernible at 1 hour.

CASE 63

History.—58-year-old man with chest pain.

Scan.—RNV at rest and during exercise.

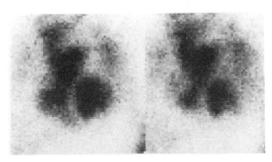

Resting end-diastole *(left)* and end-systole *(right)* in 45-degree LAO projection.

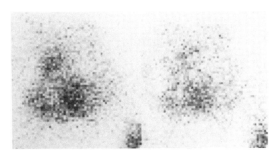

Exercise end-diastole *(left)* and end-systole *(right)* in 45-degree projection.

Findings.—Rest: decreased apicoseptal and lateral wall motion. EF = 37%. Exercise: EF = 26%.

Diagnosis.—Ischemic heart disease.

Ischemic heart disease has characteristic findings on radionuclide ventriculogram (RNV) scan, depending on whether the study is obtained at rest or during exercise. Wall motion abnormalities seen at rest indicate previous myocardial infarction. Ischemia rarely results in resting wall motion abnormalities, in the same manner that ischemia rarely produces thallium defects on resting thallium scans. The resting left ventricular ejection fraction (LVEF) is not depressed with ischemia. A depressed ejection fraction indicates previous myocardial infarction (MI).

Exercise RNV scan is the most sensitive technique for detecting ischemic heart disease. Wall motion abnormalities not present at rest that develop on exercise study are an excellent sign for coronary artery disease (CAD) with a specificity of 90% to 95%. This sign is not sensitive (50%–60%), because the exercise study can be done in only one view. The 45-degree left anterior oblique view is used to allow accurate ejection fraction calculation. Thus, only the septum, apex, and lateral walls are visible. Wall motion abnormalities that develop in other walls cannot be seen.

An abnormal response of the ejection fraction with exercise is much more sensitive than observing wall motion abnormalities because dysfunction in any wall will be reflected in a lower ejection fraction. The normal ejection fraction response to exercise is a 5-unit increase in EF at maximal exercise. A failure to increase ejection fraction 5 units or no change in ejection fraction during exercise are suggestive but certainly not diagnostic for CAD. The best sign is a fall in ejection fraction with maximal exercise. The sensitivity of exercise-induced depression of ejection fraction for CAD is approximately 90% and is highest for triple-vessel disease.

The magnitude of the drop in EF is proportional to the severity of ischemic disease. This does not always reflect the number of vessels involved. A single tight LAD stenosis might produce the same or an even greater decrease in ejection fraction compared with triple-vessel disease with less critical stenoses.

The specificity of an abnormal ejection fraction response for CAD is significantly less than the development of new wall motion abnormalities. Abnormal responses to exercise can be seen in a large number of diseases and in normal individuals.

Individuals older than 60 years may show a blunted increase, no increase, or even a drop in ejection fraction without having CAD. This may reflect a decreased cardiac reserve in older patients. Women are less likely to show a normal response to exercise.

Patients with anxiety, regardless of age, often show blunted or absent response to exercise, although their resting ejection fraction may be elevated. This is thought to be secondary to increased sympathetic tone. Patients exercised in the supine position show smaller increases in ejection fraction than patients exercised upright.

Finally, abnormal response to exercise can be seen in diseases other than CAD. These include valvular heart disease, left-bundle branch block, myocarditis, cardiomyopathies, drug toxicity, after radiation, mitral valve prolapse, chronic obstructive pulmonary disease, and thyrotoxicosis. Some investigators believe that patients with hypertension may also show decreased exercise reserve, although this is controversial.

False negative RNV exercise studies can also occur. Submaximal exercise is the most common cause. More than 25% of patients with CAD will have a normal ejection fraction response to exercise if submaximally exercised. Varying workload and including a portion of the recovery period in the maximal stress images can also cause false negative examinations.

CASE 64

History.—64-year-old diabetic man with questionable history of previous MI.

Scan.—RNV.

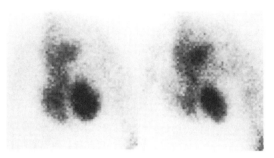

End-diastole *(left)* **and end-systole** *(right)* **in 45-degree LAO projection.**

Findings.—Akinetic or dyskinetic apex. EF = 35%.

Diagnosis.—Previous apical MI.

The three main findings of myocardial infarction (MI) on radionuclide ventriculography (RNV) are varying degrees of ventricular dilation, regional wall motion abnormalities, and reduced left ventricular ejection fraction (LVEF). Patients with inferior wall infarcts show segmental posterobasal abnormalities that may be difficult to appreciate on standard lateral anterior oblique (LAO) views. If an inferior MI is suspected, a shallow left posterior oblique view should be done. This view best shows the inferobasilar wall.

Right ventricular infarction is almost exclusively associated with inferior wall MI. Approximately 25% to 50% of patients with inferior wall MI also have right ventricular infarction. The diagnosis is important to make because therapy is altered in patients with right ventricular dysfunction. Right ventricular wall motion abnormalities and ejection fraction are difficult to evaluate on standard gated studies. Right-sided ejection fraction calculated on the same 45-degree LAO view used for left ventricular ejection fraction is inaccurate. A first-pass study, gated or ungated, done in the right anterior oblique position, is necessary to accurately evaluate right ventricular function.

LVEF is compromised most by anterior wall infarctions. Q-wave infarcts are more likely to affect function than non-Q-wave infarcts. However, patients with MI do not necessarily have a reduced LVEF; frequently it is normal (≥50%). In the first 24 hours after infarction, the ejection fraction frequently varies in both directions. It is best to use an ejection fraction determination after 24 hours to characterize left ventricular function after infarction. Finally, do not forget the ejection fraction is a reflection of the amount of tissue lost with the current event and any past events; therefore ejection fraction may not correlate well with infarct size.

Rest and exercise RNV studies may be helpful in determining prognosis in post-MI patients. A significantly lowered ejection fraction (≤35%) after MI correlates with a high 6-month mortality rate.

Left ventricular aneurysms are known complications of MI. Findings of aneurysm on RNV include an abnormal bulge in the left ventricular contour and dyskinetic wall motion.

CASE 65

History.— 27-year-old patient with rheumatic heart disease.

Scan.— ^{99m}Tc RBC RNV.

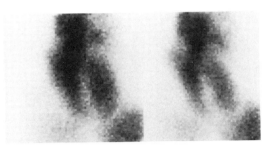

End-diastole *(left)* **and end-systole** *(right)* **in 45-degree LAO projection.**

Findings.—Elongated ventricle with decreased wall motion, especially apically. Left system is more dilated than the right.

Diagnosis.—Aortic or mitral regurgitation with diminished left ventricular function.

The radionuclide ventriculogram (RNV) is an accurate, noninvasive tool for assessing valvular regurgitation. It can be used to determine both the severity of regurgitation and the optimal time for valve replacement.

The most common cause of both aortic and mitral regurgitation is rheumatic heart disease. Mitral insufficiency also commonly occurs secondary to hypertension, cardiomyopathy, and aortic insufficiency. Less common causes of mitral insufficiency include bacterial endocarditis, Marfan's syndrome, congenital asymmetric septal hypertrophy, and papillary muscle dysfunction after myocardial infarction. Common causes of aortic insufficiency, in addition to rheumatic heart disease, include aortitis (syphilis, Takayasu's), bacterial endocarditis, Marfan's syndrome, congenital bicuspid aortic valve, and trauma.

In normal individuals, the left ventricular stroke volume equals the right ventricular stroke volume because cardiac output must be the same on both sides of the heart. In patients with either aortic or mitral valve regurgitation, the left ventricular stroke volume is greater than the right. This can be used to quantitate the degree of regurgitation.

To do this, the resting RNV is obtained in the 45-degree left anterior oblique projection. In this projection, areas of interest for both end-diastole and end-systole are drawn for both the left and right ventricles. Counts are then obtained for these regions of interest and the stroke volume for each side calculated by subtracting the end-systolic counts from the end-diastolic counts.

After this, the stroke volume index (i.e., regurgitant index) can be obtained by dividing left ventricular stroke volume count by right ventricular stroke volume count. In normal patients, the regurgitant index is 1, but can be as much as 1.15 because of technical factors. The greater the regurgitant index, the greater the degree of regurgitation.

The RNV can also be used to determine the optimal time for valve replacement. In patients with left-sided valvular regurgitation, the left ventricle progressively dilates and hypertrophies. This is reflected by elevated left ventricular end-diastolic and end-systolic volumes. Ultimately, after years of volume overload, left ventricular contractility decreases and ultimately, left ventricular failure occurs. Resting left ventricular ejection fraction (LVEF) is not a sensitive indicator of left ventricular function in cases of valvular regurgitation. Because of changes in preload and afterload, the preoperative resting LVEF may be normal, whereas the postoperative resting LVEF may be decreased with a concomitantly increased left ventricular end-systolic volume. A better indicator of the left ventricular contractile status is the LVEF response to exercise. Patients may be followed with serial stress RNV studies. The development of an abnormal response to exercise similar to ischemia indicates the beginning of significant ventricular dysfunction. At this point surgical replacement may be warranted to prevent loss of function.

CASE 66

History.— 40-year-old man with lymphoma who is taking doxorubicin (Adriamycin).

Scan.— RNV, resting.

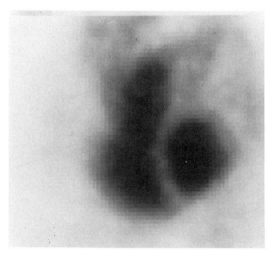

End-systole in 45-degree LAO projection.

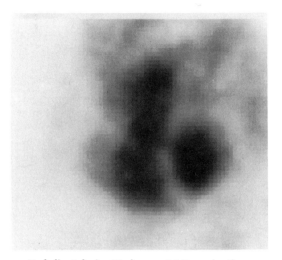

End-diastole in 45-degree LAO projection.

Findings.— Decreased global wall motion. EF = 39%.

Diagnosis.— Doxorubicin cardiotoxicity.

Radionuclide ventriculography (RNV) is useful for assessing toxic effects of drugs on cardiac function, including patients receiving cancer chemotherapy. Congestive heart failure from cardiotoxicity associated with chemotherapy is a major limiting factor of several chemotherapeutic agents, most notably doxorubicin (Adriamycin).

An initial RNV study is performed to establish baseline cardiac function. It is followed by serial scans during therapy to monitor cardiac function. The most common technique is to perform a resting RNV. Exercise studies are sometimes done to increase sensitivity for mild toxicity.

With doxorubicin, cumulative doses of up to 350 mg/m^2 of body surface area rarely produce significant cardiotoxicity. Although partially idiosyncratic in nature, at cumulative doses greater than 550 mg/m^2 one third of patients develop cardiotoxicity. Arbitrary limits on cumulative dose can be used to avoid cardiotoxicity; however, this leads to premature withdrawal of therapy in some patients. The role of the RNV scan is to detect early signs of cardiotoxicity so therapy can be stopped before the development of heart failure.

An initial "baseline" RNV scan is performed either before therapy is instituted or up to a cumulative dose no greater than 300 mg/m^2. Beginning at cumulative doses of 350 to 450 mg/m^2, repeat studies are obtained before each dose.

Cardiotoxicity is classified as mild, moderate, or severe, depending on the ejection fraction and its change from baseline. Mild cardiotoxicity is defined as a decrease in ejection fraction of 10 or more EF units and an absolute ejection fraction greater than 45%. Moderate cardiotoxicity is a decrease in ejection fraction of 15 or more units and an absolute ejection fraction of 45% or less. Severe cardiotoxicity is an absolute ejection fraction of 30% or less. Mild cardiotoxicity is an early sign of damage, but therapy may be continued with close monitoring. When moderate cardiotoxicity is seen, doxorubicin therapy should be discontinued. Follow-up studies are obtained 1 and 3 months after discontinuation of therapy, and depending on these results, therapy sometimes may be cautiously reinstituted. Drug therapy needs to be halted with severe cardiotoxicity.

CASE 67

History.—60-year-old man with new-onset congestive heart failure.

Scan.—^{99m}Tc RNV.

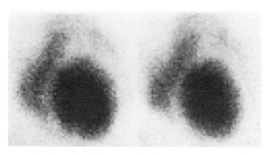

End-diastole *(left)* **and end-systole** *(right)* **in 45-degree LAO projection.**

Findings.— Dilated left ventricle with diffuse wall motion abnormalities. EF = 12%.

Diagnosis.—Idiopathic cardiomyopathy.

Distinguishing between ischemic and nonischemic cardiomyopathy can be difficult. Although both diseases have overlapping features on radionuclide ventriculography (RNV), there are characteristics that help distinguish between the two. Ischemic heart disease can be characterized by findings on both resting and exercise RNV. Ischemia is best seen on exercise RNV, causing the development of regional wall motion abnormalities and an abnormal response to exercise (inability to increase ejection fraction by 5 units). A decrease in the left ventricular ejection fraction (LVEF) is the most sensitive sign of ischemia (90%); however, it is less specific. The development of regional wall motion abnormalities is the most specific sign for coronary artery disease, but is less sensitive (60%) than a drop in ejection fraction.

RNV findings of myocardial infarction will be seen on both stress and resting RNV studies. These include regional wall motion abnormalities at rest, varying degrees of ventricular dilatation, and a reduced LVEF. Because the anterior wall makes the largest contribution to left ventricular function, anterior wall infarcts produce the most pronounced reduction in ejection fraction. However, ejection fraction is not always decreased by MI; it can remain normal. A complication of isch-

emic heart disease visible on RNV is aneurysm. They show dyskinetic wall motion.

Nonischemic cardiomyopathy can be caused by multiple etiologies. It is commonly secondary to ethanol abuse. It can also be caused by viral infection and is frequently idiopathic. Findings of dilated cardiomyopathy on resting RNV are diffuse, as opposed to segmental, wall motion abnormalities, decreased ejection fraction, and dilated left ventricle. Right ventricular dilatation and wall motion abnormalities are also present. Normal right ventricular function in the face of diminished left ventricular function is more typical of ischemic cardiomyopathy, although not pathognomonic. In contrast to ischemic heart disease, some studies have shown a more normal ejection fraction response to exercise with nonischemic cardiomyopathy.

Although these findings are more typical of either ischemic or nonischemic heart disease, none is pathognomonic. Segmental wall motion abnormalities may be seen with nonischemic disease; conversely, diffuse wall motion abnormalities and biventricular enlargement may be seen with ischemic heart disease.

CASE 68

History.—72-year-old man with history of CAD.

Scan.—RNV and phase analysis.

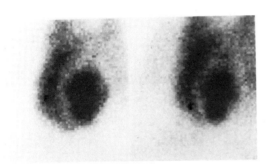

End-diastole *(left)* and end-systole *(right)* in
45-degree projection.

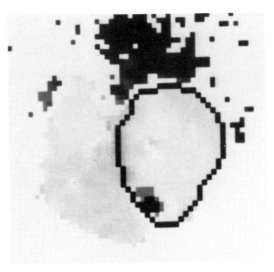

Phase image.

Findings.—Dyskinetic apex.

Diagnosis.—Left ventricular aneurysm.

Left ventricular aneurysms are known complications of MI. Aneurysms are of two types: true and false. True aneurysms are most commonly secondary to myocardial infarction. Other causes include congenital defect, erosive bacterial endocarditis, myocardial abscess, and trauma. True aneurysms are a weakening and thinning of the myocardium without myocardial rupture. They are bound by endocardium, myocardium, and epicardium. True aneurysms are located anteriorly or anteroapically. Radionuclide ventriculogram (RNV) findings are a focal bulging in the left ventricular contour with a wide mouth, dyskinetic motion, and pooling of the radiotracer.

A false aneurysm, on the other hand, represents rupture of the myocardium. They are bound only by epicardium and are more prone to catastrophic rupture than true aneurysms. Similar to true aneurysms, findings on RNV include an abnormal bulge in the left ventricular contour and paradoxical wall motion. In contrast to a true aneurysm, however, a false aneurysm is located posterolaterally and has a narrow neck.

The two most common causes of false aneurysm are transmural infarction and previous cardiac surgery. Bacterial en-

docarditis, myocarditis, and both blunt and penetrating trauma are uncommon causes. Rare causes include syphilis and tuberculosis.

Normally the ventricles contract in phase with each other and out of phase with the atria. In the case of aneurysms and pseudoaneurysms, the area involved is dyskinetic relative to the adjacent muscle. That is, an aneurysm or pseudoaneurysm moves out of phase with the remainder of the left ventricle.

The cardiac cycle can be displayed as a function of the amplitude of each point (or pixel) throughout the cycle. Because the amplitude is a measure of myocardial contractility, an amplitude image can be reconstructed demonstrating regional differences in ventricular contraction. By plotting the amplitude vs. the phase of the cardiac cycle, a phase image is produced. The phase image depicts the regional sequence of ventricular contraction. When phase analysis is used, portions of the left ventricle that contract either early or late when compared with the rest of the ventricle are said to be out of phase. Phase analysis can be useful in other clinical settings, such as with aberrant electrical pathways.

CASE 69

History.—38-year-old man after motor vehicle accident. He is a nonsmoker with a negative prior medical history.

Scan.—^{99m}Tc RBC RNV.

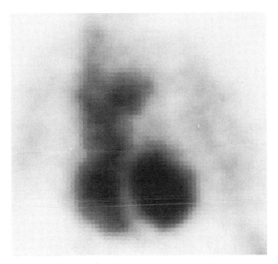

End-diastole in 45-degree LAO projection.

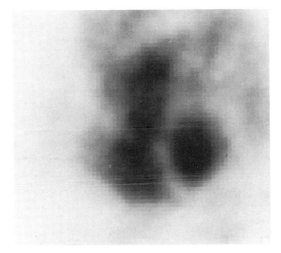

End-systole in 45-degree LAO projection.

Findings.—Decreased wall motion anteriorly.

Diagnosis.—Myocardial contusion.

Electrocardiogram–gated radionuclide ventriculography (RNV) using ^{99m}Tc labeled red blood cells is useful for evaluating ischemic heart disease, cardiomyopathy, valvular heart disease, drug-induced cardiotoxicity, cardiac transplant complications, and other conditions. The heart is evaluated from three projections: anterior 45-degree left anterior oblique (LAO), and either 70-degree LAO or left lateral views. From these three views each wall of the left ventricle may be individually examined. The anterior view demonstrates the apex and anterolateral walls. The septum, apex, and lateral walls are seen on the 45-degree LAO view. The anterior, apical, and inferoposterior walls are seen best on the 70-degree LAO or left lateral view.

For evaluation of right ventricular function, first-pass analysis from the RAO projection is required. Right ventricular ejection fraction obtained from the standard 45-degree LAO view is not accurate.

Using the 45-degree LAO projection, the RNV offers the most accurate method available for left ventricular ejection fraction (LVEF) determination. This is especially true in patients with enlarged or abnormally shaped ventricles. Angiographic and echocardiographic techniques that assume an elliptical shape are particularly inaccurate in these cases.

In a normal heart there is symmetric contraction of all walls. The septum frequently appears to have less vigorous contraction than the remaining walls. Normally the ventricular ejection fraction is more than 50%. The normal right ventricular ejection fraction (RVEF) by RNV is higher than the left ventricle because of the measuring technique. Physiologically the RVEF must be lower than the LVEF because of the larger end-diastolic volume of the right ventricle. This allows the stroke volumes on each side to be equal.

Patients with myocardial contusions may show transient wall motion abnormalities at rest, similar to the so-called stunned myocardium phenomenon described in post-MI patients. Subsequent imaging at a later date reveals restoration of normal wall motion in some patients. In addition to the transient wall motion abnormalities, these patients may also show elevation of their cardiac isoenzymes.

At one time ^{99m}Tc PYP scanning was thought to be useful in contusions. Increased deposition of ^{99m}Tc PYP was seen in the involved wall. Subsequent studies have shown the sensitivity of ^{99m}Tc PYP is low in all but severe contusions.

In addition to contusion and infarction, resting wall motion abnormalities can be seen in severe ischemic disease, nonischemic cardiomyopathies, valvular disease, endocarditis, and abscess.

CASE 70

History.—57-year-old man, 2 years after heart transplantation, clinically doing well. He has had two episodes of mild rejection in the past.

Scan.—^{99m}Tc RBC RNV.

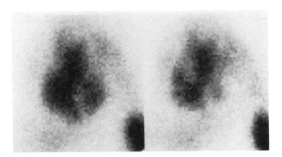

End-diastole *(left)* and end-systole *(right)* in
45-degree LAO projection.

Findings.—Normal wall motion is present in the anterior, inferior, lateral, and apical walls of the left ventricle. The septum shows less wall motion. The LVEF is 54%.

Diagnosis.—Normal posttransplant RNV. EF = 50%.

Common uses for the radionuclide ventriculogram (RNV) include gated measurement of left ventricular function and first-pass studies for judging right ventricular function. The RNV is useful for evaluating ischemic heart disease, valvular heart disease, and cardiomyopathies. Other uses include monitoring cardiac function in patients receiving chemotherapy (doxorubicin), shunt analysis, and differentiating cardiac from pulmonary dysfunction in patients with chronic obstructive pulmonary disease.

Another growing population in which RNV is useful is in patients with cardiac transplants. The RNV findings in a normal cardiac transplant patient differ in several respects from those in a patient with a native heart. In a transplanted heart, the apex is positioned more laterally than in a native heart. This is because at the time of transplant a significant portion of both native atria are left in place and the remainder of the diseased heart is removed. The residual atrial tissue is used as a base into which the transplanted heart is sutured. This leads to a more lateral orientation of the apex. This also accounts for the large size of the atria in cardiac transplant patients.

Because of the resultant more lateral position, the 45-degree LAO view may no longer show the best interventricular separation for ejection fraction determination; therefore, a 60- to 65-degree LAO view may be required. The normal transplanted heart, like the normal native heart, has an ejection fraction of 50% or greater. The septum of a cardiac transplant, however, may show decreased or paradoxical wall motion. Similar to the 45-degree LAO view, a left lateral or even left posterior oblique projection may be required for assessing anterior, apical, and inferoposterior wall motion that would normally be seen on the 70-degree LAO view.

CASE 71

History.— 72-year-old man with chest pain 4 days earlier.

Scan.— Planar ^{99m}Tc PYP scan.

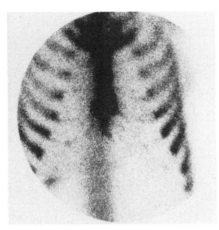

Anterior view.

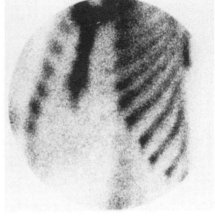

35-degree LAO view.

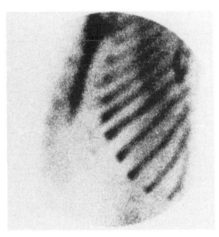

70-degree LAO view.

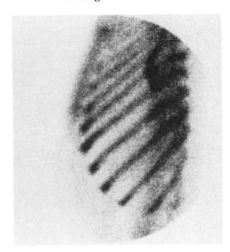

Left lateral view.

Findings.— Activity in sternum and ribs. No myocardial uptake.

Diagnosis.— Normal ^{99m}Tc PYP scan.

With the use of cardiac isoenzymes and ECGs, most myocardial infarcts (MI) are diagnosed without the need for imaging studies. The role of the ^{99m}Tc pyrophosphate (PYP) scan is in patients in whom the usual diagnostic tests have failed.

^{99m}Tc PYP, originally used for bone scanning, is the radiopharmaceutical most commonly used to detect myocardial infarction. It is a condensed phosphate compound containing two phosphate residues. Myocardial cells in infarcted tissue become permeable to calcium. It is the calcium to which the ^{99m}Tc PYP binds.

Anaerobic preparation of ^{99m}Tc PYP is required to prevent oxidation of tin. The preparation must have less than 5% reduced hydrolyzed technetium, and less than 1% free technetium. Chromatography for both free technetium and reduced hydrolyzed technetium should be performed as part of quality control.

The patient is injected with 20 mCi of ^{99m}Tc PYP, and imaging is begun 2 to 4 hours after injection. A high-resolution collimator and standard field camera are used to obtain views done for 400,000 counts each. The four views obtained are anterior, 35-degree left anterior oblique (LAO), 70-degree LAO, and left lateral projections. Single-photon emission computed tomography (SPECT) views should also be obtained. Sensitivity is improved with SPECT compared with planar imaging.

Because ^{99m}Tc PYP is a bone agent, the normal PYP scan shows skeletal uptake. If blood pool activity is present, diffuse faint activity in the region of the heart may be seen. If so, more delayed imaging may be helpful.

Normally, the ^{99m}Tc PYP scan shows no evidence of soft tissue activity in the region of the heart. Linear uptake may be seen in the costal cartilage, mimicking inferior wall infarction. Activity in the kidneys, which excrete the ^{99m}Tc PYP, may be misinterpreted as myocardial uptake, especially if the camera is positioned lower than normal.

CASE 72

History.— 57-year-old man with a history of CAD who underwent coronary artery bypass graft. His baseline ECG showed left-bundle branch block. Postoperatively he had elevated CPK levels with elevated MB fraction.

Scan.— A ^{99m}Tc PYP scan was performed 60 hours after surgery.

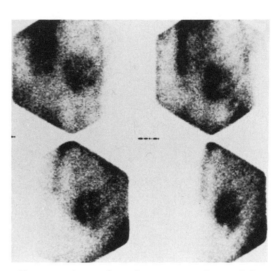

Top, anterior and 35-degree LAO views of the chest.
Bottom, 75-degree LAO and left lateral views.

Findings.—Because ^{99m}Tc PYP is a bone agent, sternum and rib uptake is seen. Activity is present in the anterior and lateral walls of the left ventricle. The intensity of myocardial uptake is more than that in the sternum (4+).

Diagnosis.—Acute anterolateral wall MI.

The ^{99m}Tc pyrophosphate (PYP) scan has a niche in the diagnosis of myocardial infarction (MI). When isoenzyme determinations and ECG are used, most MIs are diagnosed without the involvement of nuclear medicine. The role of the ^{99m}Tc PYP scan is to confirm acute MI in patients in whom the diagnosis is either difficult or uncertain by enzyme studies and ECG. For example, patients with baseline ECG abnormalities may not show new ECG changes with infarction or may have nondiagnostic changes. Other patients are admitted with infarcts more than 48 hours old, decreasing the reliability of cardiac enzyme studies.

Another group of patients who can present diagnostic difficulties are those who have recently undergone cardiac surgery. In the perioperative patient, new Q waves on ECG after coronary artery bypass surgery do not necessarily indicate new MI. Also, it is normal for the CK-MB fraction to be elevated after cardiac surgery. Like cardiac surgery patients, it is common for patients who have undergone cardioversion or chest compression to have elevated CK-MB fractions.

In the perioperative patient, ^{99m}Tc PYP scans are both highly sensitive and specific for the diagnosis of acute infarction. In patients undergoing cardiac surgery, it may be helpful to obtain a baseline ^{99m}Tc PYP scan before surgery because they may have persistently abnormal scans from old infarctions.

Increased uptake by the myocardium can be graded by comparing the degree of myocardial uptake with bone uptake using the sternum as the reference.

Grade 0:	No myocardial uptake (i.e., normal).
Grade 1+	Minimal myocardial activity secondary to either blood pool or chest wall activity.
Grade 2+	Definite myocardial activity but less than bone.
Grade 3+	Myocardial activity equal to bone.
Grade 4+	Myocardial activity greater than bone.

Scans with activity of 0 to 1+ are normal. Myocardial activity of 2+ or greater indicates MI.

Of patients with acute transmural MI, 80% will have activity of 3+ or 4+; 20% will show 2+ activity. Oblique views to localize the activity are often useful in defining the walls involved. Subendocardial, or non-Q-wave, infarcts may show diffuse myocardial uptake and can be difficult to differentiate from blood pool activity. Once scans are abnormal, 20% of them will remain persistently abnormal; the other 80% will go on to resolution.

The sensitivity of the ^{99m}Tc PYP scan for acute MI depends on the timing of the scan. If the image is obtained between 48 and 72 hours after the infarction, sensitivity is approximately 95% for transmural MIs and 80% for nontransmural MIs. Sensitivity is highest for anterior infarctions and lowest for inferior infarctions. Overall specificity for acute MI is 80+% and increases as the activity seen on the scan increases from 2+ to 4+. Specificity is also improved with focal rather than diffuse activity.

One common cause of false positive results on ^{99m}Tc PYP scan is costochondral cartilage uptake mimicking inferior infarct. Single photon-emission computed tomography (SPECT) imaging is helpful in improving both sensitivity and specificity by better localizing and characterizing the uptake.

^{99m}Tc PYP scanning may also be helpful in the evaluation of possible right ventricular infarction. From 25% to 50% of inferoposterior infarcts have associated right ventricular infarction. Because both the enzymes and ECG will be abnormal secondary to left ventricular infarction, diagnosis of right ventricular involvement is difficult. Right ventricular involvement will show a W shape on left anterior oblique projections of ^{99m}Tc PYP scans. The three parts of the W are composed of uptake in the inferior wall, lower septum, and right ventricle.

^{99m}Tc PYP can be used to size infarcts and establish prognosis. As would be expected, larger-size infarcts are associated with poorer prognosis. The pattern of uptake is also helpful. A doughnut-shaped pattern occurs with extensive tissue necrosis. Poor blood flow prevents the ^{99m}Tc PYP from entering the center of the infarct. The doughnut sign is usually seen in the left anterior descending artery distribution and is associated with extremely large infarcts. It is associated with increased mortality.

Myocardial uptake of ^{99m}Tc PYP has been described in a number of conditions other than acute MI. These include doxorubicin and radiation toxicity, pericarditis, myocarditis, myocardial contusion, cardiac injury after repeated electrocardioversion, and persistently abnormal scan from previous MI.

CASE 73

History.—44-year-old man hospitalized with chest pain. The patient had ventricular fibrillation requiring cardioversion. His creatinine kinase level was mildly elevated.

Scan.—^{99m}Tc PYP scan, planar and SPECT.

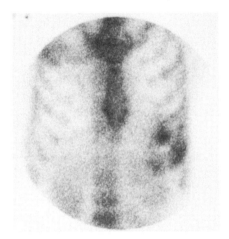

Anterior chest view.

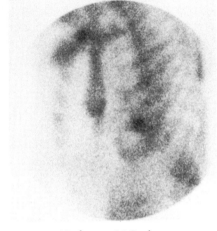

35-degree LAO view.

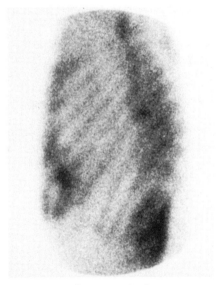

70-degree LAO view.

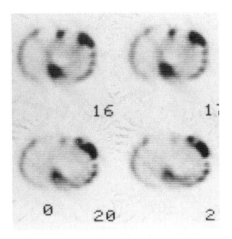

SPECT reconstruction view of the chest.

Findings.— Increased uptake over left side of chest on planar images. SPECT shows activity is confined to chest wall.

Diagnosis.—No evidence for acute MI. Cardioversion injury present.

Planar views are obtained from multiple projections in an attempt to characterize and localize abnormal chest uptake. One common cause of false positive results on ^{99m}Tc PYP scan is costochondral cartilage uptake mimicking inferior infarct. Likewise, chest wall uptake can mimic uptake in underlying structures. Single-photon-emission computed tomography (SPECT) imaging is helpful in improving specificity by better localizing the uptake.

This patient shows uptake confined to the chest wall. There is no uptake in the region of the heart. The chest uptake is from defibrillation and not from an acute myocardial infarction (MI). Electric cardioversion or defibrillation may show ei-

ther focal or diffuse uptake. It is usually caused by a "burn" injury from the electrical energy. Improper placement of the defibrillation paddles increases the likelihood of such injuries. Patients who undergo repeat cardioversion over a short period of time may show actual ^{99m}Tc PYP uptake within the heart itself.

Other causes of chest wall uptake that can mimic an MI on ^{99m}Tc PYP scan are rib fracture, postsurgical changes, breast activity (normal and in a carcinoma), penetrating wounds (knife or bullet injury), and skin lesions (pseudoxanthoma elasticum).

CASE 74

History.—57-year-old man with 4 days of intermittent chest pain; MI had been ruled out.

Scan.—^{99m}Tc PYP scan.

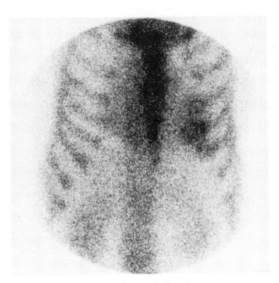

Anterior view of the chest.

Findings.—Increased uptake in anterolateral region of heart.

Diagnosis.—Unstable angina.

The diagnosis of acute myocardial infarction (MI) is generally made by the combination of serial electrocardiograms and cardiac isoenzyme fractions. ECGs show ST segment elevation in acute MI, with the evolution of Q-waves in transmural infarction. Cardiac isoenzymes show an elevated MB fraction of creatinine phosphokinase (CPK) or a reversal of the normal lactate dehydrogenase (LD_1/LD_2) ratio, which is less than 1. These tests are not always diagnostic for acute MI, however, and their sensitivity drops dramatically 48 to 72 hours after an acute MI. Patients who have had cardiac surgery or cardioversion may have equivocal enzyme changes.

^{99m}Tc PYP scanning sensitivity for acute MI depends on the timing of the scan with respect to the onset of infarction. Forty-eight to 72 hours after the infarct, ^{99m}Tc PYP sensitivity is 95% for transmural MI and 80% for nontransmural MI. Specificity varies with the intensity and focality of uptake but overall is more than 80%.

Unstable angina represents a spectrum of symptoms from chronic stable angina to frank infarction. Approximately 30% of patients with unstable angina show abnormal uptake on ^{99m}Tc PYP scintigraphy. This may reflect ongoing necrosis of a small number of myocardial cells, although uptake of ^{99m}Tc PYP has been described in ischemic but viable cells.

The myocardial uptake in unstable angina tends to be diffuse. These patients have an increased incidence of both nonfatal MI and cardiac death. The subgroup of patients with angina, abnormal ^{99m}Tc PYP scan, and ischemic ECG changes have an especially poor prognosis.

Diffuse myocardial uptake has been described in a number of conditions in addition to unstable angina. These include acute subendocardial MI, cardiomyopathy, doxorubicin cardiotoxicity, previous MI, metastatic calcification, myocarditis, pericarditis, and transplant rejection.

CASE 75

History.—58-year-old man with chest pain; MI had been ruled out.

Scan.—^{67}Ga scan.

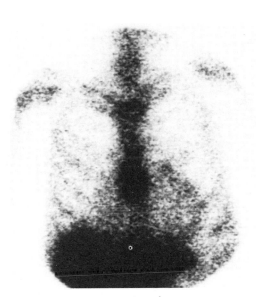

Anterior chest image.

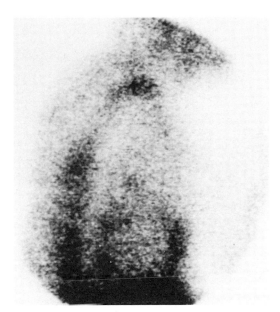

Right lateral chest image.

Findings. —There is a ring of uptake in cardiac region.

Diagnosis.—Pericarditis.

The visceral pericardium is a serous membrane separated by a small amount of fluid (a plasma ultrafiltrate) from the fibrous sac of the parietal pericardium. The pericardium restricts the anatomic position of the heart, prevents sudden dilation of cardiac chambers during exercise, facilitates atrial filling during ventricular systole, prevents cardiac displacement and kinking of the great vessels, minimizes friction between the heart and surrounding structures, and retards the spread of infection from the lungs and pleural spaces to the heart.

Pericarditis, the most common pathologic disorder affecting the pericardium, can be classified using two different schemes: acute vs. nonacute and infectious vs. noninfectious. The classic manifestation of pericarditis is chest pain, pericardial friction rub, electrocardiographic changes (ST segment elevation), and paradoxical pulse. All patients with acute pericarditis should be observed for the development of pericardial effusion and, if effusion is present, for signs of tamponade.

Viral, or idiopathic, pericarditis is an important clinical entity because of its frequency and because it may be confused with other more serious illnesses. There is no specific therapy, but treatment with anti-inflammatory agents (aspirin, nonsteroidal anti-inflammatory agents, or corticosteroids) effectively suppresses the clinical manifestations and is useful in patients in whom a purulent or tuberculous form of pericarditis has been excluded.

CHAPTER 4

Gastrointestinal

CASE 76

History.— 49-year-old woman with questionably palpable spleen on physical examination.

Scan.— ^{99m}Tc sulfur colloid liver-spleen scan.

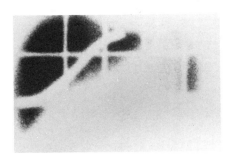

Anterior view of upper half of abdomen with 5 cm lead grid and costal margin.

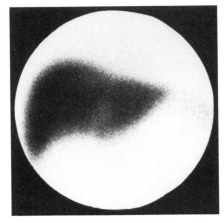

Anterior view of abdomen.

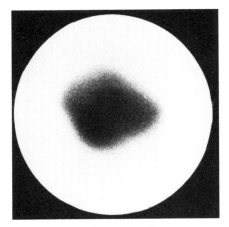

Right lateral view of abdomen.

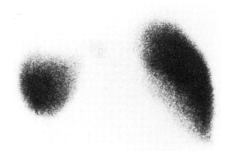

Posterior view of abdomen.

Findings.— Homogeneous uptake in liver and spleen.

Diagnosis.— Normal liver-spleen scan.

Liver-spleen scanning has many uses, including assessment of location and size of the liver and spleen, detection of metastatic disease, assessment of parenchymal disease, and investigation of abdominal trauma. Radionuclide imaging competes with computed tomography (CT) and ultrasound but is useful in selected cases, especially if single-photon emission computed tomography (SPECT) is added.

The liver-spleen scan is performed after intravenous injection of technetium 99m sulfur colloid. These particles are taken up by the reticuloendothelial system of the liver, spleen, and bone marrow, with their distribution partly dependent on particle size. Particles less than 1.5 μm are deposited mainly in the spleen. Particles up to 100 μm are preferentially taken up by the bone marrow, whereas, particles 200 to 1,000 μm in diameter localize primarily in the liver. ^{99m}Tc sulfur colloid (the most commonly used liver-spleen agent) has a 200 to 500 μm particle size. The normal distribution of this size particle is 86% in the reticuloendothelial system of the liver, 6% in the spleen, and the remaining 8% in the bone marrow.

The liver varies greatly in shape and size. It is a very soft, pliable organ, with its appearance dependent on surrounding organs and structures. On the anterior view, the right lobe is significantly larger than the left. The liver size is measured on this view as the maximum cephalocaudad distance using a lead grid over the liver and spleen. The normal liver is 17 ± 2 cm, and the normal spleen is 10 ± 3 cm. Variations in liver shape and appearance include:

1. Reidel's lobe, a marked elongation of the right lobe.
2. Falciform ligament causing a vertical line of decreased activity between the right and left lobes.
3. Central defect caused by the porta hepatis.
4. Gallbladder fossa causing a defect along the antero/inferior border.
5. Indentation in the lateral border of the right lobe caused by impression of the costal margin.

6. Photopenic areas caused by breast attenuation in the superior right lobe of the liver. (Imaging should be repeated with the breast elevated to confirm this as the cause of the defect.)
7. Prominent right renal fossa on posterior view.

The spleen normally appears equal to or less intense than the liver on both the anterior and posterior views. A reversal of this pattern is called "shunting" and usually indicates hepatocellular dysfunction, resulting in more colloid available for uptake in the spleen and bone marrow.

Some variations in spleen shape and appearance include cup-shaped spleen, persistent fetal lobulation, elongation of the anchoring ligaments of the spleen resulting in excess mobility (so-called wandering spleen), and accessory spleens.

CASE 77

History.—34-year-old man with history of trauma.

Scan.—^{99m}Tc sulfur colloid liver-spleen scan.

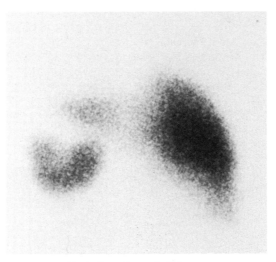

Posterior view of abdomen.

Findings.—Apparent defect in superior spleen.

Diagnosis.—Normal liver-spleen scan, cup-shaped spleen.

Like the liver, the spleen's anatomy is quite variable. The shape and position of the spleen are influenced by surrounding structures.

The spleen is normally located in the left upper quadrant of the abdomen. It is 10 ± 3 cm in vertical height measured on the posterior image. The fetal lobulations of the spleen may persist, creating notches and clefts on the borders. An accessory spleen may appear as a focal collection of activity located near the hilum.

The normal position of the spleen varies with elevation or depression of the diaphragm. Suspensory ligaments of the spleen may also be quite loose, allowing increased mobility of the spleen (wandering spleen). The cup-shaped spleen is another normal variation in spleen shape. This occurs when the hilum is oriented more superiorly. The image of a cup-shaped spleen will have an apparent defect in the superior pole.

Occasionally the left lobe of the liver will extend to the left chest wall behind the spleen. On the posterior view the liver activity superimposes on the spleen, falsely giving the appearance of a splenic defect such as an infarct, abscess, or hematoma. When the colloid study is combined with a diisopropyliminodiacetic acid (DISIDA) scan or a denatured red blood cell (RBC) study, better definition of the liver or spleen is possible.

The intensity of activity in the spleen should be equal to or less than that of the liver on the posterior image. The spleen should always appear less intense than the liver on the anterior view because of the posterior position of the spleen.

CASE 78

History.—60-year-old man with colon carcinoma.

Scan.—^{99m}Tc sulfur colloid liver-spleen scan.

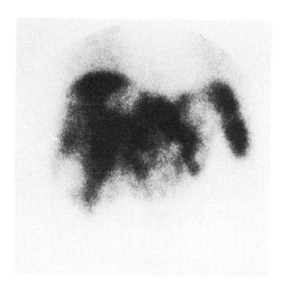

Anterior view of abdomen.

Findings.—Multiple "cold" defects in the liver and spleen.

Diagnosis.—Metastatic disease involving the liver.

With the development of computed tomography (CT) and ultrasound, radionuclide liver-spleen scanning for detection of metastatic disease is performed less frequently; however, the routine liver radionuclide study, combined with single-photon emission computed tomography (SPECT), is a sensitive study for metastatic disease to the liver.

The most common tumors that metastasize to the liver are breast, colon, lung, gastric, pancreatic, cervical, and uterine. Metastases are the most common cause of multiple cold defects on liver scan. Metastatic disease is 20 times more common than primary hepatic tumors, making metastases the most common cause of solitary defects as well. Other less specific manifestations of metastatic disease to the liver include coarsely inhomogeneous activity and hepatomegaly. Increased flow to the liver appearing as a focal "hot" spot on flow study is also seen occasionally.

The overall sensitivity of liver-spleen scanning for the detection of metastatic disease to the liver is 80% to 85%; SPECT imaging boosts this to 90%. The sensitivity varies with the size of the lesion, the number of metastases, their location, tumor type, and the type of imaging equipment used. Lesions greater than 2 cm are usually detected, whereas those of less than 1.5 cm are rarely seen. Lesions located deep within the liver or in the left lobe are more difficult to detect. Colorectal and renal cell carcinomas tend to produce large discrete lesions, making them more easy to detect, whereas breast cancer produces smaller, more diffuse, metastases. These often appear as coarse inhomogeneity on liver-spleen scan. Finally, SPECT imaging is more sensitive than planar scans for smaller lesions and those located deep in the liver.

In addition to metastatic disease, cold defects in the liver are caused by benign lesions such as focal nodular hyperplasia, hepatic abscess, polycystic disease, or biliary obstruction. Artifacts such as coins overlying the liver may simulate metastases. Recent cancer chemotherapy can cause heterogeneous colloid uptake in the liver and colloid shift.

CASE 79

History.—62-year-old alcoholic with abdominal pain.

Scan.—^{99m}Tc sulfur colloid liver-spleen scan.

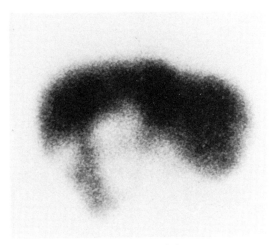

Anterior view of abdomen.

Findings.—Lobulated cold defect in right lobe.

Diagnosis.—Hepatoma.

Hepatoma, or hepatocellular carcinoma, is the most common primary malignant liver tumor. It accounts for only 1% to 2% of cancer deaths in North and South America but is responsible for 20% to 30% of malignancies in parts of Africa and Asia. Predisposing factors for the development of this tumor include:

1. Alcoholic or postnecrotic cirrhosis (most common predisposing factor in the United States)
2. Viral hepatitis
3. Chronic liver disease of any cause
4. Mycotoxin ingestion (found in high concentrations in food in Africa and Asia)

Clinical features of this tumor include hepatomegaly, right upper quadrant pain and tenderness, and, less often, blood-tinged ascites. Diagnosis is often delayed because of confusion of symptoms with the underlying disease. Serum α-fetoprotein levels greater than 500 ng/mL are found in 70% to 90% of patients with hepatoma and are helpful in diagnosis.

A solitary cold defect in the liver is most commonly caused by metastatic disease; however, two thirds of hepatomas manifest this way. Multiple cold defects can also be found in one sixth of cases, with findings of inhomogeneity, hepatomegaly, or both in the remainder. Hepatomas grow rapidly and are often quite large when the patient is first seen. The right lobe is the most common location, with occasional involvement of the left lobe as well. Isolated left lobe hepatoma is rare.

Other primary liver tumors are rare. The most common are cholangiocarcinoma and Kupffer's cell carcinomas. These are usually indistinguishable from other tumors on liver scan, although Kupffer's cell carcinomas may manifest as a hot spot.

Gallium 67 is useful in confirming the diagnosis of hepatoma. Cirrhotics, the group most likely to develop hepatomas in the United States, frequently develop cold defects on liver scan. These can be from hepatoma or from regenerating nodules and areas of necrosis. ^{67}Ga is taken up by hepatomas, whereas regenerating nodules and areas of necrosis infrequently show uptake. The sensitivity of ^{67}Ga for hepatoma is 90%. ^{67}Ga uptake is not 100% specific for hepatoma, however. In addition to uptake in occasional cases of regenerating nodules, about 15% of metastases to the liver will show uptake as well. Finally, a liver abscess should be considered, especially in solitary lesions involving the right lobe because this is the most common manifestation of abscesses.

CASE 80

History.—48-year-old man with jaundice, with elevated liver function test results.

Scan.—^{99m}Tc sulfur colloid liver-spleen scan.

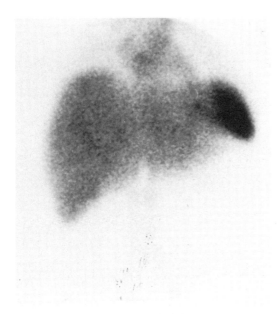

Anterior view of abdomen.

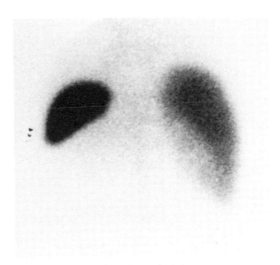

Posterior view of abdomen.

Findings.—Hepatomegaly, decreased uptake of sulfur colloid, with blood pool activity. Shunting to spleen.

Diagnosis.—Hepatitis.

The most common causes of diffuse parenchymal disease in the United States are viral and alcoholic hepatitis, fatty infiltration, and cirrhosis. The scan is quite sensitive (about 85%) for parenchymal disease of the liver, but because of similar findings with most diffuse liver disease, a definitive diagnosis is usually impossible to offer.

Scan findings depend on the degree of hepatic involvement and chronicity. With early diffuse liver disease, inhomogeneity in liver appearance (also seen in 10% of normal individuals), hepatomegaly, and shunting to the spleen and bone marrow are seen. Shunting, also referred to as "colloid shift," results from a reduction in the amount of sulfur colloid taken up by the reticuloendothelial system of the liver, leaving more available for the spleen and bone marrow.

The degree of abnormality on liver-spleen scan depends on the severity of disease. The earliest manifestation of alcoholic liver disease is fatty infiltration, which appears as mild hepatomegaly and diffusely decreased activity on liver scan. In a patient with acute alcoholic hepatitis the scan may show near absence of uptake in the liver, with prominent visualization of the spleen and bone marrow. With more chronic liver dis-

ease, scarring of the liver with areas of regeneration can produce cold defects.

In uncomplicated cases of viral hepatitis, the scan shows mild to moderate hepatomegaly, moderate inhomogeneity, and shunting. In severe cases uptake is decreased, and hepatomegaly becomes more marked. A few cases of severe hepatitis show small livers without shunting. Less commonly, small cold focal defects occur, which can be misdiagnosed as mass lesions.

Cirrhosis has many of the same findings as hepatitis except that liver size is reduced because of chronic scarring, and the spleen is significantly enlarged from portal hypertension. In alcoholic cirrhosis, the left lobe of the liver is likely to be enlarged as well. The discrepancy in the lobe size is believed to be the result of the streaming effect of high alcohol-containing portal blood from the small intestines (superior mesenteric vein) flowing to the right lobe, with low alcohol-containing portal blood from the stomach, colon, and spleen flowing to the left lobe. This results in right lobe atrophy and compensatory hypertrophy of the left lobe.

CASE 81

History.—48-year-old female alcoholic with abdominal pain.

Scan.—^{99m}Tc sulfur colloid liver-spleen scan.

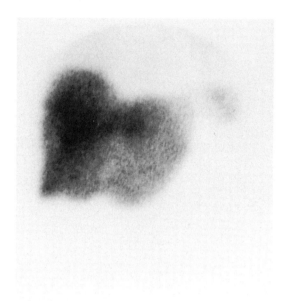

Anterior view of abdomen.

Findings.—Mild hepatomegaly and inhomogeneity.

Diagnosis.—Fatty liver.

Hepatomegaly is the most common abnormality on liver-spleen imaging. The most common causes of hepatomegaly are fatty infiltration of the liver and chronic passive congestion. Pathologically, the liver is mildly to moderately enlarged, with extensive infiltration of normal liver cells by neutral fat.

The finding of fatty liver infiltration is most often asymptomatic but may be associated with mild right upper quadrant tenderness on physical examination. Acute fatty liver after heavy alcohol consumption may manifest with severe right upper quadrant pain and tenderness and a cholestatic picture on liver function tests.

Conditions that cause or are associated with fatty infiltration of the liver include chronic alcoholism, adult-onset diabetes, and obesity. Other causes of a fatty liver are jejunoileal bypass for morbid obesity, Cushing's syndrome, corticosteroid use, chronic illness such as ulcerative colitis, chronic pancreatitis, protracted heart failure, prolonged IV hyperalimentation, hepatotoxin ingestion, kwashiorkor, and Reye's syndrome.

The liver-spleen scan finding of slight hepatomegaly, with "colloid shift" showing more activity in the spleen than the liver on the posterior view, suggests the diagnosis of fatty liver. Other scan patterns of fatty liver include diffuse inhomogeneous uptake of sulfur colloid and massive hepatomegaly. The normal liver size is determined on the anterior view and measures 17 ± 2 cm maximum cephalocaudal dimension.

Retention of radioxenon in the liver can be helpful in confirming the diagnosis of fatty liver. The xenon can be inhaled or given intravenously.

Treatment of fatty liver is generally directed at dietary modification with weight loss, reduction of alcohol consumption, and control of diabetes.

CASE 82

History.—49-year-old woman with a long drinking history, who had increasing abdominal girth.

Scan.—^{99m}Tc sulfur colloid liver-spleen scan.

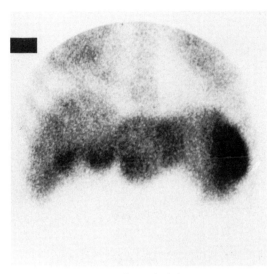

Anterior view of abdomen.

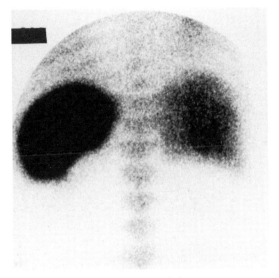

Posterior view of abdomen.

Findings.—Small, inhomogeneous liver with hypertrophy of left lobe. Splenomegaly with shunting to spine and ribs. Separation between liver activity and ribs.

Diagnosis.—Cirrhosis of the liver with ascites.

Alcoholism is the most common cause of cirrhosis of the liver in the United States today. Less common causes include biliary disease and hepatitis.

The findings of cirrhosis on liver-spleen scan depend on the severity and stage of disease. With more advanced cirrhosis, the scan findings are fairly specific; with early disease, the scan shows nonspecific findings.

Early cirrhosis produces minimal changes on liver-spleen scan. Mildly decreased uptake of tracer by the liver and mild hepatomegaly are the only findings. These findings are impossible to differentiate from those of fatty liver infiltration.

Moderate cirrhosis produces more typical changes, with atrophy of the right lobe and compensatory hypertrophy of the left lobe caused by the streaming effect of blood in the portal system. Portal blood from the superior mesenteric vein that is high in alcohol content tends to stream to the right lobe of the liver, damaging it. Blood with lower alcohol concentration from the inferior mesenteric vein tends to preferentially stream to the left lobe of the liver.

There is shunting of activity from the liver to the spleen and bone marrow because of the development of hepatic fibrosis. Portal hypertension also contributes to colloid shift by shunting portal blood to the vena cava via portacaval anastomoses (e.g., hemorrhoidal veins, esophageal varices). This decreases the amount of sulfur colloid passing through the liver, leaving higher concentrations in the blood to be extracted by the spleen and bone marrow.

Advanced cirrhosis characteristically produces a small liver with multiple cold and occasional hot areas caused by scarring and regenerating nodules. Ascites is often seen as a photopenic area around the liver and the spleen. The separation of the liver from the lateral chest wall is more apparent if increased bone marrow uptake in the ribs is present.

In the final stages of cirrhosis, hepatic uptake of sulfur colloid continues to decrease. In extreme cases, there is no visible liver activity. Increased blood pool activity and lung uptake are prominent. The latter must be differentiated from other causes of lung uptake of sulfur colloid, including poor radiopharmaceutical preparation, malignancy, or infection.

CASE 83

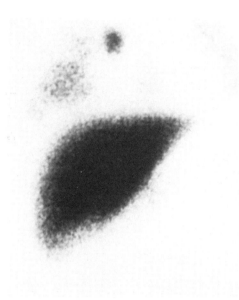

History.—45-year-old chronic alcoholic with complaints of right upper quadrant pain.

Scan.—^{99m}Tc sulfur colloid, liver-spleen scan.

Anterior image of upper half of abdomen and lower view of chest.

Findings.—This scan shows the liver is small and is separated from the body wall. There is activity above the liver.

Diagnosis.—Pulmonary uptake of sulfur colloid as a result of cirrhosis.

Pulmonary accumulation of sulfur colloid occasionally occurs during liver-spleen scanning. The proposed mechanism of uptake varies. In cirrhosis, the most common cause of pulmonary uptake, a combination of increased pulmonary macrophage phagocytosis of the isotope and increased availability because of diminished hepatic uptake is the suspected mechanism.

The metabolism of estrogenic substances is diminished in cirrhosis, causing higher concentrations of these hormones. Estrogens cause release of undifferentiated progenitor cells from the bone marrow, which enter the circulation, lodging in the capillary bed of the lung. There, they differentiate into macrophages and phagocytize the sulfur colloid, resulting in lung activity. Similar processes occur in many other diseases that demonstrate pulmonary uptake.

Another common cause of pulmonary sulfur colloid activity is faulty radiopharmaceutical production. During sulfur colloid preparation, ^{99m}Tc pertechnetate is reduced with so-dium thiosulfate in an acidified solution. Thiosulfuric acid is produced, which rapidly decomposes to sulfur colloid, to which the ^{99m}Tc adheres. If during preparation the kit is boiled too long, clumping of the particles can occur. This can cause embolization of the lungs, with resultant pulmonary activity. Aluminum ion breakthrough from the molybdenum 99–^{99m}Tc generator is another cause of sulfur colloid clumping that can result in lung uptake. Ethylenediamine tetraacetic acid (EDTA) is included in the sulfur colloid kits to bind excess Al ion and avoid this problem.

Other diseases that result in increased pulmonary uptake of sulfur colloid include metastatic disease, lymphoma, hypercoagulable state, systemic bacterial infection, collagen vascular disease, histiocytosis X, intra-abdominal abscess, and mucopolysaccharidosis type II. Rare causes include amyloidosis, anemia, Budd-Chiari syndrome, chronic passive congestion of the liver, estrogen administration, heatstroke, hepatic infarction, malaria, myelofibrosis, and some viral infections.

CASE 84

History.— 32-year-old woman taking birth control pills, who has vague right upper quadrant abdominal pain.

Scan.—⁹⁹ᵐTc sulfur colloid liver-spleen scan.

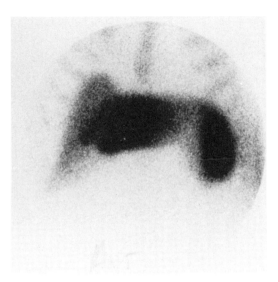

Anterior view of abdomen.

Findings.—Central area of increased uptake in liver.

Diagnosis.—Budd-Chiari syndrome.

Budd-Chiari syndrome is a rare disorder usually caused by spontaneous thrombosis of the hepatic veins. It is seen most often in patients with an underlying predisposition to thrombosis, such as polycythemia vera, paroxysmal nocturnal hemoglobinuria, renal cell carcinoma with tumor involvement of the inferior vena cava, or in patients taking oral contraceptives.

The main clinical signs and symptoms are vague upper quadrant abdominal pain, hepatomegaly, ascites, and hepatic failure. Portal hypertension is present, caused by hepatic venous obstruction elevating sinusoidal pressure; this is transmitted upstream to the portal system.

The liver-spleen scan in patients with Budd-Chiari syndrome shows marked reduction of uptake of sulfur colloid throughout most of the right lobe, with increased uptake in a small centrally located area representing the hypertrophied caudate lobe. The venous drainage of the caudate lobe is spared, being drained by multiple small tributaries that empty directly into the vena cava. The improved perfusion to the caudate lobe compared with other areas of the liver produces the hot spot.

It may take several months to develop the scintigraphic sign of increased uptake in the caudate lobe. Before that time, diffuse hepatic enlargement with overall poor or mottled uptake may be the only finding. There is marked colloid shift, with increased uptake in the bone marrow, as well as splenomegaly.

Other imaging modalities can be valuable in the diagnosis of Budd-Chiari syndrome. CT scans show enhancement or pooling of intravenous contrast material in the periphery of the liver. Ultrasound can demonstrate clot in the hepatic veins. Venography will show obstruction of the hepatic veins, often demonstrating a beaklike filling defect at the hepatic vein orifice. At the time of the liver scan, a radionuclide venogram can be performed with ⁹⁹ᵐTc sulfur colloid.

Differential considerations include cirrhosis, which can have atrophy with decreased uptake of the right lobe and compensatory hypertrophy of the left lobe. Ascites can be present with cirrhosis, but if the ascites has a rapid onset, Budd-Chiari syndrome still should be considered. A final possibility is a hepatoma replacing a large portion of the right lobe.

CASE 85

History.—29-year-old woman taking birth control pills, who has mildly elevated liver function test results.

Scan.—^{99m}Tc sulfur colloid liver-spleen scan.

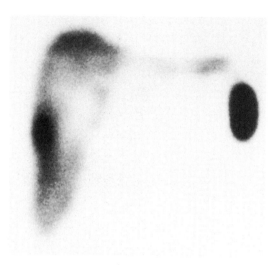

Coronal SPECT image.

Findings.—Increased focal uptake is seen in the lateral portion of the right lobe.

Diagnosis.—Focal nodular hyperplasia.

During the evaluation of a variety of medical conditions with abdominal imaging procedures, benign tumors of the liver are sometimes encountered. The most common of these are cavernous hemangiomas, followed in frequency of occurrence by hepatic adenoma and focal nodular hyperplasia. Both hepatic adenoma and focal nodular hyperplasia have an association with prolonged use of oral contraceptives in women; however, the association is much weaker with focal nodular hyperplasia. There is evidence of regression of both after discontinuation of oral contraceptive use.

Focal nodular hyperplasia is found most frequently in young women. Eighty percent of cases of focal nodular hyperplasia in the liver are solitary; 20% are multiple. Pathologically, it consists of random collections of hepatocytes, bile ducts, and Kupffer's cells. Angiographic images show increased flow to the involved areas of liver. The appearance on the delayed images is dependent on the concentration of Kupffer's cells. If there are increased numbers of Kupffer's cells in relation to normal liver (infrequent), the lesion will appear hot; if the concentration of Kupffer's cells equals that in normal liver (most frequent), the scan will be normal. If there are fewer Kupffer's cells than in normal liver (infrequent), the lesion will appear cold and indistinguishable from other causes of cold defects in the liver on liver-spleen scan.

An unsuspected mass on CT with a normal liver-spleen scan is strong evidence of focal nodular hyperplasia. In these cases, biopsy is frequently unnecessary.

CASE 86

History.—70-year-old male smoker who has elevated liver function test results.

Scan.—^{99m}Tc sulfur colloid liver-spleen scan.

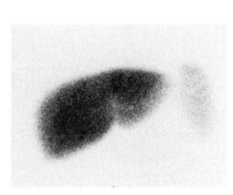

Anterior view of abdomen.

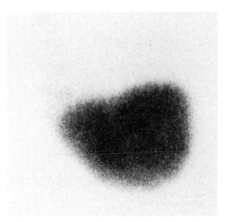

Right lateral view of abdomen.

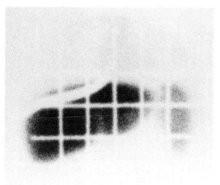

Anterior view of abdomen with 5 cm grid and costal margin marker.

Findings.—Flattening of superior liver surface with liver low in the abdomen.

Diagnosis.—COPD.

The shape of the liver is determined primarily by its surrounding structures. This case is an example of the liver shape being altered by the diaphragm of a patient with chronic obstructive pulmonary disease (COPD).

In patients with COPD, hyperinflation of the lungs commonly occurs, causing low, flat diaphragms and increased anteroposterior distance on the chest radiograph. The liver in these patients is flattened superiorly and is positioned lower in the abdomen. For these reasons it is not uncommon for a patient with COPD to be referred to the nuclear medicine department for evaluation of suspected hepatic enlargement.

The liver-spleen scan can accurately determine liver size using a lead grid on the anterior view. In addition, a costal margin marker placed over the right inferior costal margin demonstrates the position of the liver relative to the thoracoabdominal wall.

CASE 87

History.—45-year-old man with renal cell carcinoma. We are asked to evaluate for metastatic disease to the liver.

Scan.— ^{99m}Tc sulfur colloid liver-spleen scan.

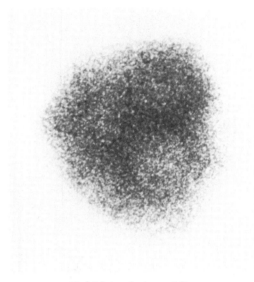

Right lateral view of liver.

Findings.—Multiple cold defects in the liver.

Diagnosis.—PM tube artifact on liver-spleen scan.

Imaging artifacts can be produced in any step from radiopharmaceutical preparation to processing the film. Critical components include the radiopharmaceutical, injection technique, the scintillation camera, collimator, formator, film, and film processor. Quality control measures are taken at each level to prevent artifacts. If, however, these quality control steps are bypassed, images may show defects not caused by disease. This can be dangerous for the patient if the error is not appreciated.

When exposed to radiation, the sodium iodide crystal in the camera scintillates, or emits light. The intensity of this light is proportional to the energy of the photon interacting with the crystal. Photomultiplier tubes behind the crystal detect the position and intensity of the emitted light. The tubes are placed in a hexagonal array optically coupled to the back of the crystal. Occasionally a single photomultiplier tube will fail or malfunction, producing a defect that is always located in the same position on the images.

For image acquisition, the energy window of the isotope being imaged is set. This allows the camera to discriminate between isotopes having different photon energies. In the peaking of a camera, a flood source is used to acquire a flood image. During acquisition, the spectral display for that isotope can be viewed and the limits of the imaging window or the photopeak can then be adjusted to assure proper peak setting. If the camera is off peak, either too high or too low, the images will often be degraded with artifacts caused by the photomultiplier tubes of the camera. The images will have a honeycomb appearance, with the photomultiplier tubes showing as areas of either increased or decreased activity. If the photomultiplier tubes appear as areas of decreased intensity, the window is usually set above the photopeak. If the photomultiplier tubes appear as areas of increased activity, the photopeak is usually set too low.

Some cameras are equipped with a microprocessor that corrects for degradation in field uniformity if the peak is offset. This can be useful, allowing imaging of the upper portion of the photopeak and thereby diminishing the contribution of Compton scatter to the image.

CASE 88

History.— 5-year-old child with elevated liver function results.

Scan.— ^{99m}Tc liver-spleen scan.

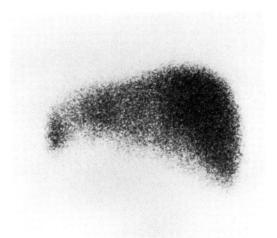

Anterior view, liver-spleen scan.

Findings.— Liver in left upper quadrant and spleen in right upper quadrant.

Diagnosis.— Situs inversus.

Situs inversus is a rare condition in which the organs of the abdomen are positioned opposite of normal. The appendix is located in the left lower quadrant, the liver in the left upper quadrant, and so forth. The condition is caused by rotation of the midgut in the embryonic period in a clockwise rather than counterclockwise direction. There are various degrees of situs inversus, with complete situs inversus often being associated with mirror-image dextrocardia.

This case illustrates the importance of careful labeling of the films. In conventional radiology, this is often done using lead markers designating left and right. In nuclear medicine, the left-right and superior-inferior orientation can be changed by simply flipping the axis change switch on the control board. It is wise practice to use a radioactive source to mark one side during image acquisition for later confirmation of the image orientation. The best imaging technique can still be negated if, after film processing, the film is incorrectly hung on the viewbox.

CASE 89

History.— 28-year-old man with history of rheumatic heart disease and positive blood cultures.

Scan.— ^{99m}Tc sulfur colloid liver-spleen scan.

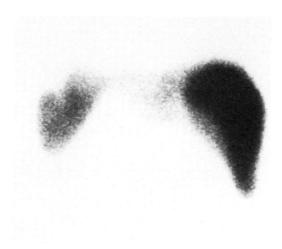

Posterior view of abdomen.

Findings.— The study shows a wedge-shaped peripheral cold defect in the spleen.

Diagnosis.— Splenic infarct.

Splenic infarcts are relatively uncommon. They usually arise in patients with hematologic disorders that produce massive splenomegaly, such as myelofibrosis, leukemia, and hemolytic anemias, or in disorders with enhanced clotting, such as sickle cell anemia. Alcoholism, subacute bacterial endocarditis, and pancreatitis are also associated with splenic infarcts.

Splenic infarcts may manifest with left upper quadrant abdominal pain that radiates to the left shoulder, abdominal guarding, and pleuritic pain. Some are asymptomatic.

If the underlying disorder causing splenic infarcts is not reversed, the process can progress and eventually infarct the entire spleen. The patient then suffers the immunologic sequella of asplenia, frequent infections caused by bacteria with a polysaccharide coat. Complete autoinfarction of the spleen is especially common in sickle cell anemia.

The typical findings of a splenic infarct on liver-spleen scan are peripheral, wedge-shaped cold defects, which may be single or multiple. The finding of a cold defect in the spleen is not specific for infarct, however. The differential diagnosis of such a defect includes hematoma, lymphoma, splenic abscess, metastatic disease (melanoma, islet cell, lung, breast), benign tumors (hemangioma, fibroma, hamartoma), and cysts.

A leukocyte scan in combination with ^{99m}Tc sulfur colloid liver-spleen scan can be used to differentiate an abscess from an infarct. An infarct will be cold on both studies. An abscess will show leukocyte uptake equal to or greater than the normal spleen in the area of the cold defect on liver-spleen scan.

Normal anatomic variations can simulate splenic infarcts. Occasionally the left lobe of the liver extends far over into the left upper portion of the abdomen ("hepatic walk"). The superimposition of activity in the elongated left lobe with the spleen can cause the appearance of a wedge-shaped "defect" on the posterior view. Examining the spleen on multiple views will help rule out an infarct. SPECT can also be helpful in these cases. A second anatomic variant that can simulate an infarct is the cup-shaped or upside-down spleen. A rounded defect is seen in the superior portion of the spleen because of the hilum.

CASE 90

History.— 27-year-old man in automobile accident who had abdominal pain.

Scan.—^{99m}Tc sulfur colloid liver-spleen scan.

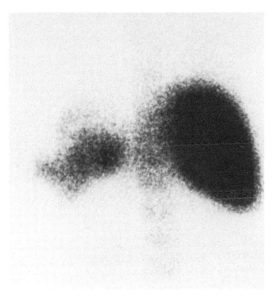

Posterior view of abdomen.

Findings.— Irregular uptake in spleen.

Diagnosis.— Splenic hematoma.

The most common cause of a splenic hematoma is blunt abdominal trauma. The trauma can be very slight, and occasionally the patient will not remember it. Patients at increased risk of splenic hematoma are those with splenomegaly secondary to thrombocytopenia, hemophilia, or infections such as Epstein-Barr virus.

The liver-spleen scan, computed tomography scan, and ultrasound are useful in the evaluation of abdominal trauma. The accuracy of liver-spleen scans in detecting splenic hematoma or fracture is 90% or better.

A splenic hematoma on liver-spleen scan is demonstrated by a photon-deficient area. The photopenic area is semilunar or round in a subcapsular or intrapulp hematoma but has a linear or stellate appearance in splenic fracture. Other less specific signs of splenic hematoma are variable degrees of splenomegaly or, in the case of diffuse intrasplenic bleeding, diffusely diminished uptake of sulfur colloid.

In cases of severe trauma, the spleen can be fragmented into several pieces. These small fragments of splenic tissue can spread through the abdomen or bloodstream, creating several scattered functional pieces of spleen, called "splenosis." These areas will concentrate sulfur colloid and can be detected with liver-spleen scans.

The use of single-photon emission computed tomography (SPECT) in the evaluation of trauma increases the sensitivity for abnormalities but requires more time, which may be difficult in the trauma patient. Standard planar views with the addition of one or two extra left anterior and posterior oblique views suffices in demonstrating most splenic abnormalities.

If the information obtained from the liver-spleen scan is inconclusive, a denatured red blood cell scan will sometimes make splenic defects more apparent.

The differentiation of a subcapsular hematoma from a splenic infarct or abscess is usually apparent by history. If an abscess is a consideration as the cause of a cold splenic defect, a scan using white blood cells labeled with indium can be performed. An abscess will be cold on liver-spleen scan and normal or hot on leukocyte images, whereas an infarct or hematoma will be cold on both studies.

CASE 91

History.— Postsplenectomy patient with fever.

Scan.—^{111}In leukocyte scan and ^{99m}Tc sulfur colloid liver-spleen scan.

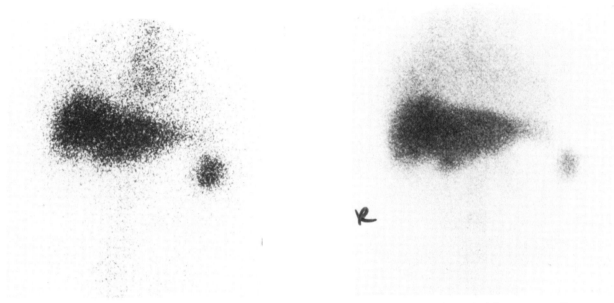

Anterior view of abdomen on leukocyte scan.

Anterior view of abdomen on sulfur colloid scan.

Findings.— Focus of activity in left upper quadrant on both studies.

Diagnosis.— Accessory spleen.

The question of whether an accessory spleen is present arises in patients who have had a splenectomy for conditions such as hereditary spherocytosis or idiopathic thrombocytopenic purpura and develop recurrence of symptoms or laboratory abnormalities. Localization of an accessory spleen before splenectomy is occasionally needed. In such cases the presence of an accessory spleen can be determined by either routine liver-spleen scanning, denatured red blood cell imaging, or ^{111}In platelet scans. Computed tomography is less specific in this clinical situation.

Accessory spleens arise embryologically when some clusters of primordial spleen cells fail to fuse. They occur in nearly 10% of people, most commonly near the hilum of the spleen and the tail of the pancreas. They may also be embedded partially or wholly within the pancreas. The average size of an accessory spleen is 1 cm.

After splenectomy, accessory splenic tissue can be seen in up to 30% of patients. This is most likely the result of hypertrophy of existing ectopic tissue; however, it has been suggested that spillage of splenic tissue during surgery can result in the development of accessory spleens as well.

Accessory spleens can cause false positive leukocyte scans. If an area of increased activity in the left upper quadrant is seen in a patient who has had a prior splenectomy, an abscess could be falsely diagnosed, when, in fact, this is uptake in an accessory spleen. A sulfur colloid scan can be performed immediately after a leukocyte scan to solve this problem. If colloid uptake is seen in the same region as the ^{111}In leukocyte activity, an accessory spleen rather than an abscess is present.

CASE 92

History.—50-year-old man with abnormal complete blood
cell count.

Scan.—^{99m}Tc sulfur colloid liver-spleen scan.

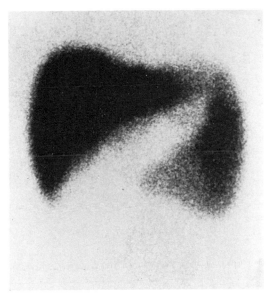

Anterior view of abdomen.

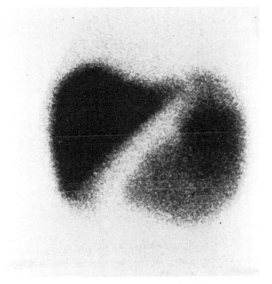

Left anterior oblique view of abdomen.

Findings.—Massive splenomegaly.

Diagnosis.—Chronic myeloid leukemia.

The accurate evaluation of splenic size is one of the uses of the liver-spleen scan. Normal adult splenic size is 10 ± 3 cm in cephalocaudad length; normal weight is 165 g. The finding of an enlarged spleen is a nonspecific finding and can be caused by a number of diseases. Important causes of splenomegaly are:

1. Massive splenomegaly (>20 cm in length)
   a. Chronic myeloid leukemia
   b. Myelofibrosis with myeloid metaplasia
   c. Gaucher's disease (glycogen storage disease)
   d. Thalassemia major
   e. Malaria
   f. Kala-azar
   g. Hydatid disease
   h. Lymphoma
2. Moderate splenomegaly
   a. Preceding causes
   b. Storage disease
   c. Hemolytic anemias
   d. Cirrhosis with portal hypertension
   e. Leukemias
   f. Metastases

3. Mild splenomegaly
   a. Preceding causes
   b. Congestive heart failure
   c. Infections
      (1) Viral: hepatitis, EBV infection
      (2) Bacterial, rickettsial, fungal
   d. Sarcoidosis
   e. Amyloidosis
   f. Rheumatoid arthritis, Felty's syndrome
   g. Systemic lupus erythematosus

Evaluation of the spleen can be confusing when the left lobe of the liver extends far to the left in the upper quadrant. If what is spleen or left lobe of liver is unclear, a heat-treated red blood cell study can be performed using denatured red blood cells labeled with ^{99m}Tc. These are sequestered by the spleen only, making it possible to clearly delineate splenic anatomy. If the liver anatomy is in question, a diisopropyl iminodiacetic acid (DISIDA) scan will provide liver detail if imaged early after injection. Images in multiple projections can be done just as with sulfur colloid.

CASE 93

History.— 14-year-old youth with sickle cell disease and Howell-Jolly bodies on blood smear.

Scan.—^{99m}Tc sulfur colloid liver-spleen scan.

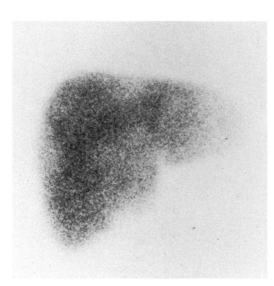

Anterior view of abdomen.

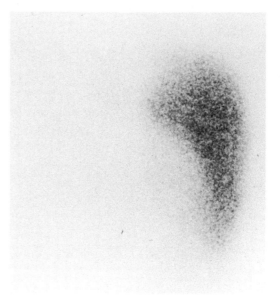

Posterior view of abdomen.

Findings.—Slight inhomogeneous liver uptake. No splenic activity was identified.

Diagnosis.—Functional asplenia secondary to sickle cell disease.

The lack of splenic uptake of sulfur colloid in patients with anatomically intact spleens is called "functional asplenia." It is important to differentiate this condition from congenital absence of the spleen, often seen in association with congenital heart disease and total splenic infarction. Individuals with functional asplenia demonstrate Howell-Jolly bodies on their peripheral blood smear, as would be expected in anatomic asplenia.

Conditions causing functional asplenia do so by impairing blood flow to the spleen or diminishing reticuloendothelial system cell function. Those that impair blood flow include sickle cell disease (most common cause of functional asplenia), and thalassemia. Conditions that diminish reticuloendothelial system cell function include tumor replacement and celiac disease.

Reversible functional asplenia can be demonstrated in sickle cell anemia. Red blood cell sickling reduces splenic perfusion, causing anoxia and diminished function. If the patient is transfused with normal red blood cells, this process is reversed by allowing adequate oxygenation of the spleen.

CASE 94

History.— 32-year-old woman with right upper quadrant pain.

Scan.—^{99m}Tc DISIDA scan.

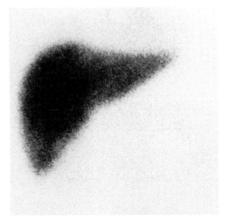

Immediate anterior image of abdomen.

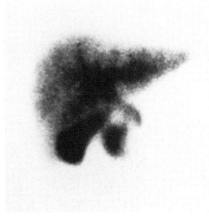

15-Minute image.

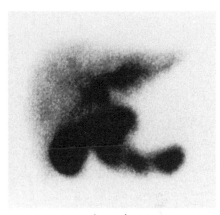

30-Minute image.

Findings.— Visualization of the gallbladder and bowel by 60 minutes.

Diagnosis.—Normal hepatobiliary scan.

Hepatobiliary imaging, or cholescintigraphy, is a physiologic test of hepatobiliary function. After the injection of a compound of ^{99m}Tc-labeled iminodiacetic acid (IDA), serial images over the liver and gallbladder show concentration of the material in the liver and its excretion through the biliary system. This test is usually performed for evaluation of suspected acute cholecystitis or obstructive jaundice; however, it is also useful for the evaluation of liver parenchymal disease and liver trauma.

Several new compounds of IDA that replace the original agent (dimethyl-IDA, or HIDA) are available. The most widely used agent at present is DISIDA. Other agents include paraisopropyl-IDA (PIPIDA) and parabutyl-IDA (BIDA). Because these agents are chemically similar to the bile acids, they compete with bilirubin for excretion. If a patient has an elevated bilirubin level, the excretion of the tracer may be delayed. Each compound's ability to be concentrated in the bile depends on the substitution group on the IDA compound.

IDA Substitution Compounds	Useful to Bilirubin Levels of:
HIDA dimethyl-IDA (first widely used agent)	8 mg/dL
PIPIDA paraisopropyl-IDA (duct visualization may be poor in normal persons)	20 mg/dL
BIDA parabutyl-IDA (slow hepatic uptake and excretion)	10–20 mg/dL
DISIDA diisopropyl-IDA	30 mg/dL

The patient must have nothing by mouth 4 to 6 hours before this study to prevent false positive nonvisualization of the gallbladder. If the patient eats during this period, the gallbladder may still be under natural cholecystokinin stimulation and in a contracted state. This prevents filling of the gallbladder with the radiotracer.

Some centers pretreat patients with cholecystokinin (CCK) 15 to 20 minutes before imaging to empty the normal gallbladder. The drug has a short duration of action; the gallbladder returns to its pretreatment state after about 15 minutes. This procedure reduces false positive studies because of inspissated bile, or "sludge," which can prevent the tracer from entering the gallbladder.

Early images of a normal hepatobiliary scan show liver, cardiac, and vascular activity that fades as hepatic uptake increases. These images allow the liver to be evaluated for filling defects such as tumors. The intrahepatic biliary tree, gallbladder, common bile duct, and small bowel normally visualize by 60 minutes. Gallbladder activity should be seen before small bowel. If the reverse is true or if the gallbladder visualizes after 60 minutes, the patient has an increased chance of having chronic cholecystitis.

A secondary route of excretion is the kidneys. This causes minimal renal activity in some patients. Patients with high bilirubin levels will show increased renal excretion similar to vicarious excretion of x-ray contrast material seen in some disorders.

CASE 95

History.—40-year-old obese woman with 1-day history of right upper quadrant pain and vomiting.

Scan.—^{99m}Tc DISIDA scan with morphine administration.

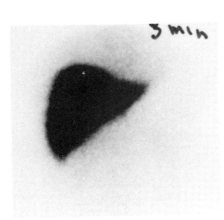
Immediate anterior view of abdomen.

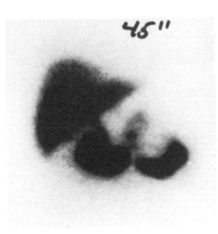
45 Minutes after injection.

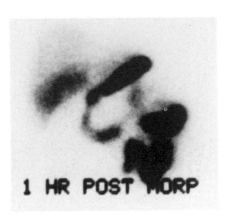
One hour 15 minutes after injection.

Findings.—DISIDA: No gallbladder visualization, with parenchymal retention of activity in gallbladder fossa. Bowel visualization with enterogastric reflux.

Diagnosis.—Acute cholecystitis.

The majority of patients with acute cholecystitis have a gallstone obstructing the cystic duct. This produces the classic symptoms of acute cholecystitis: nausea, vomiting, fever, and extreme right upper quadrant pain and tenderness. These symptoms are worse after eating a fatty meal because of cholecystokinen (CCK)-stimulated contraction of the gallbladder.

The sensitivity of hepatobiliary imaging for acute cholecystitis is 95% or more, with a specificity of 99%. The sensitivity and specificity of ultrasound for acute cholecystitis is significantly less. Oral cholecystography and intravenous cholangiography no longer are used to diagnose cholecystitis.

The scan findings of acute cholecystitis include:

1. Nonvisualization of the gallbladder at 1 to 4 hours, with normal hepatic uptake and visualization of common duct and bowel.
2. Increased activity in the region of the gallbladder fossa because of increased blood flow (secondary to inflammation) and delayed removal of tracer (because of edema). This finding is called the "rim sign."
3. A small amount of activity visible in the region of the gallbladder in as many as 7% of patients with acute cholecystitis. This can be misinterpreted as gallbladder visualization; however, comparison with ultrasound will show a size discrepancy between the gallbladder and the radioactivity. This pattern is caused by a small amount of activity in the cystic duct proximal to the obstruction.

If the gallbladder does not visualize by 45 minutes and activity is present in the small bowel, an intravenously administered dose of morphine sulfate (0.04 mg/kg) should be administered. Morphine causes spasm of the sphincter of Oddi, increasing biliary pressure. This forces bile into the gallbladder if there is a functional obstruction from chronic cholecystitis or from prolonged fasting state and parenteral nutrition (causing hyperconcentrated bile). Morphine administration dramatically improves specificity.

A second method of reducing false positive results in patients with prolonged fasting or parenteral nutrition involves intravenous administration of a dose of CCK (sincalide; 0.02–0.04 µg/kg) to empty the gallbladder 20 minutes before the DISIDA is administered. Sincalide has a short duration of action and returns the gallbladder to a noncontracted state by about 20 minutes, allowing entry of tracer.

Five percent to 15% of all patients with cholecystitis have no gallstones by ultrasound or pathology. One third of pediatric patients and 25% to 45% of postoperative patients with cholecystitis are without stones. This variant of acute cholecystitis is referred to as "acalculus cholecystitis."

Factors that predispose to acalculus cholecystitis include:

1. Chemical irritation secondary to hyperconcentrated bile (prolonged fasting)
2. Chemical toxins (same)
3. Bacterial infection (children)
4. Ischemia (diabetes, ventilator cases)

The sensitivity of hepatobiliary imaging for acalculus cholecystitis averages 80% to 85%. The findings are the same as in calculus cholecystitis, with nonvisualization of the gallbladder. Occasionally common duct obstruction is found. Acalculus cholecystitis has a much poorer prognosis than calculous disease, with one half of patients progressing to a serious complication.

CASE 96

History.— 38-year-old woman with breast cancer, right upper quadrant pain, and an equivocal ultrasound examination for acute cholecystitis.

Scan.—^{99m}Tc DISIDA scan.

Anterior image after 20 minutes.

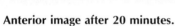

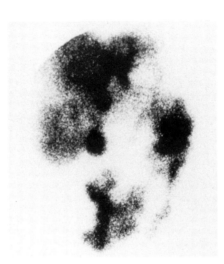

Image after 55 minutes.

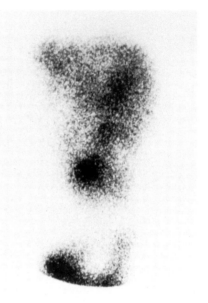

Right lateral image.

Findings.—Activity in the region of the gallbladder on early views, which is shown to be posterior on lateral images. Cold defects are present in the liver.

Diagnosis.—Duodenal activity mimicking gallbladder visualization. Acute cholecystitis. Liver metastases.

This case illustrates the potentially confusing appearances on DISIDA scan. Activity in the bowel can sometimes be focal and mimic the gallbladder.

The gallbladder is an anterior structure compared with the duodenum, which is retroperitoneal, and, therefore, a posterior structure. If it is unclear on the anterior images if gallbladder or bowel is being seen, a right lateral image should be done. If the activity angles anteriorly, it is gallbladder; if the activity is posterior, it is most likely radiopharmaceutical pooling in the C loop of the duodenum.

An alternative to doing lateral views is to have the patient drink a glass of water. If the activity in the region of the gallbladder fossa is due to radiopharmaceutical in the gastrointestinal tract, it will be washed away by the water.

CASE 97

History.— Insulin-dependent diabetic patient with fevers, chills, and abdominal pain.

Scan.—^{99m}Tc DISIDA biliary scan.

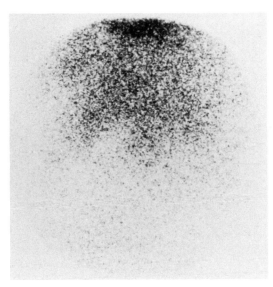

Anterior image of liver after 5 minutes.

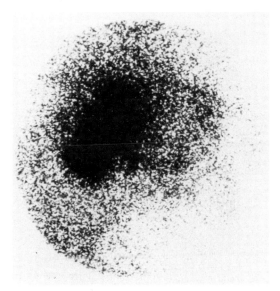

Anterior image of liver after 24 hours.

Findings.— The 5-minute image shows poor hepatic uptake, with no gallbladder or bowel visualization. Twenty-four-hour image shows large DISIDA collection in region of gallbladder.

Diagnosis.— Perforated gallbladder.

Acute cholecystitis is a common disorder that can be complicated by rupture of the gallbladder. Without prompt surgical correction, perforation carries a high mortality rate.

Those most at risk of gallbladder perforation are elderly, debilitated patients with severe atherosclerotic disease and immunocompromised patients. A perforation of the gallbladder should be suspected in toxic-appearing patients with rapidly progressive symptoms of cholecystitis associated with high fever and an elevated leukocyte count.

Gallbladder perforation occurs in about 10% of cases of acute cholecystitis. The majority of these are walled off by the body, with the development of a pericholecystic abscess. Only about 1% result in free flow of bile into the peritoneal cavity.

A third form of gallbladder rupture occurs when the inflamed gallbladder perforates into an adjacent adherent organ. This creates a cholecystenteric fistula and may involve the stomach, colon, or small bowel. The acute cholecystitis is then decompressed, with partial or complete resolution of symptoms. Occasionally gallstones may enter the bowel by this route and cause obstruction. Most cholecystenteric fistulas are discovered incidentally during cholecystectomy for symptoms of cholecystitis.

Hepatobiliary imaging is the best single study for the diagnosis of acute cholecystitis. Both the sensitivity and specificity for this disease exceed 95%. Hepatobiliary imaging of free perforation of the gallbladder demonstrates accumulation of the radiopharmaceutical in the region of the gallbladder fossa, which then flows freely into the peritoneal cavity. If the perforation is manifested by pericholecystic abscess, a pericholecystic collection of DISIDA will be seen.

CASE 98

History.— 53-year-old woman with intermittent right upper quadrant pain for 5 months.

Scan.—^{99m}Tc DISIDA scan with morphine administration at 45 minutes.

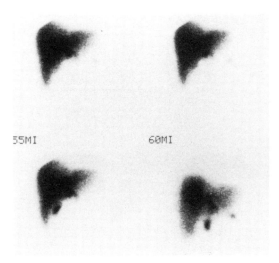

Serial images of the liver and biliary tree 45 to 60 minutes after injection; 60-minute image is in RAO projection.

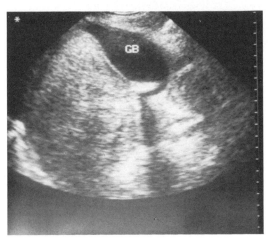

Ultrasound of gallbladder.

Findings.—DISIDA: Visualization of gallbladder at 55 minutes, 10 minutes after morphine administration. Small amount of bowel activity is present. Ultrasound: Echogenic foci in gallbladder with acoustic shadowing.

Diagnosis.—Chronic cholecystitis.

Chronic cholecystitis refers to patients with intermittently symptomatic cholelithiasis. The name implies a histologic diagnosis; however, it is more a clinical diagnosis applied to patients with biliary symptoms in whom gallstones are present. The symptoms are presumed caused by transient obstruction of the cystic duct by gallstones. The pain is usually steady and is located in the right upper quadrant. It may last minutes to hours; it begins abruptly and gradually subsides. Often, but not always, symptoms are related to meals.

The sensitivity of hepatobiliary imaging for diagnosing chronic cholecystitis ranges from 10% to 75%, varying with the population studied. Patients with severe long-standing symptoms have a higher percentage of abnormal scans.

The findings of chronic cholecystitis on hepatobiliary scans fall into three categories:

1. Delayed visualization of the gallbladder (beyond 60 minutes) because of viscous bile, stones, or fibrosis of the gallbladder, causing an anatomic or functional obstruction of the cystic duct. The isotope takes the path of least resistance through the common duct into the duodenum. The more delayed the isotope's entry into the gallbladder, the greater the specificity for chronic cholecystitis.
2. Prolonged biliary-to-bowel transit time caused by ampullitis from inflammation of the nearby gallbladder or from repeated passage of stones.
3. Visualization of the gallbladder and bowel by 1 hour, but bowel appearing before gallbladder. This finding indicates chronic cholecystitis approximately 75% of the time.

CASE 99

History.— 50-year-old man with jaundice and abdominal pain.

Scan.—^{99m}Tc DISIDA scan.

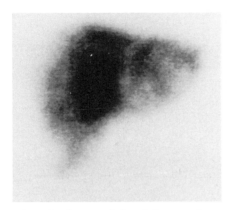

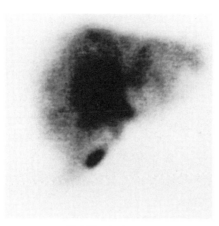

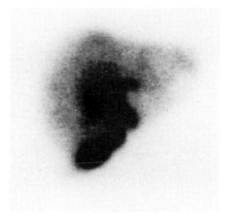

Anterior image of the abdomen after 30 minutes.

60-Minute image.

Two-hour image.

Findings.— 30 minutes: prominent hepatic ducts, no excretion or gallbladder visualization; 60 minutes: gallbladder visualization beginning; 120 minutes: gallbladder visualization without bowel visualization.

Diagnosis.—Common bile duct obstruction.

The two most common causes of common bile duct obstruction are gallstones and tumor. Gallstones are occasionally expelled from the gallbladder through the cystic duct to the common bile duct. They are often prevented, however, from entering into the small bowel by the relatively narrow sphincter of Oddi or ampulla of Vater. These stones cause symptoms by obstructing biliary flow. Of patients with cholelithiasis, approximately 15% will also have stones in the common duct.

An obstructing stone produces biliary colic and jaundice. The common duct proximal to the obstruction is subjected to a rapid rise in pressure and may dilate to 2 to 3 cm. It is this rapid rise in biliary pressure that causes biliary colic. Pancreatitis and, occasionally, ascending cholangitis can also occur.

Gradual occlusion of the common duct by a malignancy in the bile duct, ampulla, or head of the pancreas tends to manifest with painless jaundice. The degree of dilatation of the biliary tree in malignant common duct obstruction is much greater than that caused by choledocholithiasis.

Cholescintigraphy is useful in evaluating the jaundiced patient for common bile duct obstruction. It has a sensitivity of 97% and specificity of 90% for duct obstruction.

In common bile duct obstruction, no passage of activity is seen from the biliary tree into the small bowel. These structures are normally visualized by 1 hour after injection of the isotope.

Three patterns can be seen with total common duct obstruction:

1. Good hepatic uptake with visualization of gallbladder and common duct with no flow into bowel.
2. The same as no. 1, with a dilated biliary tree. Ductal width is easy to misinterpret, however, because the width of the ducts on hepatobiliary imaging is related primarily to the amount of radioactivity present rather than to the width of the duct.
3. Good hepatic uptake with no visualization of intrahepatic or common bile ducts, gallbladder, or bowel; this occurs because intraductal pressures exceed secretory pressures of the hepatocytes.

Other modalities for evaluating jaundiced patients include ultrasound and computed tomography (CT). Ultrasound is most accurate in determining intrahepatic and extrahepatic ductal dilatation. With ultrasound, the presence of gallstones in the gallbladder can be determined with a sensitivity of 85% or more. Ultrasound is limited in its ability to see common duct stones, however. If the obstruction is recent, there may not have been sufficient time for the biliary tree to dilate. In these cases the ultrasound will be incorrectly interpreted as normal. CT is helpful in evaluating for pancreatic masses. It can also be useful in measuring ductal size. Endoscopic retrograde cholangiopancreatography (ERCP) or transhepatic cholangiography should also be considered in particularly difficult cases to more fully delineate biliary tree anatomy.

Treatment of common duct obstruction is directed at the cause of the obstruction. Most patients with choledocholithiasis require systemic antibiotics and elective cholecystectomy, with common bile duct exploration. Emergent surgical intervention is sometimes necessary. In selected cases, basket stone removal and sphincterotomy with ERCP can be done.

CASE 100

History.—50-year-old man with abdominal pain. He was given intramuscular morphine just before the scan was performed.

Scan.—^{99m}Tc DISIDA scan.

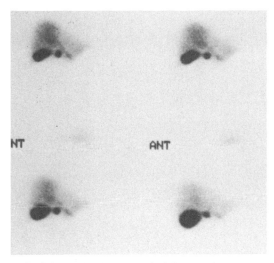

Serial anterior images of abdomen from 45 to 60 minutes.

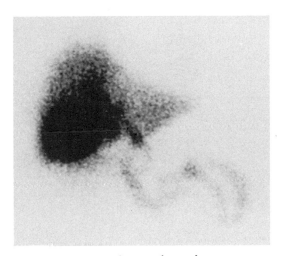

Image 10 minutes after naloxone administration.

Findings.—45- to 60-minute images: gallbladder visualization without bowel activity; postnaloxone: bowel visualization.

Diagnosis.—Narcotic-induced spasm of the sphincter of Oddi simulating common bile duct obstruction.

The two most common causes of common bile duct obstruction are choledocholithiasis and tumor. Narcotic-induced spasm of the sphincter of Oddi can simulate them on hepatobiliary scan.

The main criterion for the diagnosis of common bile duct obstruction on hepatobiliary scan is good hepatic uptake without entry of activity into the bowel. In normal individuals, common bile duct, gallbladder, and small bowel are visualized by 60 minutes.

In obstruction, common duct and gallbladder visualization depend on intraductal pressures and the duration of obstruction. The longer the obstructive process has been present, the less likely activity will enter the biliary tree.

Morphine sulfate causes spasm of the sphincter of Oddi, increasing biliary pressure to nearly 40 cm H_2O. For this reason, many physicians are trained to avoid morphine as pain medication in patients with suspected acute cholecystitis. On occasion, however, a patient taking narcotic pain medication will be referred for hepatobiliary imaging. In such patients, delayed or absent small bowel visualization is not uncommon. The nuclear medicine physician is then left with a dilemma: Does this represent pathologic obstruction of the common duct, or is it a pharmacologic effect of the narcotic?

The hepatobiliary study can be repeated with the patient off narcotic therapy or IV naloxone reversal of the morphine-induced spasm can be attempted. Naloxone is a specific opiate-competitive antagonist with no agonist effects. Its action on the sphincter of Oddi has been reported in the surgery literature as a diagnostic aid to help differentiate spasm from impacted common duct stone during intraoperative cholangiography. If the small bowel is visualized promptly after naloxone reversal of the narcotic, physiologic spasm is most likely the cause of delayed visualization. If, however, there is persistent nonvisualization of the bowel after naloxone administration, pathologic obstruction should be considered.

CASE 101

History.— 5-year-old boy with 24-hour history of painless rectal bleeding.

Scan.—^{99m}Tc Meckel's scan.

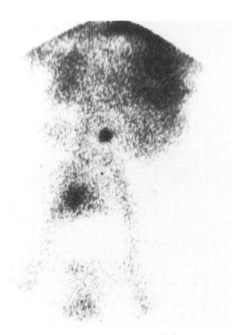

15-Minute anterior image of abdomen.

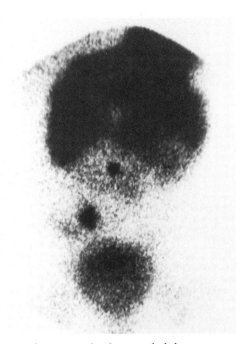

Two-hour anterior image of abdomen.

Findings.— Focal right lower quadrant activity that increased in intensity with time.

Diagnosis.— Meckel's diverticulum.

Meckel's diverticulum is the embryologic remnant of the omphalomesenteric, or vitelline, duct. It arises from the fetal yolk sac and connects the umbilicus with the fetal intestine.

Meckel's diverticulum is the most common congenital anomaly of the GI tract, occurring in about 2% of the population. It is found on the antimesenteric side of the terminal ileum, usually within 45 to 90 cm of the ileocecal valve. Its length varies from 1 to 12 cm (average, 6 cm), and occasionally it is connected to the umbilicus by a fibrous band. Twenty-five percent of Meckel's diverticula contain ectopic mucosa from the stomach, duodenum, pancreas, or colon.

Although the majority of Meckel's diverticula are asymptomatic, complications such as hemorrhage, volvulus, diverticulitis, and intussusception can occur. Only a small percentage of Meckel's diverticula have ectopic gastric mucosa, and it is these that have a propensity to cause ulceration and bleeding. The majority of symptoms related to Meckel's diverticula will occur in the patient's first 2 years of life.

Meckel's diverticula have an associated *"rule of twos"*:

- Occur in 2% of the population
- Located within 2 ft of the ileocecal valve
- Usually about 2 in. long
- 2:1 male/female predominance
- 2% become symptomatic
- Usually symptomatic before age 2 years

Radionuclide imaging is the best technique for detecting symptomatic Meckel's diverticula. ^{99m}Tc pertechnetate is injected intravenously and is concentrated in the mucous secretory cells of gastric mucosa. Serial images show concentration of ^{99m}Tc pertechnetate in the ectopic gastric mucosa identical to its concentration in the stomach. This occurs 5 to 20 minutes after injection. The activity is usually in the right lower quadrant. It may be located very close to the bladder or, rarely, in other areas of the abdomen. Postvoid images will help detect Meckel's diverticula located near the bladder.

The activity from a Meckel's diverticulum is usually small, is focal, and increases with time. Occasionally downstream wash of ^{99m}Tc pertechnetate will cause activity to decrease with time.

The scan is quite sensitive for detecting symptomatic Meckel's diverticula, with a sensitivity of 85% to 90% and a specificity of 95%.

False negative studies are caused by:

1. Small diverticuli
2. Absence of gastric mucosa
3. Autonecrosis of gastric mucosa
4. Rapid downstream wash of ^{99m}Tc pertechnetate
5. Activity in normal structures obscuring the abnormal focus

False positive studies are caused by:

1. Bladder or renal collecting system activity
2. GI tract activity
3. Ectopic gastric mucosa from gastrogenic cysts or intestinal duplications
4. Increased blood pool because of abscess, intussusception, or appendicitis
5. Hypervascularity from a tumor or arteriovenous malformation (AVM)

Pharmacologic interventions are used to increase the sensitivity of the scan. Glucagon promotes pooling and prevents downstream wash of ^{99m}Tc pertechnetate. Pentagastrin increases uptake of ^{99m}Tc pertechnetate by 30% to 60%. The combination of both glucagon and pentagastrin is often used. Cimetidine and similar agents block secretion (not uptake) by the gastric mucosa, increasing the target/background ratio.

Nasogastric suction during the test can be used to prevent activity from passing from the stomach into the small bowel. GI activity can appear focal and mimic Meckel's diverticulum.

CASE 102

History.—76-year-old nursing home resident with dizziness and bright red blood per rectum.

Scan.—^{99m}Tc red blood cell bleeding study.

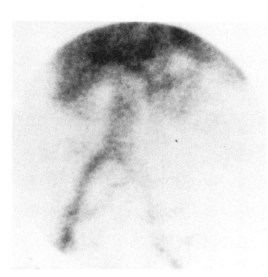

Anterior image of abdomen 5 minutes after reinjection of labeled RBCs.

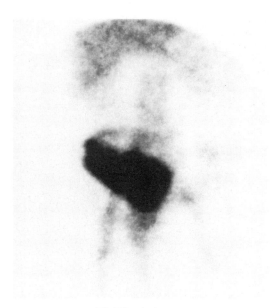

30-Minute image.

Findings.—Right lower quadrant activity intensifying over time.

Diagnosis.—Right lower quadrant GI bleed.

Gastrointestinal bleeding is usually divided into upper and lower GI bleeding, with the ligament of Treitz as the dividing point. Lower GI bleeding usually comes from the colon or rectum and is caused by diverticular disease, angiodysplasia, solitary ulcer, inflammatory bowel disease, or ischemic colitis. Other causes include benign or malignant neoplasms, coagulopathy, radiation injury, and chemotherapy toxicity.

The site of GI bleeding can be difficult to localize endoscopically. In such cases a radionuclide scan is valuable in localizing the bleeding site. This information can guide the angiographer or surgeon.

Radionuclide bleeding studies can be done using either tagged red blood cells or sulfur colloid. ^{99m}Tc sulfur colloid is injected intravenously and extravasates at the bleeding site. The remaining sulfur colloid is rapidly taken up by the liver and spleen, reducing background activity. This increases the target/background ratio. If the bleeding site is high in the abdomen, it can be obscured by colloid uptake in the liver and spleen. Delayed images will detect the bleed after the activity has moved distally by peristalsis.

At our institution, ^{99m}Tc-labeled red blood cells are the preferred technique for localizing GI bleeding. Extravasated red blood cells accumulate at the bleeding site and show up as focal hot spots. The focal area of uptake moves distally with peristalsis. If the hot spot does not move, it most likely represents activity within a vascular structure. For example, penile blood pool activity is easily misinterpreted as a low rectal bleed.

Approximately 3 mL of blood must accumulate to be detected. This fact, plus high background activity, delays detection of slow bleeds longer than with sulfur colloid.

The red blood cell tag is adequate for up to 24 hours. This allows intermittent GI bleeding to be detected without reinjecting. A possible source of confusion on red blood cell studies is free ^{99m}Tc pertechnetate. This occurs primarily with in vivo labeling rather than the in vitro techniques. Some laboratories use nasogastric suction to prevent passage of free ^{99m}Tc pertechnetate from the stomach into the bowel, reducing false positive studies.

The sensitivity of colloid and red blood cell radionuclide bleeding studies is similar in animals. Bleeding rates as low as 0.05 to 0.1 mL/minute can be detected. This is several times as sensitive as contrast angiography. However, a multiinstitutional clinical study comparing ^{99m}Tc sulfur colloid bleeding studies to red blood cell examinations found erythrocytes several times more sensitive in detecting bleeding.

CASE 103

History.— Rectal bleeding, with a hematocrit of 25%.

Scan.— ^{99m}Tc red blood cell bleeding study.

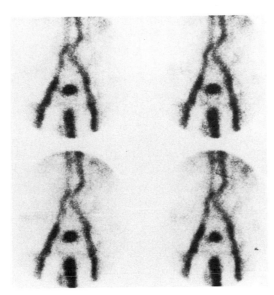

Serial anterior images of abdomen.

Findings.— Linear region of activity below bladder.

Diagnosis.— False positive low rectal bleed, penile blood pool activity.

This case illustrates one of the more common sources of error in interpreting ^{99m}Tc-labeled red blood cell or sulfur colloid gastrointestinal bleeding studies. Penile blood pool activity in the very vascular corpora cavernosa can mimic a low rectal or anorectal bleeding site.

Low rectal bleeding is more difficult to detect because there is no downstream movement of activity with time. Blood accumulates in the rectal vault and eventually is passed in a bowel movement. Attenuation of activity by the pelvic soft tissues contributes to the problem of detecting rectal bleeds.

Blood pool activity in the penis usually parallels vascular activity in adjacent blood vessels. If blood pool activity is present in the femoral vessels as well as in the low midline on early sulfur colloid images, penile blood pool is likely. If penile activity is suspected, position the penis away from midline for later images. This should clarify whether the activity is from the penis or from rectal blood. Also, any stools passed during the study should be imaged to determine if they contain radiolabeled colloid or red blood cells.

CASE 104

History.— 66-year-old woman who had bright red rectal bleeding for 2 days. Multiple colonic diverticuli were noted on a barium enema done 3 months earlier.

Scan.— After IV administration of 15 mCi of ^{99m}Tc sulfur colloid, serial angiographic and delayed images were obtained over 60 minutes.

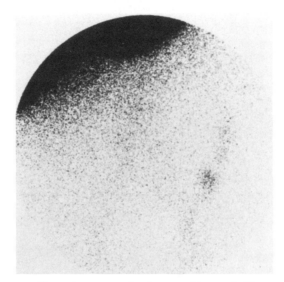

Five-minute anterior image of lower half of abdomen and pelvis.

Findings.— Angiogram not shown. Increased uptake in the left lower quadrant on delayed images.

Diagnosis.— Diverticular bleed.

^{99m}Tc sulfur colloid is less commonly used for gastrointestinal bleeding studies than ^{99m}Tc-labeled red blood cells. Sulfur colloid does have some advantages over red blood cell studies, however.

Because any sulfur colloid that is not extravasated at the bleeding site is rapidly taken up by the reticuloendothelial system, the target/background ratio is higher than with labeled red blood cells. This allows a more rapid diagnosis to be made. Sulfur colloid studies become abnormal within a few minutes of injection even with slow bleeds. ^{99m}Tc red blood cell studies, on the other hand, often do not become abnormal for 45 minutes to several hours after injection.

Because sulfur colloid images are usually taken more frequently than red blood cell studies, it can be easier to localize a bleeding site with colloid. This is especially true when delayed images on red blood cell study become abnormal 6 or 24 hours after injection. All one can say in these cases is that some time during the preceding hours the patient bled from a site more proximal than the activity's current location.

Although red blood cell studies have been advocated for imaging intermittent GI bleeds, ^{99m}Tc sulfur colloid studies can also be used. Repeat injections can be done if it appears the patient is bleeding again.

The main theoretical disadvantage of sulfur colloid is that upper GI bleeds can be difficult to detect because of liver and spleen uptake in the reticuloendothelial system. However, if imaging is continued for 1 hour or more, activity that is hidden by the liver and spleen will move distally by peristalsis and become visible in the lower portion of the abdomen. Oblique views can also be helpful in detecting activity behind the liver and spleen.

CASE 105

History.—43-year-old man with melanotic stools for 2 days.

Scan.—^{99m}Tc red blood cell bleeding study and ^{99m}Tc DMSA renal scan.

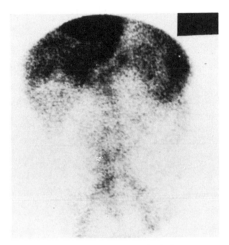

Anterior early image of abdomen.

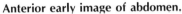

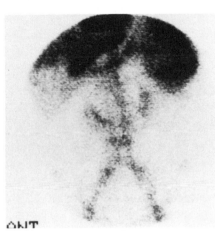

Delayed image.

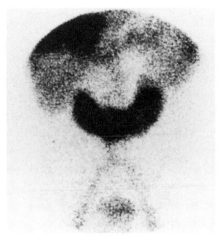

DMSA scan of anterior view of abdomen.

Findings.—Red blood cells: central focus of activity increasing with time; DMSA: U-shaped area of uptake in region of red blood cell activity.

Diagnosis.—Horseshoe kidney mimicking a GI bleed.

When one is interpreting gastrointestinal bleeding studies, it is important to be familiar with the normal structures that can mimic bleeding sites. The causes of false positives for GI bleeding using ^{99m}Tc red blood cells fall into two main groups: vascular structures and areas of concentration of free ^{99m}Tc pertechnetate.

In distinguishing between GI hemorrhage and normal structures it is important to evaluate how activity changes over time. Blood that has been extravasated within the bowel acts as an irritant, increasing peristalsis. Because of this, focal activity that moves with time is much more likely to represent GI bleeding than fixed activity.

Depending on the method of red blood cell labeling, free ^{99m}Tc pertechnetate may be present. This is secreted by the stomach and salivary glands and can be passed into the intestines, mimicking an upper GI bleed. Placing a nasogastric tube is helpful both to test for blood and to remove the free ^{99m}Tc pertechnetate.

Free ^{99m}Tc pertechnetate is also excreted by the kidneys, and collections of activity in the upper or lower portion of the abdomen may represent free ^{99m}Tc pertechnetate in the kidney, collecting system, or bladder.

Possible causes of false positives using ^{99m}Tc-labeled red blood cells are:

1. Normal or abnormal vascular structures
    a. Penile activity
    b. Kidney (normal or ectopic position)
    c. Left ovarian vein
    d. Hepatic cavernous hemangioma
    e. Varices
    f. Aneurysm
    g. Arterial graft
    h. Arteriovenous malformation
    i. Cutaneous hemangioma
2. Concentration of free ^{99m}Tc pertechnetate
    a. GI tract
    b. Gallbladder
    c. Kidney
    d. Bladder
    e. Abscess

CASE 106

History.— 27-year-old with hepatic mass found incidentally during pelvic ultrasound.

Scan.—^{99m}Tc-labeled red blood cell planar and SPECT study.

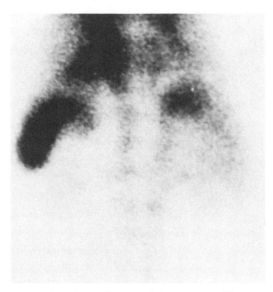

Posterior planar image of abdomen at 1 hour.

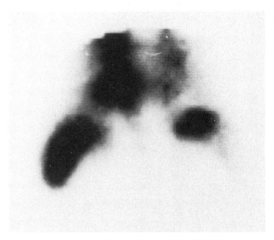

Two-hour coronal reconstructed SPECT image of abdomen.

Findings.— Planar: focal activity posterior right lobe; SPECT: same.

Diagnosis.—Cavernous hemangioma of the liver.

Cavernous hemangiomas are the most common benign tumors of the liver. The skin and mucous membranes are the other common locations for hemangiomas. Hemangiomas are much more common in females; the female/male ratio is 6:1.

Microscopically, cavernous hemangiomas consist of dilated, tortuous, closely packed veins. They are usually small, subcapsular, and solitary. Hemangiomas enlarge by dilation of existing vessels; because of this, they are considered congenital anomalies rather than true neoplasms.

Liver hemangiomas are usually asymptomatic. They are often found incidentally and are important because they can mimic a malignant process on computed tomography (CT) or ultrasound. Percutaneous biopsy can cause bleeding complications.

Occasionally a cavernous hemangioma can become massive and replace a large portion of one lobe of the liver. Large hemangiomas function as an arteriovenous shunt and result in congestive heart failure.

Surprisingly, cavernous hemangiomas are not hypervascular on hepatic angiography. They have increased blood volume but not increased perfusion. This is an important characteristic used in imaging. When a solitary lesion is found in the liver on CT or ultrasound, patients are often referred to nuclear medicine to further define the characteristics of the lesion. Blood pool imaging agents such as ^{99m}Tc-labeled red blood cells are useful in these cases. Hemangiomas show increased blood pool activity on delayed images in the face of normal or decreased early flow. A combination of planar and single-photon emission computed tomography (SPECT) images (both early, after injection of the labeled RBCs, and at 2 hours) are needed to demonstrate these characteristic findings.

Liver hemangiomas show a cold defect on ^{99m}Tc sulfur colloid liver-spleen scans. This defect will "fill in" over time if the patient is then administered ^{99m}Tc-labeled red blood cells. The CT appearance of a hemangioma depends on whether contrast has been given and with the stage of enhancement after contrast administration. Progressive enhancement from the periphery to the center is seen frequently; this appearance is characteristic of a hemangioma.

CASE 107

History.—60-year-old chronic alcoholic with LeVeen shunt for ascites, who had increasing abdominal girth.

Scan.—LeVeen shunt patency study performed by placing 5 mCi of ^{99m}Tc MAA into the peritoneum.

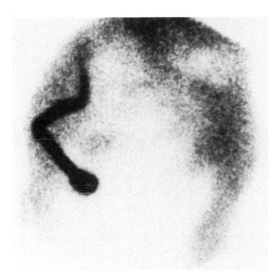

Early anterior image of abdomen.

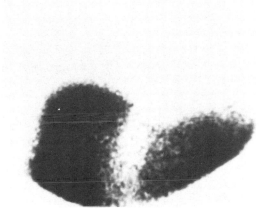

Two-hour image of upper half of abdomen and lower half of chest.

Findings.—Abdomen: activity diffusely distributed throughout abdomen; chest: no uptake.

Diagnosis.—Blocked LeVeen shunt.

The LeVeen shunt is used in patients with intractable ascites. It consists of a synthetic tube connecting the peritoneal cavity to the bracheocephalic vessels. It has a pressure-sensitive, one-way valve that allows flow of ascitic fluid into the superior vena cava. This type of shunt can be associated with significant complications, including occlusion, infection, and disseminated intravascular coagulation. If ascitic fluid reaccumulates after shunt placement, the patient is often referred to nuclear medicine for evaluation of shunt patency.

The shunt patency study is performed by placing ^{99m}Tc macroaggregated albumin (MAA) in the peritoneum via paracentesis. The patient is asked to roll side to side to uniformly distribute the material. An image over the abdomen is taken to be sure the injection is not into a loculation. Serial images are then obtained over the upper part of the abdomen and the chest. If the shunt is patent, MAA will traverse the LaVeen shunt, gaining access to the inferior vena cava. The MAA then embolizes in the lungs as in a V/Q scan. Activity in the lungs implies patency of the shunt. If activity fails to reach the lung over a sufficient imaging period, shunt blockage is likely.

To determine if the blockage is in the proximal or distal limb, MAA sometimes is directly injected into the tubing. Patency of the vena caval portion implies proximal blockage.

At one time ^{99m}Tc sulfur colloid was used as the radiopharmaceutical for shunt patency studies. It was sometimes difficult to tell if the liver and spleen visualized because of the background of activity in the ascitic fluid.

CASE 108

History.— 58-year-old woman with solitary hepatoma in right lobe. A chemotherapy catheter was placed. This study is performed to confirm correct catheter placement.

Scan.— 3 mCi of ^{99m}Tc MAA was injected in the infusion port and multiple images obtained.

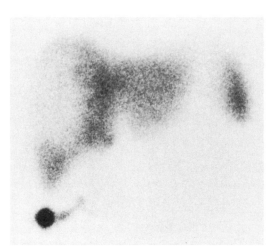

^{99m}Tc sulfur colloid liver-spleen scan, anterior image.

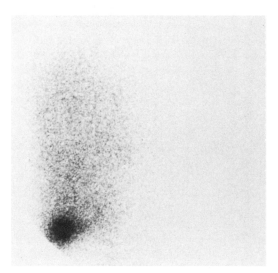

Anterior image of abdomen after MAA injection through hepatic artery catheter.

Findings.— Sulfur colloid: cold defect right lobe; MAA: activity in distribution of mass.

Diagnosis.— Correct catheter placement.

Selective intra-arterial chemotherapy can be beneficial in patients with hepatic primary or metastatic malignancies. The technique allows high concentration chemotherapy to be delivered directly to the tumor. The tip of the catheter is placed into a vessel perfusing the portion of the liver containing the tumor, avoiding as much normal liver as possible. One method of confirming the catheter's position is a radionuclide catheter placement study.

^{99m}Tc-labeled macroaggregated albumin particles (MAA) are injected in the infusion catheter port under conditions identical to chemotherapy infusion. These embolize the capillary bed of the perfused portion of the liver on the first pass. The distribution of these particles closely resembles the distribution of the chemotherapeutic agent.

The distribution of MAA particles is compared with that of ^{99m}Tc sulfur colloid. The liver tumor will appear as an area of decreased uptake on sulfur colloid scan because there are no reticuloendothelial cells in liver malignancies. It is important that no GI uptake be seen. Perfusion of the GI tract can cause necrosis.

The radionuclide method has significant advantages over x-ray contrast studies. Small volumes are injected under conditions identical to those used for chemotherapy infusion. This more closely demonstrates the true distribution of treatment. Contrast studies require a larger volume and must be injected at a higher rate, which can distort the distribution of flow.

An additional benefit of this study is the ability to qualitatively identify arteriovenous fistulas in the tumor. Following injection of MAA, images over the lungs will show any MAA that may have passed through the liver without passing through a capillary bed (arteriovenous shunt). This has implications regarding systemic toxicity of the chemotherapy agent.

CASE 109

History.— 57-year-old man with a 25-year history of insulin-dependent diabetes mellitus who complains of frequent nausea and vomiting after eating.

Scan.—A 300 g meal, labeled with 100 μCi of ^{111}In DTPA (liquid phase), and 600 μCi of ^{99m}Tc sulfur colloid (solid phase) was ingested. Serial images were then obtained over the stomach and recorded on computer.

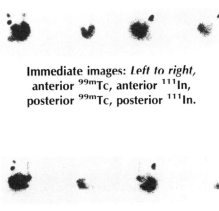

Immediate images: *Left to right, anterior ^{99m}Tc, anterior ^{111}In, posterior ^{99m}Tc, posterior ^{111}In.*

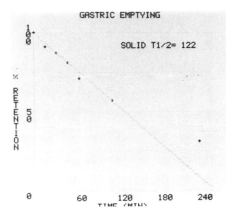

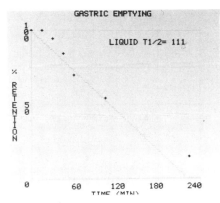

225-minute images: *Left to right, anterior ^{99m}Tc, anterior ^{111}In, posterior ^{99m}Tc, posterior ^{111}In.*

Time-activity curve for liquid emptying.

Time-activity curve for solid emptying.

Findings.— This study shows prolonged liquid and solid gastric emptying. The normal t½ for solid gastric emptying is 45 to 109 minutes. Normal liquid t½ ranges from 12 to 64 minutes.

Diagnosis.—Diabetic gastroparesis

Decreased gastric motility may occur in patients with diabetes mellitus. This autonomic neuropathy is part of a more generalized polyneuropathy that affects several organ systems. Diabetic gastroparesis results from damage to the vagus nerve. Other factors such as hyperglycemia may also play a role. It occurs in about 20% to 30% of diabetic patients. In the majority, symptoms are mild. Symptoms include early satiety, bloating, nausea, postprandial fullness, and epigastric pain. As the disease progresses, recurrent vomiting may mimic gastric outlet obstruction.

Diagnosis of diabetic gastroparesis is difficult using conventional fluoroscopic studies. Upper GI x-ray studies can detect anatomic abnormalities but are insensitive for physiologic abnormalities such as impaired gastric motility. A dilated stomach with retention of food is an indirect sign of gastroparesis sometimes present on upper GI radiographs.

The radionuclide gastric emptying study is an ideal way to confirm gastroparesis in a symptomatic patient. After an overnight fast, a meal tagged with a radioactive tracer is ingested. In our department, the solid portion of the meal is labeled with 600 μCi of ^{99m}Tc sulfur colloid and the liquid is labeled with 100 μCi of ^{111}In diethylenetriaminepentaacetic acid (DTPA). With the patient in the upright position, serial images over the stomach are then obtained in the anterior and posterior views using separate photopeaks for ^{111}In and ^{99m}Tc.

The findings of delayed liquid and solid gastric emptying suggest the diagnosis of gastroparesis. A high-grade gastric outlet obstruction can show similar values; however, mechanical obstruction usually shows more normal liquid emptying. Other causes of delayed gastric emptying include drugs, surgery, scleroderma, chronic ideopathic intestinal pseudo-obstruction, amyloidosis, and anorexia nervosa.

CASE 110

History.—42-year-old woman with nausea and vomiting and a history of peptic ulcer disease.

Scan.—Gastric emptying scan using 100 μCi of ^{111}In orange juice (liquid phase) and 600 μCi of ^{99m}Tc liver pate (solid phase).

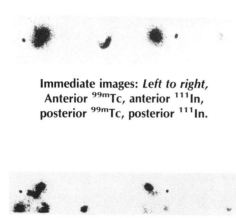

Immediate images: *Left to right,* Anterior ^{99m}Tc, anterior ^{111}In, posterior ^{99m}Tc, posterior ^{111}In.

Images 150 minutes after ingestion: *Left to right,* anterior ^{99m}Tc, anterior ^{111}In, posterior ^{99m}Tc, posterior ^{111}In.

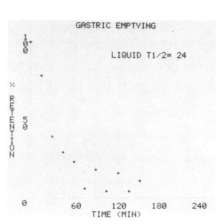

Time-activity curve of stomach for liquids (^{111}In).

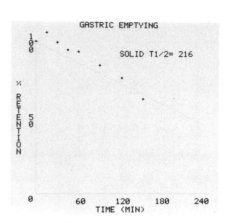

Time-activity curve of stomach for solids (^{99m}Tc).

Findings.—Delayed solid (normal, 45–109 minutes) and normal liquid emptying (normal, 12–64 minutes).

Diagnosis.—Mechanical gastric outlet obstruction.

There is a wide range of normal gastric emptying rates. The rate at which the stomach empties depends on meal volume, weight, caloric content, whether solids or liquids are ingested, and the patient's age and sex. Even the time of day the study is performed (circadian rhythm) and the patient's psychologic state are important.

A variety of disease states affect gastric emptying. Symptomatic gastric emptying abnormalities are often seen in diabetes, peptic ulcer disease, after surgery, and in a variety of less common disorders such as scleroderma, amyloidosis, anorexia nervosa, and chronic idiopathic intestinal pseudo-obstruction. Some of these will respond to drugs such as metoclopramide or erythromycin.

Nuclear medicine offers the ability to simultaneously measure liquid and solid gastric emptying by having the fasting patient ingest a meal of orange juice tagged with ^{111}In DTPA (liquid phase) and ^{99m}Tc sulfur colloid–labeled liver pate (solid phase) in a standardized 300 g beef stew meal. Serial anterior and posterior images are then obtained using the 140 keV photopeak of ^{99m}Tc and the 247 keV photopeak of the ^{111}In. The information obtained must be corrected for "crosstalk" or downscatter of counts from the ^{111}In peak into the ^{99m}Tc window. A correction for decay is important in patients with delayed emptying. A time-activity curve over the stomach is then constructed from which the time to half-emptying (t½) for both solids and liquids can be obtained.

Liquids normally empty with a biphasic curve. The initial portion of the curve usually has a steeper slope, with the later portion of the curve approximating solid emptying. The liquid t½ should be obtained from the initial slope of the curve. Solid gastric emptying is more linear.

In our department, the normal liquid emptying t½ is 12 to 64 minutes. Normal solid gastric emptying t½ ranges from 45 to 109 minutes. Patients with prolonged liquid and solid emptying usually have gastroparesis. Gastric outlet obstruction will be manifested by prolonged solid gastric emptying; however, liquid emptying may be normal. Dumping syndrome will show very rapid liquid and solid emptying.

CASE 111

History.—47-year-old woman with a history of peptic ulcer disease who underwent a vagotomy and pyloroplasty 8 months earlier. She had symptoms of weakness, abdominal pain, sweating, and dizziness 30 minutes after eating.

Scan.—A 300 g meal labeled with 600 μCi of ^{99m}Tc sulfur colloid (solid phase) and 100 μCi of ^{111}In DTPA (liquid phase) was ingested. Serial images were then obtained over the stomach.

Immediate images: *Left to right,* anterior ^{99m}Tc, anterior ^{111}In, posterior ^{99m}Tc, posterior ^{111}In.

Images 30 minutes after ingestion: *Left to right,* anterior ^{99m}Tc, anterior ^{111}In, posterior ^{99m}Tc, posterior ^{111}In.

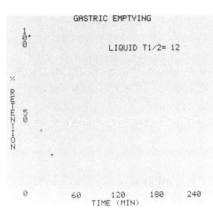

Liquid emptying curve.

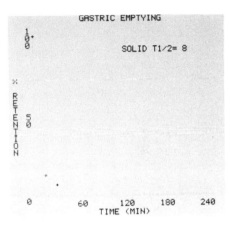

Time-activity curve for solid emptying.

Findings.—The study demonstrates rapid solid and liquid gastric emptying.

Diagnosis.—Dumping syndrome.

In patients who have undergone peptic ulcer surgery, the normal control mechanisms for gastric emptying are altered. This can result in the dumping syndrome. Symptoms consist of postprandial palpitations, tachycardia, sweating, weakness, flushing, nausea, abdominal discomfort, vomiting, postural hypotension, and occasional syncope. The onset of symptoms is usually within 30 minutes after eating and is thought to be caused by rapid emptying of hyperosmolar gastric contents into the small bowel. Fluid shifts into the bowel result in small bowel distention and intravascular hypovolemia. Another proposed mechanism is an autonomic reflex that follows small bowel distention. This syndrome has been reproduced in normal individuals by infusing hypertonic solutions into the proximal small bowel and by distention of the jejunum.

The usual treatment consists of avoiding simple sugars and carbohydrates, with more caloric intake in the form of fats and protein, and alterations in meal size. Occasionally a second surgical procedure is required.

Another syndrome also referred to as dumping syndrome, or delayed dumping syndrome, is actually thought to be reactive hypoglycemia and occurs 2 to 4 hours after eating. The pancreas overshoots in its release of insulin, causing temporary hypoglycemia and its associated symptoms.

Gastric emptying studies document rapid gastric emptying in dumping syndrome patients. Both liquid and solid gastric emptying values are accelerated.

CASE 112

History.—50-year-old man with heartburn.

Scan.—The patient fasted for 6 hours before the study. He ingested 300 μCi of ^{99m}Tc sulfur colloid in 300 mL of acidified orange juice (150 mL of orange juice and 150 mL of 0.1N HCl) was ingested. An initial image was obtained at 10 to 15 minutes in the upright position to assure passage of material into the stomach. Serial images of the stomach and esophagus with the patient supine were then obtained. After the initial image, an abdominal binder was used to increase intra-abdominal pressure in 5 mm Hg steps to 100 mm Hg. Images were recorded on the computer.

Findings.—Study showed increased esophageal counts beginning at 5 mm Hg, greater than 3%.

Diagnosis.—Gastroesophageal reflux.

Heartburn is a common complaint in patients with symptomatic gastroesophageal reflux (GER). Such patients receive significant relief with conventional measures, including H$_2$ antagonists. Occasionally GER has very confusing presenting symptoms such as chronic pulmonary disease or chest pain, mimicking cardiac disease. In such cases, additional diagnostic studies are needed.

Radionuclides provide an attractive way to evaluate patients with suspected GER. The procedure involves ingestion of 300 μCi of ^{99m}Tc sulfur colloid in 300 mL of acidified orange juice. An upright image at 10 to 15 minutes is obtained to assure that all activity is in the stomach. After this, an abdominal binder is used to increase the pressure on the lower esophageal sphincter.

GER is then calculated by using the formula:

$$R = \frac{(Et - Eb)}{Go} \times 100$$

where R = percent GER, Et = esophageal counts at time t, Eb = esophageal background counts, and Go = gastric counts at the beginning of the study. GER is considered significant if R is greater than 3%.

This procedure is very sensitive (90%) for detecting GER. Sensitivity is similar to the acid reflux test but does not require intubation of the esophagus. It is much more sensitive than fluoroscopic studies, endoscopy, or lower esophageal sphincter manometry. Barium swallow studies are best used to evaluate for anatomic lesions and complications of reflux, such as stricture.

Because most patients who reflux and aspirate do so at night while sleeping, an overnight test can be done. Delayed images over the chest the next morning are performed. Any activity in the chest is considered abnormal.

CASE 113

History.—50-year-old man with dysphagia.

Scan.—15 mL of water labeled with 300 μCi of ^{99m}Tc sulfur colloid swallowed in a single bolus, followed by dry swallows every 15 seconds.

Findings.—At 15 seconds, 30% transit.

Diagnosis.—Achalasia.

Achalasia is a disorder of esophageal motility manifested by absence of primary peristalsis and dysfunction of the distal esophageal sphincter. In these patients, the esophagus dilates and hypertrophies without organic stenosis. The underlying defect is absence or destruction of the ganglion cells of Auerbach's myenteric plexus; this causes failure of lower esophageal sphincter relaxation during swallowing. The etiology of the disorder is unknown.

Males are affected more often than females. It may occur at any age, but the incidence is highest between the ages of 30 and 60 years. There is a slightly increased incidence of esophageal carcinoma in patients with achalasia.

The evaluation of esophageal motility should include a barium swallow for anatomic resolution; however, if quantitative information is needed, such as following a patient's response to therapy, radionuclide esophageal transit studies can be performed. One significant advantage of the radionuclide study is its low radiation dose to the patient compared with radiographic studies.

Radionuclide esophageal transit studies are performed by measuring the transit of an orally administered liquid labeled with ^{99m}Tc sulfur colloid through the esophagus. The patient should fast for 6 hours before the study. Fifteen milliliters of water labeled with 300 μCi of ^{99m}Tc sulfur colloid is swallowed in a single swallow from the supine position. The patient then dry-swallows every 15 seconds for 5 to 10 minutes. Serial 1-second images of the anterior chest, which include the esophagus and proximal side of the stomach, are obtained for the first 15 seconds and then at 15-second intervals for the next 10 minutes. These are recorded on the computer.

Esophageal transit is then calculated using the formula:

$$E(t) = \frac{E(max) - E(c)}{E(max)} \times 100$$

where $E(t)$ = percent of esophageal transit at time t, $E(max)$ = maximum counts in esophagus, and $E(c)$ = esophageal counts at time t.

Normal patients pass 90% of the activity through the esophagus by 15 seconds or eight swallows; patients with achalasia will show transit of only 20% to 40% in the same time. Patients with scleroderma have similar levels. Patients with diffuse esophageal spasm have markedly decreased transit in the first half of the study, but most will have normal values after about 20 swallows.

CHAPTER 5

Genitourinary

CASE 114

History.— Kidney transplant donor evaluation.

Scan.— ^{99m}Tc DTPA and ^{131}I hippuran renal scan.

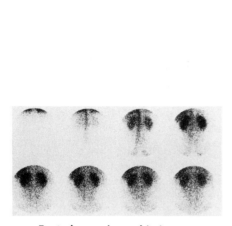

Posterior angiographic images.

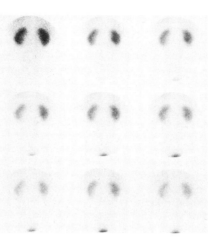

Serial delayed ^{99m}Tc DTPA images.

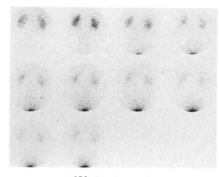

Serial ^{131}I hippuran images.

Findings.— Prompt symmetric flow and excretion are present.

Diagnosis.— Normal renal scan.

The radionuclide renal scan is primarily a physiologic rather than anatomic imaging study. After intravenous administration of a radiopharmaceutical, the appearance time, concentration and excretion of the tracer into the collecting system can be followed to evaluate renal blood flow and function. The specific information obtained depends on the radiopharmaceutical injected.

Glomerular filtration is normally evaluated using technetium 99m diethylenetriaminepentaacetic acid (DTPA). After IV injection, ^{99m}Tc DTPA rapidly distributes in the extracellular space. ^{99m}Tc DTPA is completely filtered by the kidney (except for 3%–5%, which is protein bound) and is not resorbed or secreted by the tubules. After bolus injection, serial images at 2-second intervals for 30 seconds are done to evaluate renal perfusion. Delayed images at 2-minute intervals show relative function early; later images demonstrate the patency of the collecting system. By 20 to 30 minutes, most activity has washed out of the kidney. A time-activity curve of each kidney shows a peak at 3 to 5 minutes, followed by a downsloping curve.

Tubular function can be evaluated using hippuran (o-iodohippurate) labeled with iodine 131 or iodine 123. This agent is chemically similar to p-aminohippuric acid (PAH), which is the gold standard for measuring renal plasma flow. The ^{131}I hippuran should have less than 1.5% unbound ^{131}I to minimize thyroidal radiation. Saturated solution of potassium iodide (SSKI) can be administered before ^{131}I hippuran is used to block uptake by the thyroid gland.

Hippuran is extracted from blood primarily by tubular secretion (80%); only 20% is removed by glomerular filtration. Its clearance is dependent on renal blood flow and the renal extraction efficiency for hippuran. Ninety-six percent of hippuran in renal arterial blood is extracted as it passes through the kidney, making this agent ideal for calculation of effective renal plasma flow. After IV injection, hippuran equilibrates in the extracellular space over 4 to 5 minutes. Seventy percent of the injected dose is excreted in urine by 30 minutes. The maximum concentration in the kidneys is reached about 3 minutes after injection, with subsequent washout of activity over the next 30 minutes.

^{99m}Tc mertiatide (MAG-3) has recently been made available for renal imaging. It is rapidly excreted by the kidneys via active tubular secretion and glomerular filtration. It can provide split-function excretion curves similar to hippuran with superior image quality and much lower radiation dose. Renal angiograms are also possible.

An agent used for static cortical imaging is ^{99m}Tc dimercaptosuccinic acid (DMSA). ^{99m}Tc DMSA is highly bound to plasma proteins, which prevents significant glomerular filtration. It is taken up into the renal cortex in the proximal convoluted tubule; the cortex/medullary ratio is 22:1. Fifty percent of the injected dose is localized in the kidney at 1 hour. It is cleared slowly, with 30% excreted in the urine by 14 hours. ^{99m}Tc DMSA is the agent of choice when high-resolution images of the renal cortex are needed. The main disadvantages of ^{99m}Tc DMSA are the high radiation dose it delivers to the kidneys and its short 30-minute shelf-life after preparation.

CASE 115

History.— 41-year-old man with edema, proteinuria, hypertension, and elevated creatinine levels.

Scan.—^{99m}Tc DTPA and ^{131}I hippuran renal scans.

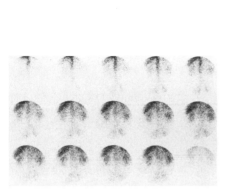

^{99m}Tc DTPA flow study.

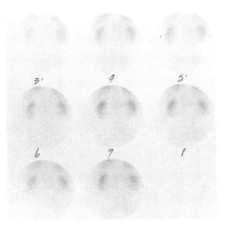

^{99m}Tc DTPA function scan.

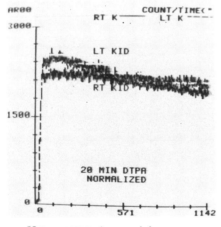

^{99m}Tc DTPA time-activity curve.

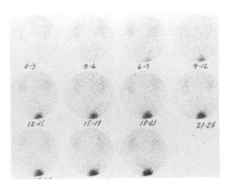

^{131}I hippuran function scan.

Findings.—^{99m}Tc DTPA: diminished flow bilaterally and decreased uptake and excretion; hippuran: decreased uptake and excretion.

Diagnosis.—Chronic renal failure.

Chronic renal failure is the end result of a host of insults to the kidney. Frequent causes of renal failure are chronic obstruction, recurrent infection, vesicoureteral reflux, glomerulonephritis, hypertension, and diabetes. Renal scan cannot determine the cause of renal failure in most patients. Chronic renal failure patients usually have diminished flow and tubular function on renal scan regardless of cause.

Because the radionuclide renal scan avoids the use of iodinated contrast, it is often used in preference to an intravenous pyelogram or contrast-enhanced computed tomography to evaluate chronic renal failure. Ultrasound can delineate the anatomy of the kidneys, but lacks physiologic information.

Glomerularly filtered agents such as ^{99m}Tc DTPA are poorly concentrated in the kidneys of patients with renal failure. Agents excreted by the renal tubules (e.g., ^{131}I hippuran, are more useful. With ^{131}I hippuran, visualization of the kidneys is possible with as little as 3% of normal renal function.

Blood urea nitrogen (BUN) levels ranging from 62 to 146 mg/dL and creatinine levels of 3.5 to 17.2 mg/dL have been successfully imaged with ^{131}I hippuran. ^{99m}Tc DMSA that binds to the renal tubules frequently yields images superior to ^{131}I hippuran in uremic patients.

When noncortical agents are used in severe renal failure patients, the kidneys are more likely to be seen after dialysis. It is thought that during dialysis organic anions that compete with the radiopharmaceutical for renal excretion are removed.

Some added information regarding the etiology of renal failure can sometimes be obtained by calculating the filtration fraction. When the filtration fraction (glomerular filtration rate/effective renal plasma flow) is elevated, the tubular function is usually more severely affected than the glomerular filtration (e.g., in acute tubular necrosis). Prerenal states cause a decreased filtration fraction.

CASE 116

History.—62-year-old man with abnormal urinalysis.

Scan.—^{99m}Tc DTPA renal scan.

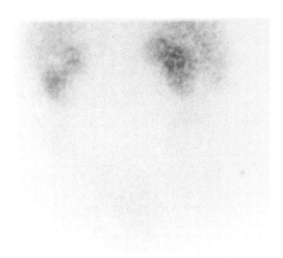

Posterior 2-minute ^{99m}Tc DTPA image.

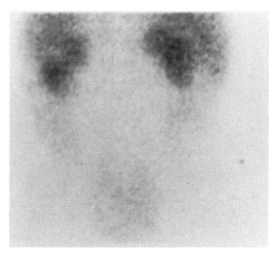

Posterior 6-minute ^{99m}Tc DTPA image.

Findings.—Cold defect in the superior left kidney.

Diagnosis.—Left renal mass.

The role of the renal scan in the evaluation of a renal mass is somewhat limited because of the low-resolution images obtained and the availability of ultrasound, computed tomography, and angiography. However, the renal scan is a useful screening tool for renal abnormalities.

The most common renal neoplasm in adults is hypernephroma, or renal cell carcinoma. This tumor constitutes 85% of all renal malignancies. The highest incidence is in the sixth decade; it almost never occurs in patients less than 20 years of age. Two thirds of patients with von Hippel–Lindau disease will eventually develop renal cell carcinoma.

Hypernephroma often manifests as painless hematuria or with symptoms of metastatic disease to bone, lung, and liver.

On renal scan, increased flow to the tumor is seen in the angiographic phase, with an area of decreased activity present on delayed images. Because benign masses cannot be differentiated from malignant ones on delayed renal scan, all renal abnormalities should be further evaluated.

The most common renal neoplasm in children and the sec-

ond most common malignant tumor of the kidney overall is Wilms' tumor, or nephroblastoma. This tumor often reaches a large size and may be bilateral, manifesting as a palpable mass in one half of cases. The findings of Wilms' tumor on renal scan are similar to those of hypernephroma.

Pseudotumors of the kidney can appear as renal masses on radiologic studies but differ from true tumors in that they are composed of normal renal tissue. They are capable of accumulating and excreting radiopharmaceuticals, whereas true renal tumors are not. There are three main causes of pseudotumors. First is a dromedary hump, a humplike mass of the lateral margin of the left kidney composed of normal renal cortex. The two other pseudotumors are hypertrophied columns of Bertin and focal compensatory hypertrophy.

In evaluation for possible pseudotumor, a DMSA scan can be done to prove the mass is composed of functional renal cortex. Multiple planar views or single-proton emission computed tomography (SPECT) imaging is necessary.

CASE 117

History.— 46-year-old woman with renal insufficiency.

Scan.— A flow study and renal scan using ^{99m}Tc DTPA were performed.

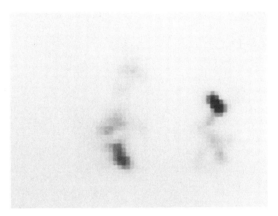

Posterior view of abdomen.

Findings.— Multiple cold defects in bilaterally enlarged and poorly functioning kidneys.

Diagnosis.— Polycystic renal disease.

Polycystic renal disease is characterized by multiple cysts in the kidneys. It occurs in two age groups. An adult form, inherited as an autosomal dominant trait, usually becomes symptomatic in the third or fourth decades. Signs and symptoms include flank pain, hematuria, renal colic (from kidney stones), hypertension, and chronic renal failure, with less fluid overload and anemia than occurs in other causes of renal failure. Renal failure is accelerated by obstruction from stones, clots, or cysts, and frequent infections.

Liver cysts are found in about 30% of patients. Of those with hepatic cysts, however, only 50% will have cystic disease of the kidneys. Hepatic insufficiency is rarely a problem with adult polycystic disease. Cysts are also found occasionally in the thyroid, spleen, pancreas, lungs, ovaries, and testicles. Intracranial aneurysm with hemorrhage is common in polycystic disease, accounting for 9% of deaths.

The infantile and childhood forms of the disease are inherited as an autosomal recessive trait. The infantile form manifests at birth with enlarged kidneys, oliguric renal failure, and hypertension. The childhood form has milder renal abnormalities but is associated with hepatic fibrosis, which frequently is fatal.

The renal scan in polycystic disease shows enlarged kidneys, with multiple cold defects in the renal cortex on the angiographic and delayed images. DMSA is probably the best agent for determining the amount of functional renal tissue and the location of the cysts. If a cyst becomes infected, a leukocyte scan will show focal uptake corresponding to a photopenic defect on DMSA scan.

Hepatic cystic disease can be diagnosed using ^{99m}Tc sulfur colloid scans, ultrasound, or CT. Hepatic cysts appear as photopenic defects on liver-spleen scan. When patients with polycystic disease are evaluated, it is best to avoid agents that cause renal toxicity.

CASE 118

History.— 60-year-old man with chronic atrial fibrillation, now with the acute onset of left flank pain.

Scan.— ^{99m}Tc DMSA SPECT renal scan.

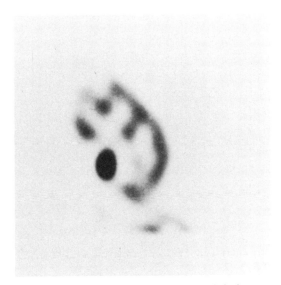

Coronal SPECT reconstruction of left kidney.

Findings.— The scan shows a wedge-shaped defect involving the superior pole.

Diagnosis.— Renal infarct.

Renal infarction is a common problem in patients prone to emboli because of the large percentage of the cardiac output (20%) that these very vascular organs receive. The most common source of emboli is the heart as a result of atrial fibrillation, rheumatic fever, bacterial endocarditis, valvular heart disease, and myocardial infarction. Atherosclerotic disease of the aorta is another common source of emboli. Thrombosis of a renal artery accounts for only 4% of renal infarcts.

The symptoms of renal infarction depend on the amount of renal cortex involved. The more proximal the vessel occluded by the embolism, the larger the infarct and the more severe the symptoms. A large renal infarct often causes the acute onset of constant flank pain. Hematuria is present in about 50% of patients. Fever, elevated white blood cell count, and variable degrees of oliguria or renal insufficiency may also be present. Renal infarction is bilateral in about 50% of cases. Even with infarction of an entire kidney, the patient may be left with normal renal function if the contralateral kidney is unaffected and is able to hypertrophy.

The cortical imaging agent ^{99m}Tc DMSA is the best radiopharmaceutical to evaluate suspected renal infarction. This agent binds to the proximal convoluted tubule of the renal cortex, with about 50% of the dose localized to the kidney by 1 hour. In renal infarcts, planar and single-photon emission computed tomography (SPECT) images will show wedge-shaped cortical defects. Flow and serial delayed images obtained with ^{99m}Tc DTPA or ^{99m}Tc MAG-3 will also demonstrate an area of absent flow and function in renal infarction. In children, ^{99m}Tc glucoheptonate is frequently used. It has a lower renal radiation dose than DMSA.

CASE 119

History.— 45-year-old patient with recurrent pyelonephritis, who is allergic to IV contrast material.

Scan.—^{99m}Tc DMSA renal scan.

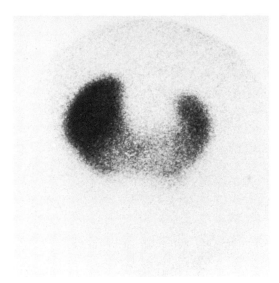

Anterior ^{99m}Tc DMSA image of abdomen.

Findings.—U-shaped uptake in midabdomen.

Diagnosis.— Horseshoe kidney.

Horseshoe kidney is the result of fusion of the kidney's lower poles. It occurs in 0.01% to 0.25% of the population. The anomaly can vary from a single band of nonfunctional fibrous tissue connecting the lower poles to a true horseshoe appearance, with the bridge consisting of renal parenchyma. The fusion occurs during the second month of gestation before the ascent of the kidneys from the pelvis. The fused kidney then ascends and is usually located anterior to the aorta. Because the ureter courses anteriorly over the connecting bar, urine flow can become partially obstructed.

Horseshoe kidney should be suspected whenever the normal axis of the kidneys becomes vertical or reversed (lower poles more medial than the upper poles). The diagnosis is important because of the increased incidence of urinary obstruction, stone formation, vesicoureteral reflux, infection, and trauma.

Other congenital ectopic anomalies of the kidneys include crossed renal ectopia, pancake kidney, pelvic kidney, and unilateral genesis.

In crossed renal ectopia, one kidney is located across midline with its upper pole fused to the lower pole of the more normally positioned kidney. This occurs in 0.1% to 0.05% of the population and is often considered a variant of horseshoe kidney.

A pancake or disk kidney results from complete fusion of the kidneys in the pelvis. They can assume a variety of configurations. The fused renal mass is usually found to have two ureters, each entering the bladder in the normal position.

The pelvic kidney, also referred to as congenital ectopia of the kidney, is caused by failure of ascent of a normally formed kidney. The ureter length is shorter than that of a normal kidney, and the kidney size is usually smaller. A pelvic kidney can sometimes be mistaken for a pelvic tumor.

Unilateral agenesis is the congenital absence of one kidney. This uncommon anomaly results from failure of the primitive embryologic precursor of the kidney to develop.

The renal scan can be useful in delineating renal anatomy and position. If an ectopic kidney is suspected, it is important to obtain anterior views of the abdomen and pelvis during the renal scan. The bladder may mimic or obscure a pelvic kidney, so postvoid images should also be done. Complications of anomalous locations of the kidney, such as obstruction to urine outflow, can be evaluated with a diuretic renal scan.

CASE 120

History.—54-year-old man 3 days after cadaveric renal transplantation, with ascites and an elevated creatinine level.

Scan.—^{99m}Tc bone scan.

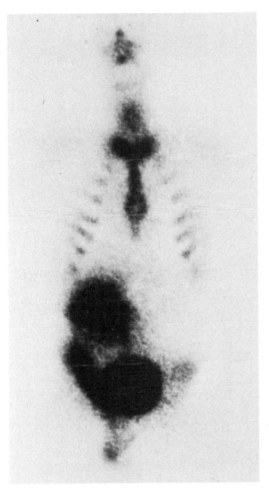

Anterior bone scan.

Findings.—This scan shows activity in kidney, bladder, and along right pelvic wall.

Diagnosis.—Urinoma.

The transplanted kidney is normally placed in the iliac fossa. The transplant's renal artery is connected to the native internal iliac or hypogastric artery, and the renal vein is grafted into the native iliac vein. A ureteroneocystostomy is performed using an oblique submucosal tunnel through the bladder wall.

A postoperative complication occurring in less than 5% of renal transplant patients is a urine leak. Leaks may be free into the abdomen, producing urine ascites, or they may be walled off, producing a urinoma. The most common site of leakage is at the anastomosis of the ureter to the bladder. Ureteral necrosis because of an inadequate blood supply or rejection is the usual cause. Technical error at the time of donor nephrectomy or transplantation can also result in urine

leaks. With rejection, the urine leak is more delayed than with other causes. Whatever the etiology, it is a serious problem usually requiring reoperation. A feared complication of a urine leak is graft infection, which may result in loss of the graft.

The most typical finding of urinoma on a radionuclide renal scan is a photopenic area on early images, which fills in on delayed images. It may take 2- or 4-hour delayed images to appreciate fill-in, so if a urine leak is suspected, delayed images are important. It is helpful to obtain postvoid images as well, to differentiate bladder activity from urinoma. Decubitus views can be helpful in evaluating patients for urine ascites.

CASE 121

History.— 14-year-old youth injured in a bicycle accident, who complains of left flank pain.

Scan.—^{99m}Tc DTPA furosemide (Lasix) renal scan.

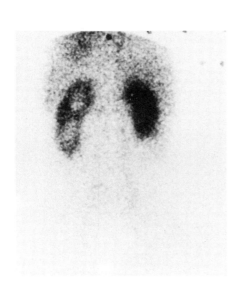

Early posterior images of abdomen before furosemide administration.

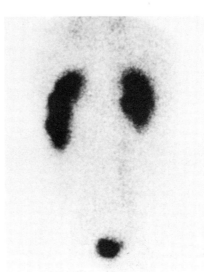

Images after furosemide administration.

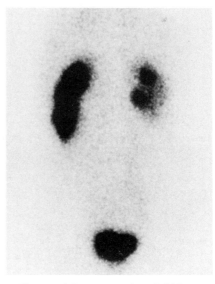

Time-activity curve of each kidney.

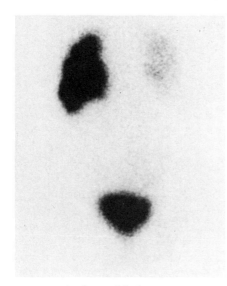

Angiographic images.

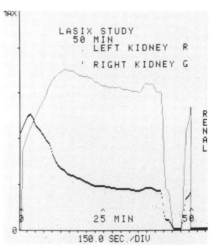

Static ^{99m}Tc DTPA images.

Findings.—Accumulation of activity in dilated left renal pelvis. Washout of activity from right kidney.

Diagnosis.—Ureteropelvic junction obstruction of the left kidney.

After surgery to relieve obstruction, the collecting system of a kidney can remain chronically dilated. If such a patient should develop a urinary tract infection, the clinician is left with a question of recurrent obstruction. Progressive accumulation of activity in a kidney or its collecting system during a renal scan can be confusing because it can be seen in both obstructed and dilated but nonobstructed systems.

The classic technique to evaluate for renal obstruction is the Whitaker test. This is an invasive examination requiring percutaneous cannulation of the renal pelvis and the infusion of saline solution. In obstruction, the increase in renal pelvic pressure is greater than in normal systems.

If a diuretic is administered during a radionuclide renal scan, an obstruction can usually be differentiated from a dilated but nonobstructed collecting system. Intravenous furosemide (Lasix) is administered about 20 minutes after DTPA or MAG-3 injection. Following this, serial images are continued at 2-minute intervals for another 30 minutes. Time-activity curves over the kidneys and ureters are then generated.

The dose of furosemide administered is as high as possible without harming the patient. For pediatric patients, this is 0.3 to 1 mg/kg. For adults, we generally use 20 to 40 mg. If the patient has renal insufficiency, it is best to consult the patient's physician to arrive at a dose large enough to assure adequate diuresis.

The scan of a patient with a dilated but nonobstructed system will show washout of activity from the area of suspected obstruction after furosemide administration. The kidney time-activity curve will show a short segment of continued upslope, representing increased urine flow in response to the diuretic, followed by a downsloping curve. Normal and nonobstructed systems drain with a half-time of 10 minutes or less.

With a high-grade obstruction of urinary flow, the scan will show progressive accumulation of activity, with a continued upslope or flattening of the kidney's time-activity curve over the kidney. Obstructed systems drain with a half-time of 20 minutes or more.

A potential problem arises if there is little change or a gradual decrease in activity after furosemide administration. This pattern can be seen in patients with impaired renal function who respond poorly to furosemide or in partial obstruction.

CASE 122

History.—60-year-old man with hypertension poorly responsive to medical management.

Scan.—^{99m}Tc DTPA and ^{131}I hippuran renal scans were performed as baseline. Repeat studies were done 1 hour after oral administration of 50 mg of captopril.

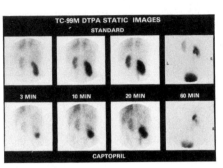

^{99m}Tc DTPA images.

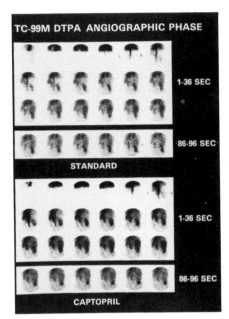

^{99m}Tc DTPA flow studies.

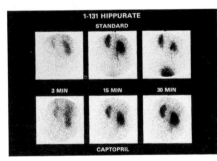

^{131}I hippuran images.

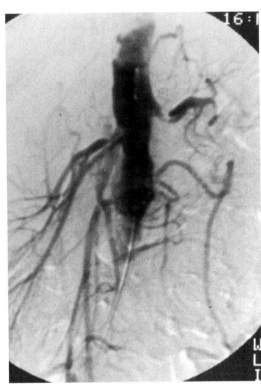

Anterior aortogram.

Findings.—Renal scan: poor flow to left kidney. Delayed washout of activity after captopril, right greater than left. Aortogram: bilateral renal artery stenosis.

Diagnosis.—Bilateral renovascular hypertension.

Renal scans before and after administration of captopril are used as a screening examination in patients with suspected renovascular hypertension. The majority of patients with hypertension have essential hypertension. Renovascular hypertension accounts for only about 1% to 2% of hypertensive patients. For this reason, only patients with risk factors for renovascular hypertension should be studied. These include younger patients and those with a history of vascular disease, severe hypertension, or hypertension that is difficult to control.

In renovascular hypertension, glomerular filtration pressure is maintained in the affected kidney by vasoconstriction of the efferent arteriole mediated by the renin-angiotensin-aldosterone system. Captopril is a specific competitive inhibitor of angiotensin I converting enzyme and blocks efferent arteriolar vasoconstriction. The result is a decrease in glomerular filtration in the affected kidney.

DTPA is removed from the blood by glomerular filtration. With unilateral renal artery stenosis there is no significant change in the normal kidney after captopril administration. However, a noticeable drop in glomerular function occurs in the affected kidney. This is manifested on the renal scan by decreased uptake and prolonged excretion of the radiopharmaceutical compared with the normal side. A baseline study for comparison is useful in differentiating renovascular stenosis from other nonreversible causes of diminished function.

^{131}I hippuran scans are also useful in renovascular hypertension even though hippuran is cleared by tubular secretion. After captopril administration there is progressive accumulation of hippuran in the affected kidney; hippuran is extracted from the blood and enters the urinary space, but there is little or no urine flow to wash it out because of the decreased glomerular filtration rate (GFR).

In addition to the visual signs of renovascular hypertension, measurement of GFR before and after captopril administration can be useful to detect bilateral renovascular hypertension. This is done by a one- or two-serum sample technique; two-sample techniques are more accurate. In our experience, a 20% or greater drop in GFR is significant.

The sensitivity and specificity of precaptopril and postcaptopril scans for detecting renovascular hypertension is about 85% and 95%, respectively. This study is also useful in evaluating patients for restenosis after angioplasty.

CASE 123

History.—24-year-old man 1 day after living related renal transplantation for treatment of end-stage renal failure from reflux nephropathy.

Scan.—^{99m}Tc DTPA flow study and renal scan and ^{131}I hippuran renal scan.

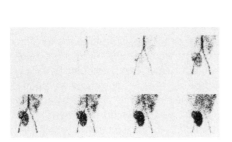

^{99m}Tc DTPA flow study.

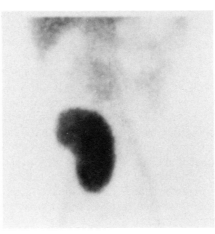

Early ^{99m}Tc DTPA image.

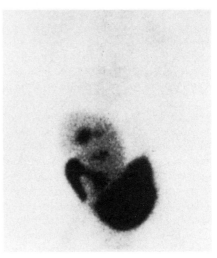

Late ^{99m}Tc DTPA image.

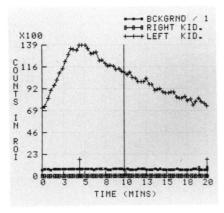

20-Minute ^{99m}Tc DTPA time-activity curve.

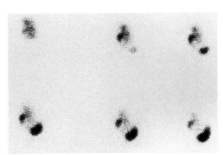

^{131}I hippuran study.

148

Findings.— The scan shows normal flow to the right pelvic allograft. Serial delayed images demonstrate normal function, with no evidence of obstruction, urine leak, or other complication.

Diagnosis.— Normal renal transplant.

Renal transplantation has become an accepted and fairly common alternative to hemodialysis in the treatment of end-stage renal failure. Renal transplantation is most successful when the kidney donor and recipient are identical twins. Immunosuppressive drugs are not necessary, and the grafts do extremely well. This is, however, a rare situation. A living related donor is the next best alternative. In this situation, ischemic damage to the kidney is minimized, and the transplant has a 90% chance of surviving 10 years.

After transplantation, the function of the allograft is monitored with frequent blood tests, physical examination, and urine output monitoring. In our institution, radionuclide renal scans are routinely obtained immediately after transplantation (in the recovery room) to confirm the presence of flow to the kidney. On the first postoperative day, another renal scan is done as a baseline and to evaluate for any evidence of obstruction, leak, or vascular impairment. Thereafter, scans are obtained to monitor for rejection, cyclosporine toxicity, acute tubular necrosis, urinomas, renal artery stenosis, and renal infarction. Subsequent renal scans should be interpreted using the baseline scan for comparison.

For transplant monitoring, the renal scan can be performed in several different ways. Our current method is to use ^{99m}Tc DTPA. In the past, ^{131}I hippuran scans were performed after the DTPA study to measure tubular function. However, we believe that the function of the kidney as measured by excretion of DTPA rarely varies from the functional information obtained with hippuran. The patient is thus spared the radiation exposure of repeated ^{131}I hippuran doses. In cases of very poor renal function, hippuran is still used because of its better concentration in renal failure. ^{99m}Tc MAG-3 may be the best choice for evaluating renal transplants. Cost is its main disadvantage.

The normal transplant renal scan shows peak renal activity coincident to peak iliac artery activity. Activity in the kidney rapidly increases to clearly define the maximum level and then falls. Various computer-generated values can be of help but are dependent on the quality of the bolus injection. These include time-to-peak activity, time to reach peak activity and then fall to half peak, mean slope of upstroke of the time-activity curve, maximum slope of upstroke, and integral of the time-activity curve.

Serial delayed images over the kidneys should be interpreted in the same manner as native kidneys. Maximum ^{99m}Tc DTPA activity should be about 4 to 6 minutes, with visible washout of activity thereafter. Maximum hippuran activity in the kidney is about 3 to 4 minutes after injection, with a downsloping time-activity curve. MAG-3 shows similar findings.

History.— 14-year-old youth 2 weeks after transplantation, who has a rising creatinine level.

Scan.—^{99m}Tc DTPA renal scan.

Flow study.

20-Minute delayed ^{99m}Tc DTPA image.

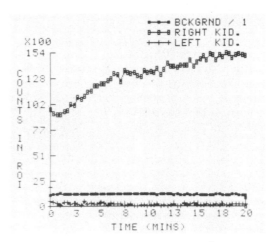

Time-activity curve over transplant.

Findings.— Decreased flow and function.

Diagnosis.— Acute renal transplant rejection.

Transplant rejection is divided into four categories according to the part of the immune system mediating the rejection and the time interval after transplantation:

1. **Hyperacute:** Caused by the presence of preformed antibodies in the recipient's circulation. It occurs within the first 1 to 12 hours after transplantation and leads to rapid thrombosis of the vascular bed of the graft, with functional destruction within minutes to hours.
2. **Accelerated acute:** Predominantly cell-mediated rejection, occurring 1 to 5 days after transplantation.
3. **Acute:** A cell-mediated process caused by sensitized lymphocytes migrating into the graft and destroying cells without participation of humoral antibodies, usually occurring 1 to 3 weeks after transplantation.
4. **Chronic:** Humoral antibody-induced injury to the endothelial and interstitial cells, causing compromise of the vascular bed, decreased graft size, hyperten-sion, and, ultimately, renal failure. This probably occurs in all allografts to varying degrees.

The scintigraphic findings of allograft rejection in all types of rejection are similar; they are decreased flow and function. The decreased flow seen on the angiographic portion of the scan is caused by decreased microvascular perfusion. This finding usually worsens with time if the rejection episode is not treated. Decreased function is manifested by decreased uptake and delayed excretion into the collecting system.

Increased sulfur colloid uptake is also seen in rejection. Unfortunately, ATN sometimes also shows uptake. This makes separation of ATN from mild to moderate rejection difficult. Other radiopharmaceuticals that can show uptake in rejection are gallium 67, leukocytes labeled with indium 111, and ^{111}In platelets.

Note that ^{67}Ga uptake in a transplanted kidney is normal in the immediate postoperative period; it is only after approximately 3 months that uptake is considered abnormal.

CASE 125

History.— 35-year-old 1 day after cadaveric renal transplantation.

Scan.—^{99m}Tc DTPA renal scan.

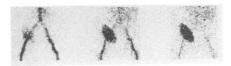

Angiographic images.

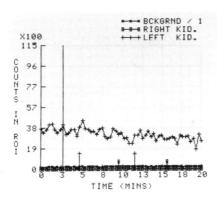

Time-activity curve of kidney.

Two-minute delayed ^{99m}Tc DTPA image.

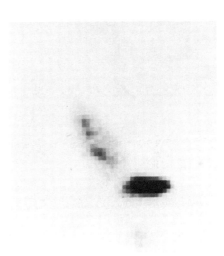

20-Minute ^{99m}Tc DTPA image.

Findings.— Normal flow and decreased function.

Diagnosis.—ATN after cadaveric renal transplantation.

The two most common causes of parenchymal failure after renal transplantation are ATN and allograft rejection. Acute tubular necrosis (ATN) is common after cadaveric renal transplantation but uncommon after living-related transplantation. The higher incidence of ATN after cadaveric renal transplantation is caused by an extended ischemic period. This can be warm ischemia in a hypotensive donor before harvesting or cold ischemia during storage and transport of the organ before transplantation.

ATN is manifested by diminished urine output immediately after transplantation or after an initial period of normal graft function. The recovery period is usually 3 weeks but can last as long as 6 weeks. Rejection often occurs at some point during the period of recovery from ATN; this can produce a confusing picture. Because rejection results in diminishing perfusion, serial renal scans can be helpful in differentiating rejection plus ATN from ATN during this period.

ATN in the first 24 hours after transplantation is characterized by normal flow in the presence of significantly depressed uptake and poor or absent excretion of radiotracer. In ATN occurring after 24 hours, the flow can be somewhat diminished; however, it is much better than might be expected with such poor tubular function. These findings can be confused with rejection; however, untreated rejection will show progressively worsening flow, whereas in ATN, flow remains unchanged or improves with time.

CASE 126

History.— Patient with anuria 2 days after cadaveric renal transplant into right side of pelvis.

Scan.—^{99m}Tc DTPA renal scan.

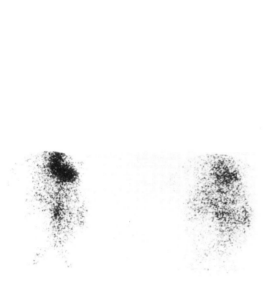

Anterior angiographic images.

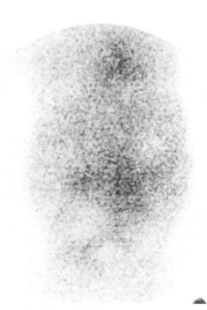

10-Minute ^{99m}Tc DTPA
anterior image of abdomen.

Findings.— Flow and delayed images: photopenic area in right lower quadrant.

Diagnosis.— Renal artery occlusion complicating cadaveric renal transplantation.

Renal artery occlusion is a catastrophic complication of renal transplantation. The renal scan's findings are identical to those of renal vein thrombosis and severe rejection. Therefore, these diseases cannot be distinguished by renal scan.

In renal artery occlusion, the renal scan shows a photopenic area in the region of the graft on the angiographic images; the photopenia persists on delayed images. This should be differentiated from nonvisualization of the kidney, which implies perfusion to the kidney equal to that of adjacent tissues. Such a kidney has very diminished flow but still has some chance for recovery. Severe rejection and renal vein thrombosis can also appear as a photopenic defect.

The finding of a photopenic area in the transplant fossa usually means irreversible damage to the kidney and warrants surgical excision. Further evaluation is performed in some centers with arteriography, renal biopsy, or both before transplant nephrectomy.

Segmental infarction is occasionally seen when a segmental artery is compromised. This occurs intraoperatively with ligation of a vessel or postoperatively with vascular thrombosis. The renal scan will show a wedge-shaped defect on delayed imaging in the involved area. The best examination for defining the extent of renal infarction is a DMSA scan with SPECT.

CASE 127

History.— 18-year-old woman with rising creatinine level after renal transplantation. Patient is taking cyclosporine.

Scan.— ^{99m}Tc DTPA renal scan.

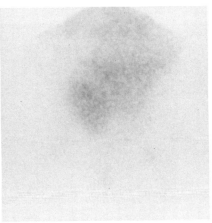

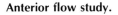

| Anterior flow study. | Two-Minute delayed image. | 20-Minute image. |

Findings.— Normal flow and decreased function.

Diagnosis.— Cyclosporine toxicity.

Cyclosporine is an immunosuppressive agent derived from fungi that has been shown to improve graft survival in transplant patients. It is well known that cyclosporine can cause nephrotoxicity if prolonged excessive blood levels are maintained. This is an important cause of decreased function in cadaveric renal transplants and in the native kidneys of cardiac transplant patients.

The tubular cells are primarily affected. With chronic use, cyclosporine causes glomerulosclerosis manifested histologically by interstitial fibrosis and arteriopathy with intimal hyperplasia. Initially this injury was thought to be reversible; however, studies have shown it can be irreversible. End-stage renal failure has occurred in a small number of heart transplant patients.

Cyclosporine toxicity can be minimized by careful monitoring of cyclosporine blood levels. The desired blood level of cyclosporine is that high enough to achieve effective immunosuppression but low enough to prevent cyclosporine renal damage.

Cyclosporine toxicity has three clinical manifestations. The acute episode is thought to be caused by vasoconstriction, and is mediated by prostaglandin and thromboxane. The second is subacute renal failure lasting longer than 1 week, with incomplete recovery after withdrawal of cyclosporine. The third is a chronic nephropathy with elevated creatinine levels after 1 year or more.

Classically, cyclosporine toxicity is manifested on renal scan by preserved flow with decreased function. It can decrease flow to the kidney, however. The findings on renal scan vary even with similar cyclosporine levels. It is difficult to differentiate cyclosporine toxicity from acute tubular necrosis or rejection, and often the answer is clear only when renal function improves after a decrease in cyclosporine dosage.

CASE 128

History.— 29-year-old diabetic patient 1 day after renal transplantation with decreased urine output and a persistently elevated creatinine level.

Scan.—^{131}I hippuran renal scan.

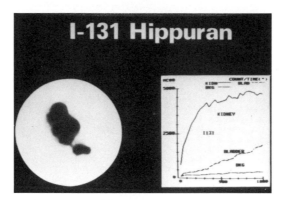

Left, late ^{131}I hippuran image. *Right,* time-activity curve of kidney.

Findings.— The scan shows progressively increasing activity.

Diagnosis.— Ureterovesical junction obstruction after renal transplantation.

It is important to quickly recognize obstruction of a transplanted kidney to minimize the degree of permanent damage. Monitoring urine output may not be a good method for detecting obstruction because persistent urine output from native kidneys may mask blocked transplant ureteral flow.

A mild degree of obstruction of the distal transplant ureter after surgery is common because of transient edema at the site of the ureteroneocystostomy. Persistent obstruction at the ureterovesical junction may be caused by a variety of processes. A ureteral scar may form at the site of the anastomosis. Kinking of the ureter, blood clots, renal calculi, or extrinsic pressure caused by lymphocele, abscess, or hematoma can also occur. The findings on renal scan of urinary tract obstruction in transplants are similar to those found in native kidneys. A problem in evaluating transplants with diuretic renal scans is that there is no normal kidney for comparison.

With an obstructed system, there is delayed and diminished flow to the kidney with delayed cortical visualization and prolonged transit time. There is also activity in the collecting system of the kidney that increases with time. Remember that a prominent collecting system can also be seen in a dilated but nonobstructed system. With long-standing or complete obstruction, nonvisualization of the kidney may occur.

A diuretic renal scan can be helpful in differentiating a dilated but nonobstructed system from an obstructed system. A dose of furosemide sufficient to assure a diuretic response is administered intravenously. Serial images of the kidney are obtained, and a time-activity curve over the kidney is constructed. In a dilated but nonobstructed system, diuretic administration causes the curve to slope downward with a washout half-life of less than 10 minutes. If a high-grade obstruction exists, the curve will be upsloping both before and after the diuretic administration.

CASE 129

History.— 3-year-old girl who has had multiple urinary
tract infections.

Scan.— 1 mCi of ^{99m}Tc is instilled in the patient's bladder via a
catheter. Images were obtained during filling and micturition.

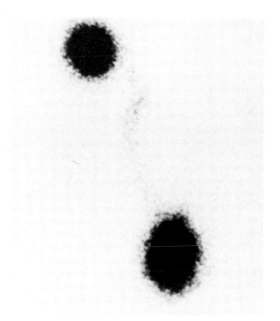

**Posterior image of abdomen and pelvis during
bladder filling.**

Findings.— Activity extending to kidney on left.

Diagnosis.— Left vesicoureteral reflux.

Vesicoureteral reflux can lead to irreversible renal damage
if not diagnosed and treated early. The usual cause of vesicoureteral reflux is a failure of the vesicoureteral valve mechanism. A competent valve is dependent on the oblique entry
of the ureter into the bladder, an adequate intramural length,
and contraction of the ureterotrigonal muscle during mictura-
tion. The long-term failure of this one-way valve mechanism
leads to reflux of urine, with frequent infections and renal
scarring. This can cause hypertension and, eventually, renal
failure.

Approximately 50% of children with urinary tract infections in the first year of life will have reflux. This incidence
decreases with age.

Radionuclide cystography (RNC) is becoming more widely
used in the evaluation of children with urinary tract infections. Its popularity as a diagnostic tool stems from two advantages over radiographic voiding cystourethrography
(VCUG). First, RNC is more sensitive for vesicoureteral reflux.
As little as 0.25 mL of refluxed urine can be detected. Second, the radionuclide technique exposes the patient to
less radiation. In fact, the radiation dose is almost 100 times
less than that from radiographic VCUG.

An advantage of the radiographic VCUG over RNC is the
anatomic information provided about the renal pelves, ureters, and urethra. For this reason, some radiologists perform
an initial radiographic study. These radiologists reserve RNC
for monitoring vesicoureteral reflux in patients with known
reflux. Because low-grade reflux will resolve with conserva-
tive therapy, serial studies to follow these patients are frequently done.

The degree of reflux is graded in radiographic VCUG using
five classes. The grading system for RNC is similar but separates patients into three classes:

1. *Mild, or RNC severity 1 reflux* (grades 1 and 2 radiographically): activity confined to ureter.
2. *Moderate, or RNC severity 2 reflux* (grade 3): activity
   extending to pelvicalyceal system.
3. *Severe, or RNC severity 3 reflux* (grades 4 and 5):
   distended redundant collecting system.

In the majority of patients reflux occurs during micturition.
Eighty percent will show reflux during both filling and micturition and 20% during the filling phase only.

CASE 130

History.— 19-year-old man with 1-day history of painful right testicle.

Scan.— Testicular scan.

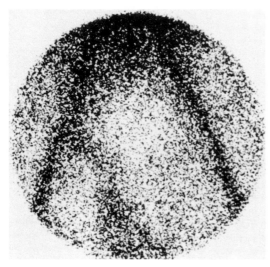

Early angiographic anterior image of pelvis and scrotum.

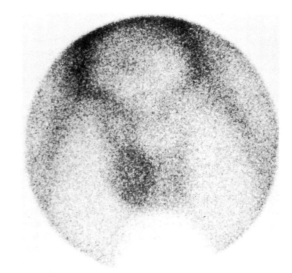

Blood pool image of scrotal area.

Findings.— Increased flow and blood pool to right side of scrotum.

Diagnosis.— Epididymo-orchitis.

The testicular scan is used to differentiate epididymitis from torsion in patients with acute onset of testicular pain.

The epididymis is a comma-shaped structure lying on the posterolateral surface of the testes. Epididymitis is an inflammatory process involving the epididymis and can be bacterial or posttraumatic. Most cases of epididymitis are caused by bacteria entering the epididymis from the prostate, seminal vesicles, or urethra or, less frequently, by hematogenous spread. It is usually found in adults, with symptoms of tender enlargement of the epididymis, leukocytosis, and pyuria. The pain of epididymitis is usually relieved with elevation of the testicle (Prehn's sign). These symptoms are sometimes difficult to isolate to the epididymis because of varying degrees of testicular involvement with infection.

The scan findings of epididymitis include:

1. Increased flow through the spermatic cord vessels on the involved side.
2. Curvilinear laterally placed increased activity on the perfusion study corresponding to the posterolateral location of the inflamed epididymis. This can be more midline if the epididymis is displaced medially.
3. Delayed images showing increased activity in the region of the epididymis.
4. With acute epididymo-orchitis, the findings are similar but show more medial testicular involvement as well.

This study is most often used to evaluate patients with the acute onset of unilateral scrotal pain and swelling. It has little utility in the evaluation of chronic scrotal masses because testicular cancers have a variable appearance on scan.

The testes receive arterial flow from the testicular arteries, which originate from the aorta just below the level of the renal arteries. These arteries enter the spermatic cord above the internal inguinal ring. The deferential and cremasteric arteries also travel within the spermatic cord to supply the vas deferens and the cremasteric muscle.

The scrotal vessels arise from the internal, superficial, and external pudendal arteries, which originate from the femoral vessels. These vessels do not travel through the spermatic cord or anastomose with vessels supplying the testes. They cannot, therefore, support testicular viability.

Testicular scanning is performed with the patient in the supine position, with the penis taped up on the patient's abdomen. The scrotum is suspended in a towel or with a tape sling; care is taken so the testicles do not overlap. A converging collimator is used for adolescents and a pinhole collimator is used for pediatric patients, and 15 to 20 mCi of ^{99m}Tc pertechnetate is injected as a bolus. Serial angiographic images at 2- to 5-second intervals are obtained for 60 seconds, followed immediately by several delayed images, each acquired for 700,000 counts. Because free ^{99m}Tc pertechnetate is used, a discharging agent such as perchlorate is sometimes used to lower thyroid irradiation.

A normal testicular scan shows smooth medial borders of each iliac artery. No significant activity is seen in the area of testicular, deferential, or pudendal arteries. The scrotal perfusion, if visible at all, is seen only as a minimally intense area of activity. The delayed images show the scrotum and its contents as a homogenous area of activity similar in intensity to the thigh.

CASE 131

History.— 15-year-old youth with painless right scrotal enlargement over 6 months, now with vague scrotal pain.

Scan.— Testicular scan. A lead shield was used.

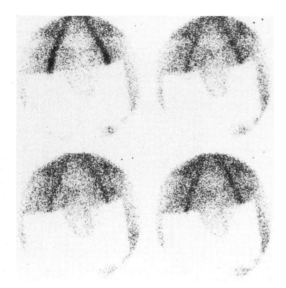

Angiographic images.

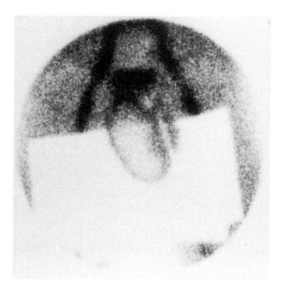

Blood pool image of scrotum.

Findings.— This scan shows a photopenic area on the right on both flow study and delayed images.

Diagnosis.— Hydrocele.

The processus vaginalis is the evagination of the peritoneum created as the testis passes from the abdominal cavity through the inguinal canal into the scrotum. A hydrocele is a collection of fluid confined by the processus vaginalis of the scrotum. This condition is common in newborns; the processus vaginalis remains patent in 80%.

A hydrocele may be communicating or noncommunicating. Communicating hydroceles occur when the processus vaginalis communicates with the peritoneal cavity, allowing peritoneal fluid to accumulate in the scrotum. Indirect inguinal hernias are also increased in this condition. Noncommunicating hydroceles occur when the neck of the processus vaginalis becomes obliterated, leaving trapped fluid within the cavity of the tunica vaginalis near the testis. Normally this fluid is absorbed within the first year of life. Occasionally after trauma or inflammatory conditions of the scrotum, fluid will accumulate within this space, causing a hydrocele. Surgical correction is often required.

The diagnosis of a hydrocele is suggested by a smooth, oblong, nontender scrotal mass, which transilluminates. Occasionally hydroceles mimic more acute conditions, such as an incarcerated inguinal hernia, epididymo-orchitis, or testicular torsion.

At times hydroceles are confused with torsion on testicular scan. A hydrocele appears as a photopenic area within the scrotum. The testis may appear as an area of increased activity within the photopenic hydrocele. Angiographic images of an uncomplicated hydrocele are usually normal. Careful physical examination with scrotal transillumination is helpful to prevent misinterpretation of the scan. If a hydrocele is present in addition to another process such as epididymitis or trauma, the scan is especially confusing. In such cases, the scan will demonstrate the findings of the underlying process with the addition of a photopenic area.

CASE 132

History.— 13-year-old youth with right scrotal pain for 1 hour.

Scan.— Testicular scan.

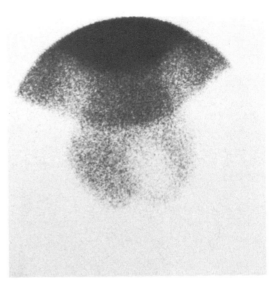

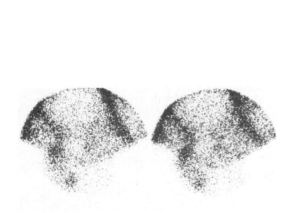

Flow study.

Immediate image.

Findings.— Decreased flow and blood pool activity in the right scrotum.

Diagnosis.— Testicular torsion.

Testicular torsion is a medical emergency caused by twisting of the testicle on its pedicle; this results in compromised circulation to the testicle. Without prompt surgical correction or spontaneous detorsion, the testicle infarcts.

Torsion usually occurs in pubertal boys, with the peak occurrence at 14 years of age; however, it may occur before birth through age 30 years. Torsion in older patients is rare.

The two forms of testicular torsion are intravaginal and extravaginal. Intravaginal torsion is much more common and results from complete envelopment of the testes by the tunica vaginalis. Normally the tunica vaginalis only partially envelops the testicle and epididymis, allowing these structures to adhere to the scrotal wall, preventing torsion. Extravaginal torsion is much rarer and involves torsion of the spermatic cord near the external ring. This occurs primarily in newborns.

With either type of torsion, the venous supply is occluded first. Later, sufficient pressure builds to shut off arterial flow as well. This results in edema, congestion of the compromised testicle, and, eventually, infarction.

The primary clinical finding is the acute onset of pain localized to the scrotum. Physical examination reveals a swollen tender testicle, which appears higher than the normal side. Elevation of the testicle does not relieve the pain (Prehn's sign). Another physical finding suggesting torsion as the cause of scrotal pain is an abnormal position of the non-

involved testis. Normally when the patient is standing the long axis of the testicle is more vertical. If the patient has complete envelopment of the testicle and epididymis by the tunica vaginalis (the condition, usually bilateral, which predisposes one to torsion), the testicle assumes a more horizontal lie in the scrotum. If this so-called bell clapper deformity is found in the nonpainful testicle, the patient is more likely to have torsion.

Therapy of testicular torsion is emergent surgical exploration of the scrotum, with detorsion and orchiopexy, or surgical anchoring of each testicle to the scrotal wall to prevent any future chance of recurrence. If the diagnosis is delayed more than 4 to 6 hours, irreversible damage occurs.

Radionuclide testicular scanning done acutely shows decreased or absent perfusion to the affected side; delayed images show a photopenic area with activity less than the opposite testicle and less than that of the thigh. Increased activity may be seen high in the cord. It is essential to correlate the scan findings with physical examination of the patient in the position of scanning.

If spontaneous detorsion occurs before imaging, the perfusion and delayed images show increased activity on the affected side. This pattern simulates epididymitis.

Other causes of unilaterally decreased activity on testicular scan include hydrocele and hematocele. Palpation and transillumination are helpful in excluding these causes.

CASE 133

History.— 13-year-old youth with 5-day history of left scrotal pain.

Scan.— Testicular scan.

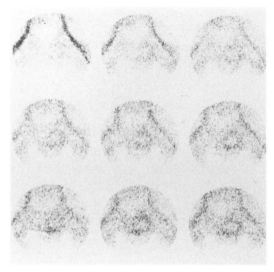

Anterior angiographic images of scrotum.

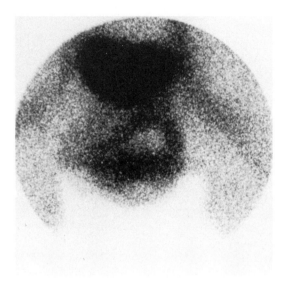

Anterior blood pool image of scrotum.

Findings.— Left scrotal halo of increased uptake on flow and blood pool images.

Diagnosis.— Missed testicular torsion.

Radionuclide imaging has a sensitivity and specificity in excess of 90% for testicular torsion. "Missed torsion" refers to the later phases of untreated testicular torsion 24 hours after onset of symptoms. In these cases, irreversible damage to the involved testicle has occurred.

The findings of missed torsion on radionuclide imaging are:

1. Variable amount of hyperemia around the ischemic testicle on perfusion imaging. (Scrotal blood supply arises from the pudendal vessels and does not course through the spermatic cord.)

2. Delayed images show the classic bull's-eye, or halo, pattern, with increased activity around the testicle and a central photopenic area. The photopenic area usually but not always has less activity than the opposite testicle or the thigh. When the bull's-eye pattern is seen, salvage of the testicle is unlikely. Other causes of the bull's-eye sign include abscess, hematocele, and hematoma.

CASE 134

History.—22-year-old woman with chills, fever, and back pain.

Scan.—^{67}Ga scan.

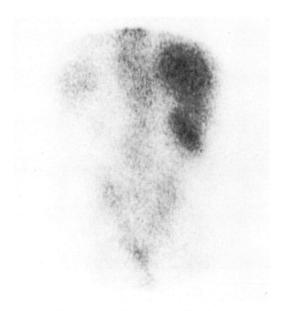

**72-Hour posterior image of abdomen
and pelvis.**

Findings.—Marked uptake below right lobe of liver, with less intense activity below spleen on left.

Diagnosis.—Bilateral pyelonephritis.

Acute urinary tract infections (UTI) can be subdivided into those that affect the lower tract (urethritis, prostatitis, cystitis) or the upper tract (acute pyelonephritis). Many different organisms can infect the urinary tract, but the most common are the gram-negative rods, which cause more than 80% of all UTIs in patients with no anatomic abnormalities or stones. *Escherichia coli* accounts for most infections; other less common gram-negative organisms include *Proteus, Klebsiella, Enterobacter, Serratia,* and *Pseudomonas.* Gram-positive organisms play a less important role, although *Staphylococcus saprophyticus* accounts for 10% to 15% of UTIs in young girls, and *Staphylococcus aureus* may be seen in patients with stones or previous instrumentation.

In acute pyelonephritis, the clinical symptoms include fever, chills, nausea, vomiting, flank pain, and sometimes diarrhea. Physical signs include tachycardia, tenderness on deep abdominal palpation, and the classic sign of exquisite tenderness over one or both costovertebral angles. Some patients, especially if they are older, have sepsis. Most patients have leukocytosis, bacteruria, and pyuria, with leukocyte casts in the urine.

Pyelonephritis, either acute or chronic, shows intense ^{67}Ga uptake. Numerous other renal lesions can show ^{67}Ga accumulation, including other infections (renal abscess, perinephric abscess, tuberculosis), neoplasm (renal cell carcinoma, lymphoma, Wilms' tumor, leukemia, melanoma), systemic diseases (sarcoidosis, polyarteritis nodosa, amyloidosis, hepatic failure, tuberous sclerosis), iatrogenic conditions (chemotherapy, radiation therapy, renal transplantation), and saturated iron binding sites from multiple transfusions, iron injections, and hemachromatosis.

CHAPTER 6

Pulmonary

CASE 135

History.—22-year-old woman with chest pain.

Scan.—^{133}Xe and ^{99m}Tc lung scan.

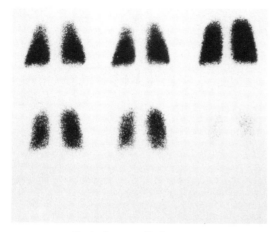

Posterior ventilation scan.

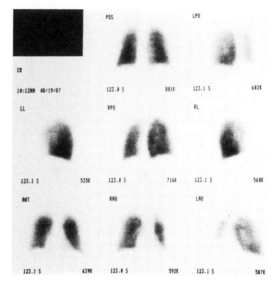

**Eight-view perfusion scan. *POS*-posterior,
LPO-left posterior oblique, *LL*-left lateral,
RPO-right posterior oblique, *RL*-right lateral,
ANT-anterior, *RAO*-right anterior oblique,
LAO-left anterior oblique.**

Findings.— Ventilation: normal. Perfusion: normal.

Diagnosis.—Normal V/Q scan. No evidence of
pulmonary embolism.

The appearance of the normal ventilation scan depends on the agent used. With xenon 133, the two lungs appear as mirror images. The costophrenic angles are not as well seen as in perfusion scans. Because of the lower energy of ^{133}Xe compared with technetium 99m, activity in the anterior portion of the lung gives rise to fewer counts than on a ^{99m}Tc scan; therefore, in contrast to a perfusion scan, the heart causes almost no defect on posterior images. However, if an anterior image is obtained, a very prominent heart defect is seen.

During washout the lower lung zones clear quicker than the upper zones. By 3 minutes, the lung activity will clear to background levels, although occasional patients will show slightly longer retention.

The normal perfusion scan shows a smooth outline with a gradient of decreasing activity from the base to the apex. The heart makes a prominent defect on anterior views, with a less distinct defect on posterior and lateral views.

There are a number of normal variations in the appearance of the perfusion scan. Women may show decreased basilar activity because of breast attenuation. Occasionally a prominent defect is seen in the upper lung field on oblique views because of attenuation by the scapula and overlying musculature. This can be very distinct and can simulate a pulmonary embolism. The fact that this defect is not well seen on other views can help differentiate it from a true abnormality.

Decreased activity is sometimes seen in the right apex, and in the azygous lobe if present. Obese patients with small lung volumes often have blunted, even absent costophrenic angles.

Cardiomegaly, ectatic aortas, increased atrial size in valvular diseases, pectus excavatum, and kyphoscoliosis all can cause perfusion defects. Comparison with chest x-ray film is helpful in preventing misinterpretation in these cases.

CASE 136

History.—48-year-old woman with pleuritic chest pain.

Scan.—Krypton 81m ventilation and ^{99m}Tc MAA lung scan.

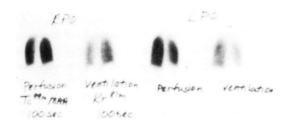

Perfusion and ventilation scans in right and left posterior oblique projections.

Findings.—Ventilation normal. Perfusion normal.

Diagnosis.—No evidence of pulmonary embolism.

The ventilation portion of the lung scan can be performed using a variety of inhaled isotopes. ^{133}Xe gas is the most widely used agent and gives information about pulmonary vital capacity (single-breath phase), accessory ventilation (equilibrium), and airway obstruction (washout).

Because of its low energy (81 keV), ^{133}Xe studies must be performed before the perfusion study. Xenon 127 gas has a more favorable energy (172 and 203 keV) for imaging, allowing the ventilation study to be acquired after the perfusion study. This allows the views that best show perfusion defects to be chosen for the ventilation scan, improving accuracy. However, because of its long half-life (36.4 days compared with 5.3 days for ^{133}Xe) and its higher energy, using storage for disposal is a significant problem.

^{81m}Kr gas has a favorable imaging energy (190 keV), allowing the ventilation study to be done after the perfusion scan. However, because of its exceedingly short half-life (13 seconds), only single-breath/equilibrium data are obtained. Ventilation studies may also be performed with aerosols that can be labeled with a number of isotopes, including ^{99m}Tc, indium 111, and indium 113m. Aerosols also allow imaging to be performed after perfusion. They can be nondiagnostic in patients with severe chronic obstructive pulmonary disease (COPD) because they tend to deposit centrally rather than penetrate peripherally.

All of these ventilation techniques require an awake, cooperative patient to complete. The ventilator-dependent patient with possible pulmonary embolus cannot have his or her ventilation evaluated by these methods. Ventilation studies on the patients with intubated airways may be performed using ^{133}Xe dissolved in saline solution. The ^{133}Xe saline solution is injected intravenously, and posterior images over the lungs are then obtained.

Although single-breath and equilibrium information is not obtained with ^{133}Xe saline solution, the relatively insoluble ^{133}Xe comes out of solution into the alveolus and is then expired through the airways, giving washout information.

Because the ^{133}Xe is delivered intravenously, it is possible gas would not enter areas blocked by pulmonary embolism. However, collateral air drift through the canals of Lambert and pores of Kahn usually allow gas to enter these areas. Also, it is retention that one is looking for rather than single-breath information. It should be stressed, however, that no formal data are available for this technique, and results should be interpreted with caution. Expelled gas must be collected for radiation safety.

A more common use of ^{133}Xe in saline solution is for diagnosing inhalational injuries. Areas of retention beyond 90 to 120 seconds are abnormal. This use of ^{133}Xe is well documented in the literature.

CASE 137

History.— 22-year-old woman taking birth control pills, who has chest pain.

Scan.— ^{133}Xe and ^{99m}Tc MAA lung scan.

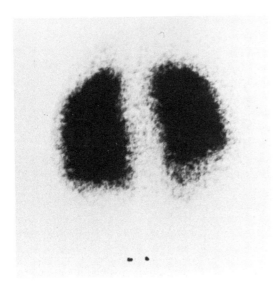

Posterior single-breath ventilation image.

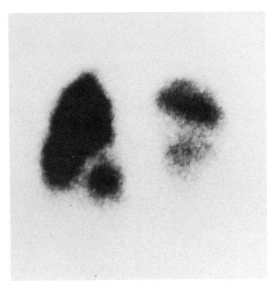

Posterior perfusion image.

Findings.— Normal ventilation with multiple large perfusion defects. V/Q mismatch.

Diagnosis.— High probability for acute pulmonary embolism.

The clinical diagnosis of pulmonary embolism is difficult because the signs and symptoms are often either nonspecific or absent. Studies indicate the clinical diagnosis of pulmonary embolism is correct in only 25% to 45% of patients. The classic triad of hemoptysis, thrombophlebitis, and pleural friction rub infrequently is seen. The most common symptoms are dyspnea (86%), cough (70%), and pleuritic chest pain (58%). Physical examination findings include tachypnea, tachycardia, accentuation of S2, and pulmonary rales. Hypoxemia, hypocarbia, and respiratory alkalosis may be present on arterial blood gas analysis. The electrocardiogram usually is normal, although evidence of right ventricular strain is sometimes seen. Most commonly, the chest x-ray film is normal. Often nonspecific findings will be present, such as atelectasis, effusion, elevated hemidiaphragm, and, rarely, oligemia. Infiltrates secondary to pulmonary infarction are seen in less than 10% of cases. Although pulmonary artery angiography has good sensitivity and excellent specificity for pulmonary embolism, it is invasive, expensive, and carries a small but definite risk of morbidity and mortality. For this reason, the V/Q (ventilation-perfusion) scan is the primary test for PE.

The classic perfusion scan findings of pulmonary embolism are multiple, peripheral, segmental, wedge-shaped perfusion defects, more often in the lower lung fields. The perfusion defects tend to be segmental because pulmonary blood flow corresponds to segmental pulmonary anatomy. This may involve the entire lung, lobe, segment, or portion of a segment. Eighty percent of defects caused by COPD are nonsegmental. One study of angiographically proved emboli showed 75% of emboli caused segmental defects. Multiple defects are usually present, because as the thromboembolus passes through the right atrium and ventricle it fragments into smaller emboli.

Angiographic studies show the average patient with pulmonary embolus has 11 emboli. The greater the number of emboli, the higher the sensitivity of the V/Q scan. Although 20% to 25% of emboli will produce no perceptible perfusion change, 97% of emboli that completely occlude vessels 2.0 mm or more in diameter are detectable. Only about 25% of emboli that cause partial occlusion to blood flow are seen. Because of the segmental vascular anatomy and its branching pattern, the defects are peripheral and wedge shaped. If a stripe of peripheral activity is seen lateral to a perfusion defect, a pulmonary embolus is less likely because defects from emboli are pleural based (stripe sign). Occasionally multiple very small emboli lodge peripherally, causing the lung to appear small, the so-called shrunken lung sign. The "fissure" sign, a defect along a pulmonary fissure, may be seen with

TABLE 6–1.
Scheme for Interpretation of V/Q Scans

Interpretation	Pattern	Pulmonary Embolism Frequency (%)
Normal Probability of pulmonary embolism	Normal perfusion	0
Low	Small V/Q mismatches	0
	Focal V/Q matches with no corresponding radiographic abnormalities	4.8
	Perfusion defects substantially smaller than radiographic abnormalities	7.7
Intermediate	Diffuse, severe airway obstruction	20
	Matched perfusion defects and radiographic abnormalities	27
	Single moderate V/Q mismatch without corresponding radiographic abnormality	33
High	Perfusion defects substantially larger than radiographic abnormalities	87
	≥1 large or ≥2 moderate sized V/Q mismatches with no corresponding radiographic abnormalities. (Many nuclear medicine physicians categorize single mismatched defects as intermediate regardless of size)	92

either effusion or with small emboli that lodge along the pleural surface.

Emboli show a predilection for the lower lobes. In contrast, perfusion defects from COPD often involve the upper lobes even in the absence of significant lower lobe defects.

The ventilation study is usually normal in cases of pulmonary embolus. Occasionally, however, reflux bronchospasm occurs with pulmonary embolus leading to retention of Xe. Bronchoconstriction has been seen in 1.5% of experimentally induced emboli in dogs. Generally, though, this is a transient phenomenon, lasting only 4 to 8 hours.

No patterns on V/Q scan are pathognomonic or exclusive for pulmonary embolus, other than a normal perfusion scan. For this reason, V/Q scans are interpreted as normal, low, indeterminate (intermediate), or high probability for acute pulmonary embolus. The three main interpretation schemes are the Biello, the McNeill, and the recently introduced PIOPED (prospective investigation of pulmonary embolus diagnosis) criteria. At our institution, we use the Biello criteria to interpret V/Q scans (Table 6–1).

CASE 138

History.— 29-year-old woman with a past history of pulmonary embolism developed new shortness of breath.

Scan.—^{133}Xe and ^{99m}Tc MAA lung scan.

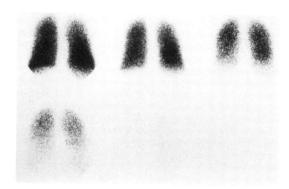

Posterior ventilation images.

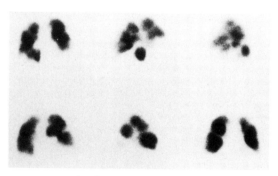

Six-view perfusion images.

Findings.— Ventilation: normal. Perfusion: multiple perfusion abnormalities.

Diagnosis.— Acute vs. old pulmonary embolism.

Pulmonary emboli show varying rates of resolution. Most resolution occurs in the first few days; by 3 months virtually all resolution is complete. The majority of young, otherwise healthy patients will regain normal perfusion. However, some patients do not; the elderly and those with preexisting lung disease are the most likely not to resolve their perfusion defects.

Previous pulmonary embolism frequently shows a V/Q mismatch, making it indistinguishable from acute pulmonary embolism. The best way to differentiate acute from old PE is to compare the present V/Q scan with a previous one. If the patient does not have any new perfusion defects, it is unlikely he or she has had recurrent PE. The previous emboli cause vascular narrowing, which raises the pulmonary vascular resistance in these areas. Thus, when new emboli enter the lung, they tend to go to the normal regions of the lung rather than to the higher resistance sites of previous PE. To allow comparison, it is a good idea to obtain a second "baseline" V/Q scan before discharging patients being treated for pulmonary embolism.

From 30% to 60% of patients receiving anticoagulation will develop new perfusion defects. This may occur through three mechanisms. First, proximal emboli may fragment and shower more distal vessels. Second, emboli may resolve at different rates, changing the relative pulmonary resistance. When macroaggregated albumin (MAA) is injected, it may preferentially flow away from previously perfused areas to the new sites of relatively lower vascular resistance. Finally, different rates of vascular relaxation rather than clot resolution may cause pulmonary resistance changes, resulting in redistribution of particles as described earlier.

CASE 139

History.—40-year-old woman with chest pain.

Scan.—^{133}Xe and ^{99m}Tc MAA lung scan.

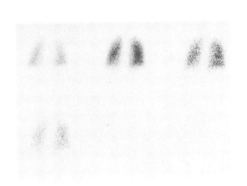
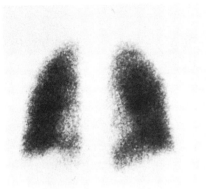
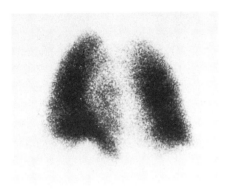

| Posterior ventilation scan. | Posterior perfusion image. | Left posterior oblique perfusion image. |

Findings. Ventilation: normal; perfusion: single moderate defect in left base. There is a V/Q mismatch.

Diagnosis.—Indeterminate for acute pulmonary embolus.

The three main sets of criteria used to interpret ventilation-perfusion lung scans are the Biello, PIOPED (prospective investigation of pulmonary embolism diagnosis), and McNeil criteria. At our institution we use the Biello criteria for V/Q scan interpretation, with one modification. A single large V/Q mismatch classifies the scan high-intermediate probability by the modified Biello criteria, as opposed to high-probability in the unmodified Biello criteria.

Findings that lead to an indeterminate V/Q classification by the Biello criteria are severe diffuse obstructive pulmonary disease (diffuse xenon retention) with perfusion defects (20% probability), perfusion defect equal in size to chest radiograph abnormality (27%), and single moderate-sized perfusion defect (25%–75% of a segment) in an area of normal ventilation and normal radiographic appearance (33% probability of pulmonary embolus).

Biello has a separate set of criteria for interpreting studies with chest radiograph infiltrates. This is done by comparing the size of the perfusion defect on scan to the size of the chest radiograph infiltrate. As previously mentioned, a perfusion defect equal in size to a chest radiograph infiltrate makes a V/Q scan indeterminate, with a 27% probability of being

pulmonary embolus. If the perfusion defect is smaller than the corresponding chest radiograph abnormality, the scan is low probability for acute pulmonary embolus (7%). A perfusion defect larger than its corresponding chest radiograph abnormality carries a high probability of representing acute pulmonary embolus, assuming normal ventilation.

In the appropriate clinical setting, a high-probability scan is sufficient to institute anticoagulation; likewise, a low-probability scan usually excludes the diagnosis of clinically significant pulmonary embolism. Pulmonary angiography is generally reserved for patients having indeterminate lung scans.

Not all patients with indeterminate scans need angiograms, however. McNeil showed that when the clinicians have a low clinical suspicion of pulmonary embolus, only 4% of indeterminate V/Q scan patients have pulmonary embolus. With an "average" suspicion, 13% have emboli.

Her work also shows that patients with indeterminate scans should not be treated with anticoagulants without angiography in cases in which clinicians have a high clinical suspicion of pulmonary embolus. Only about half of these patients actually have pulmonary emboli.

CASE 140

History.—63-year-old man with 80-pack-year history of smoking complained of increased shortness of breath.

Scan.—^{133}Xe and ^{99m}Tc MAA lung scan.

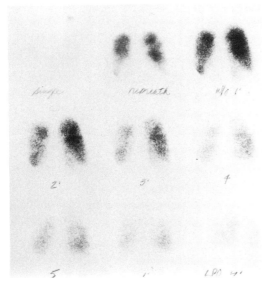

Ventilation study, posterior view
of chest.

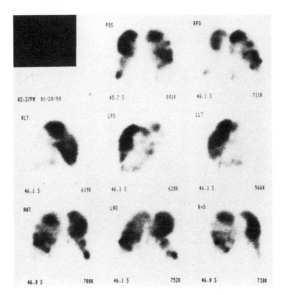

Eight-view perfusion scan.

Findings.—Ventilation: bilateral retention, right greater than left.
Perfusion: multiple perfusion defects.

Diagnosis.—Severe COPD. Indeterminate probability scan for
acute pulmonary embolus.

Chronic obstructive pulmonary disease (COPD) includes emphysema, chronic bronchitis, and bronchial asthma. All three produce both ventilation and perfusion abnormalities.

Emphysema usually is caused by prolonged tobacco smoking, and is seen more commonly in older patients. There is dilatation and destruction of alveoli, causing loss of alveolar surface area and the pulmonary capillary bed. Because alveoli support neighboring small airways, loss of this support leads to narrowing and irregularity of these airways. Increased airway resistance, decreased elastic recoil, and reduced gas exchange all lead to poor ventilation.

Findings of emphysema on ventilation scans vary, depending on the type of emphysema and the extent of involvement. There may be areas of decreased ventilation on single-breath images, because tidal volumes may be decreased and bronchial dead space increased. For the same reason, retention of ^{133}Xe is seen if ventilation occurs through accessory pathways. Clearance of ^{133}Xe correlates with forced expiratory volume in 1 second (FEV$_1$), which is often decreased in these patients.

Centrilobular emphysema affects the upper lobes predominantly. Panlobular emphysema affects the lungs diffusely.

The ventilatory defects seen in emphysema are usually patchy and nonsegmental, although discrete segmental defects may be seen. Emphysematous bullae usually fail to fill on both single-breath and equilibrium images.

Perfusion shows little change in early emphysema, and the changes are less than ventilatory abnormalities. About 80% of perfusion defects are patchy and nonsegmental, whereas 20% are segmental. Segmental defects are seen in the areas of most severely compromised ventilation.

Chronic bronchitis is a common disease of smokers. There is thickening of the bronchial mucosa, with an increase in mucous glands and excessive mucous secretion. This leads to irregular narrowing of airways. The earliest changes are seen in the small airways. Bronchial infections produce inflammation and sometimes even bronchospasm. These changes lead to increased airway resistance and reflex hypoxic vasoconstriction. Although both ventilation and perfusion abnormalities are seen in bronchitis, matched V/Q abnormalities are less frequent than in emphysema. Because bronchitis and COPD coexist in most patients, distinguishing between the two is difficult on scan.

Bronchial asthma is another form of COPD seen in a

younger patient population. In asthma, airflow obstruction is caused by bronchospasm, mucosal edema, and mucous plugging. During an asthma attack, the ventilation study may show single-breath and washout abnormalities, often more pronounced than corresponding perfusion abnormalities. Perfusion scans may show subsegmental, segmental, and even lobar perfusion abnormalities identical to those caused by pulmonary emboli. As the asthma attack subsides, both ventilation and perfusion abnormalities improve, mimicking resolving pulmonary emboli. Scan findings may be abnormal between attacks.

CASE 141

History.—34-year-old man with fever, leukocytosis, and left-sided chest pain.

Scan.—^{133}Xe and ^{99m}Tc MAA lung scan.

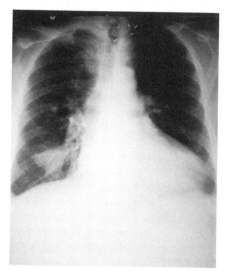

Posteroanterior chest radiograph.

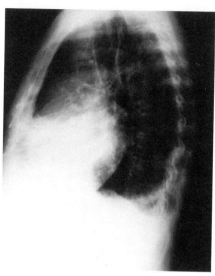

Lateral chest radiograph.

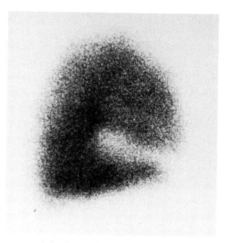

Right lateral perfusion image.

Findings.—Chest x-ray film: right lower lobe infiltrate. Ventilation and perfusion absent in area of chest film abnormality.

Diagnosis.—Indeterminate probability for acute pulmonary embolus.

The segmental or subsegmental perfusion defect in an area of corresponding chest film abnormality (infiltrate or effusion) presents an interesting problem in the interpretation of V/Q lung scans. It also reiterates the importance of reviewing chest films before interpreting lung scans.

When the chest x-ray is normal, perfusion defects are compared with ventilation in the region to determine the probability of pulmonary embolus. However, when an infiltrate is present on chest x-ray film in the area of perfusion abnormality, the ventilation study is less important. Even if the infiltrate is caused by a pulmonary infarct, the ventilation in the area is usually abnormal. Pulmonary infarcts result in hemorrhage into the alveoli; this prevents the normal influx of ^{133}Xe. Rarely, normal ventilation is seen in an infarct. This happens early in the infarct's course when alveolar hemorrhage has not yet occurred in all the alveoli; the remaining normal alveoli allow gas entry. In fact, normal ventilation in an area of chest x-ray infiltrate should be classified as high probability.

Whether the Biello or PIOPED criteria are used for interpreting the V/Q scan, the size of the perfusion defect is compared with the size of the chest infiltrate. If the perfusion de-

fect is smaller than the chest x-ray infiltrate, it is unlikely the chest film abnormality is caused by a pulmonary infarct, and the scan is classified as low probability for acute pulmonary embolus. If the perfusion defect and chest film abnormality are equal in size, the scan is indeterminate for pulmonary embolus and carries a 27% probability of representing acute PE. When the perfusion defect is larger than the corresponding chest film infiltrate, the probability for pulmonary embolus is high. One study showed angiographically proved pulmonary embolus in 16 of 18 patients (89%) with these findings.

It is common practice to interpret perfusion defects in areas of pleural effusion as indeterminate for pulmonary embolus. However, data from a series of 54 consecutive patients with perfusion defects in areas of effusions support lowering the probability. In this study, when the remainder of the perfusion study was unremarkable for pulmonary embolus, a perfusion defect that is matched to a pleural effusion on chest x-ray carried a less than 4% probability of representing pulmonary embolus.

CASE 142

History.—65-year-old man with history of COPD, now with chest pain.

Scan.—^{133}Xe and ^{99m}Tc MAA lung scan.

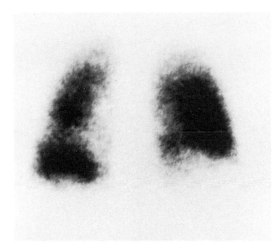

Posterior perfusion image.

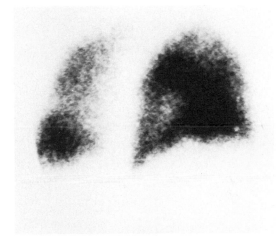

Right posterior oblique perfusion image.

Findings.—Ventilation scan (not shown) revealed retention in the left base, with borderline retention in the right base. Bilateral perfusion defects with a stripe sign were seen in the right base.

Diagnosis.—Stripe sign, low probability for pulmonary embolus.

V/Q mismatches are the basis for the lung scan diagnosis of acute pulmonary embolus. The classic perfusion defect caused by pulmonary embolus is peripheral and corresponds to pulmonary segmental or subsegmental anatomy. An embolus blocks arterial flow to all pulmonary parenchyma distal to the occlusion. The segmental, wedge-shaped nature of the defect is caused by the branching pattern of the pulmonary arteries, which follows the bronchial tree anatomy. Most pulmonary emboli defects are pleural based as well.

The perfusion study sometimes shows a defect that does not extend completely to the pleura. A rim of activity is seen peripheral to the defect. This is known as the "stripe sign." The stripe sign decreases the likelihood that the corresponding defect is due to pulmonary embolism. Planar images reduce a three-dimensional structure to two dimensions, and theoretically a connection to the pleura could be missed; however, in practice, the stripe sign has been shown to be quite reliable in excluding pulmonary embolus. Cases in which the stripe sign is present are usually classified as low probability.

CASE 143

History.— 54-year-old man with a history of ischemic heart disease is being evaluated for possible acute pulmonary embolism.

Scan.—^{133}Xe and ^{99m}Tc MAA lung scan.

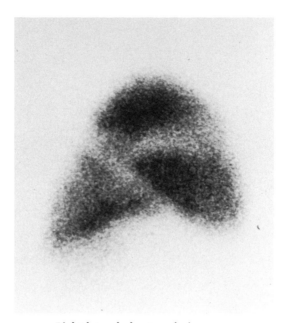

Right lateral chest perfusion scan.

Findings.— Ventilation (not shown) was normal. Perfusion shows decreased linear activity.

Diagnosis.— Fluid in the fissures; low probability of pulmonary embolus.

Acute pulmonary emboli are characteristically peripheral and pleural based because of the pulmonary vascular anatomy; an occlusion blocks blood flow to all parenchyma distal to it. Thus, perfusion defects with complete absence of perfusion extending to the pleura are characteristic of acute pulmonary embolism. If a rim of parenchymal perfusion exists distal to a perfusion defect (the stripe sign), the probability of that defect representing acute pulmonary embolism is lowered.

Fluid that is occupying a fissure, as occurs in congestive heart failure or pleural effusion from other causes, often creates perfusion defects (pseudotumors). Perfusion defects that correspond to the fissures are by definition peripheral and pleural based; therefore, they resemble pulmonary emboli. However, defects caused by pleural fluid are very broad based and are not wedge shaped. They do not correspond well to the pulmonary bronchovascular tree anatomy. These characteristics are atypical of acute pulmonary embolism.

If the fluid is loculated, the perfusion defect will remain unchanged on both supine and upright studies. These defects can be difficult to differentiate from pulmonary emboli. Free-flowing fluid will move as the patient changes position from supine to upright or vice versa. Lateral views of both lungs in the upright and the supine projections are often helpful in determining if fluid is loculated or free flowing.

CASE 144

History.—25-year-old woman with chest pain.

Scan.—^{133}Xe and ^{99m}Tc MAA lung scan.

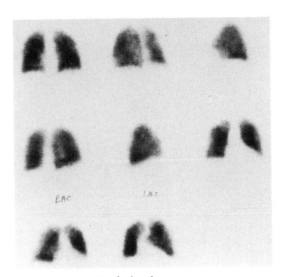

Perfusion images.

Findings.—Ventilation (not shown) was normal. Multiple small perfusion defects are present.

Diagnosis.—Low probability for acute pulmonary embolism.

The three most widely used schemes for the interpretation of V/Q scans are the Biello, McNeil, and PIOPED criteria. Although there are differences in each, all give results expressed as normal, low, indeterminate or intermediate, and high probability for acute pulmonary embolus. The PIOPED criteria add a very low probability category. All three sets of criteria classify multiple peripheral, wedge-shaped perfusion abnormalities in areas of normal ventilation as high probability for pulmonary embolus. The size and location of the defects in relation to the bronchopulmonary segments are important, however. With the Biello and PIOPED schemes, perfusion defects are categorized as small, moderate, or large. The definitions for these vary between criteria and are somewhat subjective. Regardless, only moderate and large perfusion defects are considered worrisome for pulmonary embolism.

The McNeil criteria consider a subsegmental defect to be anything less than a segment. No sizing is done. By the McNeil criteria, multiple V/Q mismatches of subsegmental defects in areas normal on chest radiograph can carry a probability of low to moderate. Both the Biello and PIOPED criteria define a small defect as 25% or less of a bronchopulmonary segment. By the Biello criteria, small V/Q mismatches are considered low probability, regardless of number. The PIOPED criteria are more complex. Three or fewer small perfusion defects in areas normal on chest radiograph are very low probability, regardless of ventilation. Greater than three small perfusion defects are low probability, regardless of the chest radiograph and ventilation.

Low probability scans generally mean the patient has less than a 15% to 20% chance of having a pulmonary embolus. Does this mean pulmonary angiography is necessary in these cases? Usually it does not. McNeil has shown that when the clinical suspicion of pulmonary embolus is low or average, only a few patients with low probability scans will have pulmonary embolus. Second, it appears that emboli with a low probability pattern may have a different significance than other pulmonary emboli. Follow-up of patients with low probability scans who were not treated with anticoagulants have shown virtually no evidence of morbidity, mortality, or recurrence of deep vein thrombosis or pulmonary embolus.

CASE 145

History.— 22-year-old man involved in motorcycle accident 3 days earlier, who sustained multiple fractures. He now has increased shortness of breath.

Scan.—^{133}Xe and ^{99m}Tc MAA lung scan.

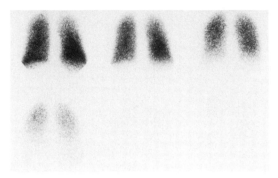

Ventilation scan.

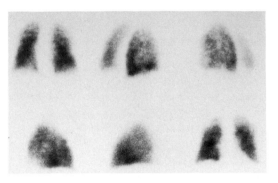

Perfusion scan.

Findings.— Ventilation: homogeneous single-breath without retention. Perfusion: multiple small defects.

Diagnosis.— Low probability for thromboembolic disease; multiple fat emboli.

Nearly all fat emboli result from trauma. Fat embolism is most common in young people with leg fractures sustained in motor vehicle accidents, the elderly with hip fractures, and in patients after arthroplasty. Less common causes of fat embolism include pancreatitis, severe burns, acute fatty liver from alcoholism, corticosteroid therapy, and sickle crisis with bone marrow infarction.

Fat embolism after acute trauma is common. Histologically proved (intra-alveolar hemorrhage and edema, lipid vacuoles in alveoli and alveolar capillaries) but clinically insignificant fat emboli may be present in 67% to 97% of cases of acute fracture patients. Clinically significant fat emboli occur in only about 6% of cases.

Fat emboli originate in the bone marrow, entering the circulation via torn veins at the fracture site. The fat is transported to the lungs as neutral triglycerides. Within the lungs, lipases convert the triglycerides into chemically active fatty acids, leading to congestion, edema, and intra-alveolar hemorrhage. Hydrolysis of coalesced chylomicrons into free fatty acids by pulmonary lipases may also play a role in the pathogenesis of fat emboli. From the lungs, fat droplets enter the systemic circulation and form emboli in other organs, especially the brain, kidneys, and skin.

The clinical manifestations of fat emboli can be divided into those arising from the lungs and those arising from other involved viscera, usually the central nervous system. Symptoms usually become manifest 1 to 2 days after the trauma. Signs and symptoms of pulmonary involvement include cough, dyspnea, tachypnea, hemoptysis, pleuritic pain, tachycardia, rales, and rhonchi. Manifestations of CNS involvement include confusion, restlessness, stupor, delirium, and coma. Petechiae are seen with skin involvement, most commonly along the anterior axillary folds, conjunctiva, and retina. The classic clinical triad of petechial rash, cerebral manifestations, and pulmonary symptoms approximately 1 to 2 days after trauma are virtually pathognomonic for fat embolism. Laboratory findings include hypoxemia, hypocalcemia, and lipiduria, all of which are variably present.

The chest radiograph is frequently normal in patients with fat emboli syndrome. When abnormal, the chest film shows widespread airspace consolidation (due to alveolar hemorrhage and edema), often with discrete acinar shadows. The distribution is predominantly peripheral and basilar, and signs of cardiogenic edema are usually absent. The time lapse between trauma and radiographic findings is the same as for the development of clinical signs and symptoms, generally 1 to 2 days.

The radionuclide lung scan may show perfusion abnormalities in the involved parenchyma, leading to V/Q mismatches. The perfusion defects tend to be small and peripheral.

Posttraumatic V/Q scans to evaluate for acute pulmonary thromboembolism are common. The above findings on V/Q scan should alert one to the possibility of fat emboli, especially on the second and third posttrauma days.

CASE 146

History.— 37-year-old man with progressive dyspnea and the onset of pleuritic chest pain. The patient's family had a history of "lung problems." We are asked to evaluate for acute pulmonary embolus.

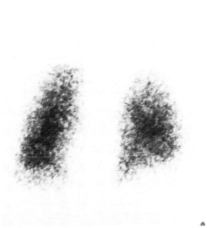

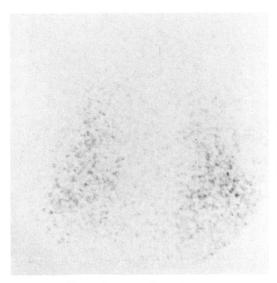

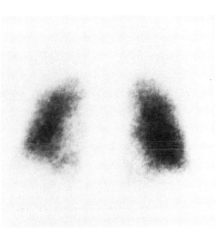

Single-breath image.   **Five-minute washout image.**   **Posterior perfusion image.**

Findings.— Ventilation: Retention at both lung bases. Perfusion: normal.

Diagnosis.—α_1-Antitrypsin deficiency.

Chronic bronchitis and emphysema are common conditions that fall under the classification of chronic obstructive pulmonary disease (COPD). These diseases are generally caused by cigarette smoking.

Alpha-1-antitrypsin deficiency (α_1-ATD) is an inherited disorder associated with α_1-AT levels less than 50 mg/dL and COPD. Although the homozygous form of the disease is rare, heterozygotes are common and have been reported in between 2% and 14% of the general population.

α_1-ATD is associated with the panacinar form of emphysema. In emphysema, widely varying patterns of ventilatory abnormalities have been described. They range from predominantly upper lobe disease in centrilobular emphysema, to predominantly lower lobe disease in panlobular emphysema, to diffuse involvement in severe disease. Because α_1-ATD is associated with panlobular emphysema, it is not surprising that the predominant ventilation abnormality is retention of ^{133}Xe in the lung bases. This finding is present in virtually all homozygotes, as well as in a significant portion of heterozygotes (α_1-AT levels, 50–150 mg%) with known or suspected lung disease. In asymptomatic heterozygotes, a substantial percentage aged 34 years or older will also show retention in the lung bases, whereas asymptomatic heterozygotes younger than 27 years old do not.

Slow pulmonary clearance of xenon is also present in patients with α_1-ATD. Slow clearance is a slightly more common finding than basilar retention, and like basilar retention, it is frequently seen in homozygotes, heterozygotes with known lung disease, and asymptomatic heterozygotes 34 years or older. Like basilar abnormalities, slow clearance is uncommon in younger asymptomatic heterozygotes.

Basilar retention of ^{133}Xe and slow pulmonary clearance are not limited to patients with α_1-ATD; these findings are also seen in emphysema patients with normal levels of α_1-AT. Basilar perfusion abnormalities corresponding to the ventilatory abnormalities are frequently seen in patients with α_1-ATD, although abnormalities in perfusion may be present elsewhere as well.

CASE 147

History.—Obese woman with right-sided pleuritic chest pain.

Scan.—^{133}Xe ventilation scan and^{99m}Tc MAA lung scan.

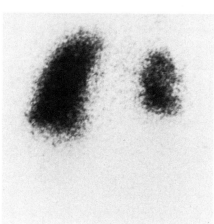

Posterior single-breath image.

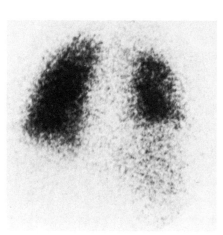

Posterior 1-minute washout image.

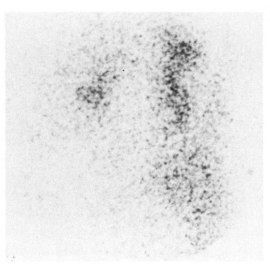

Posterior 4-minute washout image.

Findings.—Prolonged retention of ^{133}Xe in the region of the right lung base. Perfusion scan (not shown) was normal.

Diagnosis.—Hepatic steatosis.

Hepatic steatosis is associated with a variety of diseases. Lipid infiltration of the liver may have a variable symptom complex ranging from no symptoms to a picture simulating acute surgical abdomen. Obstructive jaundice and portal hypertension can occur; these can lead to the development of cirrhosis. Liver biopsy is the only definitive technique for establishing the diagnosis.

^{133}Xe retention in the fatty liver during the washout phase of a V/Q scan can simulate ^{133}Xe retention in the right lung base. When there is doubt as to the cause of this uptake, standard hepatic views in multiple projections can be obtained. The extent of ^{133}Xe uptake in the liver is closely correlated with the amount of histologically evident fatty infiltration.

Alcoholic fatty infiltration is a common cause of hepatic ^{133}Xe uptake. Other causes of fatty liver and hepatic ^{133}Xe activity include diabetes mellitus, obesity, and total parenteral nutrition. Patients with hypercholesterolemia or hypertriglyceridemia may show mild ^{133}Xe uptake in the liver as well. The more prominent the hepatic uptake, the more likely the cause is alcoholic or diabetic fatty infiltration (or both).

The patient had no alcoholic history and was not diabetic. In this case, the hepatic ^{133}Xe uptake was the result of obesity.

CASE 148

History.—59-year-old woman with new onset of pleuritic chest pain and shortness of breath. Injection of MAA was difficult, requiring several attempts.

Scan.—^{133}Xe and ^{99m}Tc MAA lung scan.

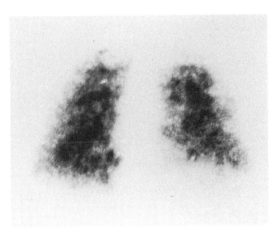

Anterior chest perfusion image.

Findings.— The ventilation study (not shown) was normal. The perfusion study is markedly abnormal. There are focal areas of intensely increased uptake at the periphery. There are also multiple perfusion defects.

Diagnosis.—This is a nondiagnostic perfusion study, secondary to "hot" clots of ^{99m}Tc MAA and too few particles.

Technical artifacts may be easily missed on ventilation scans because they mimic disease processes. Occasionally ^{133}Xe is retained in the spirometer tubing or the patient's oropharynx, which can be misdiagnosed as chronic obstructive lung disease. Hangup of a bubble of intravenously injected ^{133}Xe dissolved in saline solution can occur in central vessels, simulating retention. Repeating the study can be helpful if an artifact is suspected.

Perfusion studies may be affected by several technical problems. The first problem, as seen here, is hot clots of ^{99m}Tc MAA. Hot clots are produced by drawing back blood into the syringe containing ^{99m}Tc MAA, forming radioactive clots, and then reinjecting into the patient. They can be prevented by gently shaking the syringe to resuspend the particles before injection and by not drawing blood into the MAA-containing syringe. Hot clots may also be produced by injecting the MAA through a vein involved with thrombophlebitis.

As seen here, hot clots can produce perfusion defects that mimic pulmonary emboli. When this occurs, interpretation of the V/Q scan is difficult, and the scan has a higher likelihood of being falsely positive. Repeating the perfusion study 18 to 24 hours later is recommended.

Another potential technical problem with ^{99m}Tc MAA perfusion scans involves particle number. The minimum number of particles required to obtain homogeneous distribution of radioactivity in the pulmonary vascular bed is 60,000. With most instant kits, approximately 500,000 particles of MAA are labeled unless steps are taken to reduce the number of particles (e.g., for children, patients with severe pulmonary hypertension, and right-to-left shunt). Infiltration of a normal dose can result in too few particles being delivered to the pulmonary capillary bed. In this situation, the perfusion scan appears grossly mottled, with numerous small perfusion defects throughout both lungs, and a generalized decrease in pulmonary uptake. An image over the injection site will confirm infiltration of a portion of the dose. It is not necessary to wait before repeating the perfusion scan.

CASE 149

History.— 58-year-old man with a history of lung carcinoma.

Scan.—^{133}Xe and ^{99m}Tc MAA lung scan.

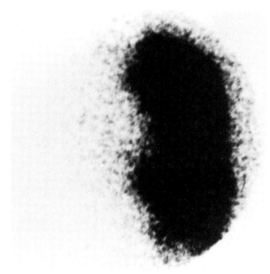

**Posterior view of chest during
single-breath ventilation.**

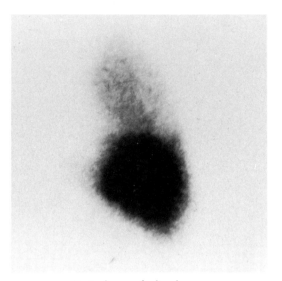

Posterior perfusion image.

Findings.— Ventilation: absent ventilation on left; perfusion: no
perfusion to left lobe.

Diagnosis.— Postpneumonectomy.

Bronchogenic carcinoma can produce abnormal ventilation and perfusion on a standard V/Q lung scan. Because virtually all lung cancer patients have a long history of heavy tobacco use and COPD, their ventilation studies often show retention of ^{133}Xe. Tumors that obstruct the airway also produce abnormal ventilation. When airway obstruction is present, decreased uptake on the single-breath image and retention on the washout images are seen, just as would occur with foreign body obstruction.

Lung cancers derive their blood supply from the bronchial arteries, not the pulmonary arteries. Because the perfusion lung scan assesses pulmonary artery flow, vascular compression from lung tumors can cause perfusion defects. When the involved vessels are near the hilum, segmental, lobar, or even whole lung, defects can be produced. Because extrabronchial spread of lung cancer is generally more widespread than endobronchial obstruction, the perfusion study is usually more affected than the ventilation study.

As mentioned, complete absence of perfusion to one lung can be produced by lung cancer; it may show also unilaterally decreased perfusion. The differential diagnosis for unilaterally decreased perfusion includes congenital heart disease after shunt procedure, postpneumonectomy, severe pleural or parenchymal disease, and, less frequently, pulmonary embolus.

CASE 150

History.—61-year-old man with COPD and newly diagnosed lung cancer involving the left lobe. A quantitative V/Q scan was done to determine if pneumonectomy was clinically possible. Preoperative FEV_1 was 3.0.

Scan.—^{133}Xe and ^{99m}Tc MAA lung scan.

**Posterior and right posterior oblique
perfusion images.**

Findings.—Ventilation (not shown) matched perfusion. MAA scan shows small area of perfusion to left upper lobe, with good perfusion to the right lobe. Split perfusion was 85% right and 15% left.

Diagnosis.—Operative candidate.

The V/Q lung scan is most often used to evaluate patients with suspected pulmonary embolism. However, the V/Q scan is also helpful in the preoperative evaluation of patients scheduled for pneumonectomy. Generally these patients have a long history of heavy tobacco use, leading to chronic obstructive pulmonary disease (COPD) and bronchogenic carcinoma. Patients with advanced disease are considered inoperable; however, surgical cure is attempted in patients with early disease that has not yet spread. The quantitative V/Q scan is part of the preoperative evaluation of patients for pneumonectomy and can determine if the patient's remaining diseased lung is adequate for the patient's survival.

The scan is acquired similarly to the usual V/Q scan for pulmonary emboli but is recorded on a computer. The ventilation study is acquired using ^{133}Xe gas. Single-breath, equilibrium, and washout images are obtained from the posterior projection. The perfusion study is then acquired with ^{99m}Tc MAA using the eight standard projections.

Regions of interest are then drawn over the left and right lungs in the anterior and posterior projections for both the ventilation (single-breath) and perfusion studies. The geometric mean is calculated for each lung. Thus, the amount of ventilation and perfusion going to each lung is quantitated. In addition, V/Q matches or mismatches are recorded.

The interpretation of the quantitative V/Q scan is different from that of the scan done for acute pulmonary embolus. Given the patient population on which the quantitative V/Q scan is performed, ventilation, perfusion, and chest radiograph abnormalities are all commonly seen; therefore, no comment is made on the probability for acute pulmonary embolus. The quantitative V/Q scan is obtained to assess regional pulmonary blood flow and viability. Because these patients generally have decreased pulmonary reserve, they are at high risk for operative and postoperative pulmonary complications. Often their oxygen-exchanging capabilities are marginal before surgery, and removal of the diseased lung segment may itself be life-threatening or even fatal. By multiplying the percentage of lung function in the noncancerous lung by the forced expiratory volume at 1 second, the forced expiratory volume in 1 second (FEV_1) after surgery can be determined. FEV_1 values less than 0.8 to 1.0 L/sec are not considered adequate for survival. These patients are not surgical candidates in spite of their small lung cancers.

CASE 151

History.—Burn patient with respiratory symptoms.

Scan.—^{133}Xe in saline solution scan.

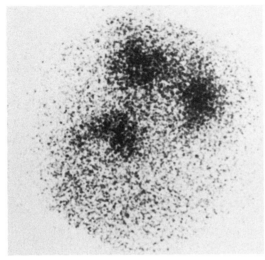

^{133}Xe saline solution ventilation washout
image at 4 minutes.

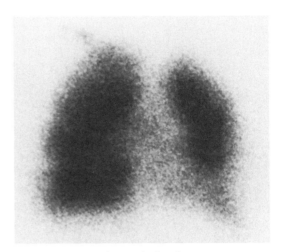

Anterior perfusion image.

Findings.—Focal areas of ^{133}Xe retention.

Diagnosis.—Smoke inhalation injury.

Smoke inhalation is a syndrome characterized by acute laryngotracheobronchitis, with bronchospasm and bronchorrhea. These effects are thought to be caused by combustion products, including sulfur dioxide, nitrogen dioxide, toluene dioxocyanate, hydrocyanide, and hydrochloric acid, which, like smoke itself, are potent bronchoconstrictors and tissue irritants. The severity of the injury is related to both the concentration and duration of exposure to the offending agents.

Inhalation injury predisposes the respiratory tract to infection and causes a significant increase in the mortality associated with burns. Generally, early diagnosis is made on the basis of clinical findings (e.g., the presence of facial, neck, or shoulder burns, singed nasal hairs, intraoral burns, carbonaceous sputum, wheezing). Although the pulmonary damage may be obvious on initial examination, signs of inhalation injury often do not become evident until later in the postburn period, and occasionally they are seen only at autopsy. Early diagnosis allows immediate therapy, helping to minimize complications.

Because inhalation injuries affect primarily the airways, the ^{133}Xe ventilation study is useful in diagnosing the disease. It is most useful when done before the fourth postburn day when clinical and radiographic signs of inhalation injury are often absent.

If the patient is cooperative, the ventilation study can be performed in the usual manner, with the patient inhaling ^{133}Xe gas. Single-breath, equilibrium, and washout images are obtained in the posterior projection. Pediatric patients and those with intubated airways can be studied using intravenous injection of ^{133}Xe dissolved in saline solution.

The predominant finding of inhalation injury on ventilation study is prolonged focal retention of ^{133}Xe. Inhalational injuries rarely cause diffuse retention. An abnormal ventilation study indicates a poor prognosis for patients with inhalation injury because their mortality approaches 60%, whereas the mortality of burn patients with normal ventilation studies is slightly less than 30%.

CASE 152

History.—63-year-old man with adenocarcinoma of the colon metastatic to the liver. He had recurrent right-sided pleural effusions and ascites. We were asked to evaluate for transdiaphragmatic communication.

Scan.—One millicurie of ^{99m}Tc MAA was injected intraperitoneally. Images over the abdomen and chest were obtained after thoracentesis.

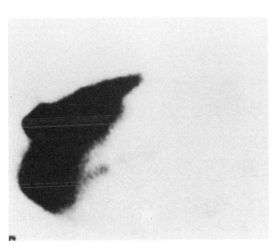

Immediate postinjection image of upper half of abdomen and lower half of chest.

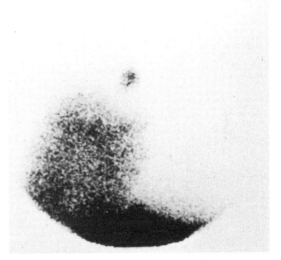

Two-hour anterior image of chest.

Findings.—The initial image shows widespread activity corresponding to the peritoneal cavity. A 2-hour delay image of the anterior chest and abdomen shows activity throughout the right hemithorax, in addition to abdominal activity.

Diagnosis.—Abnormal diaphragmatic communication between the right hemithorax and the peritoneal cavity.

Recurrent pleural effusions can result from a variety of causes. Frequently these patients have either a primary thoracic or abdominal malignancy, or they suffer from severe liver disease, such as cirrhosis. Clinically the effusions reaccumulate rapidly and can be significant management problems. If the patient has ascites, nuclear medicine imaging can determine if peritoneal fluid is crossing the diaphragm into the thoracic cavity, causing the recurrent effusions.

Isotope is injected into the peritoneum and then followed to see if it moves into the chest. ^{99m}Tc MAA commonly is used. Imaging of the abdomen is performed to check for appropriate placement of the isotope. If the activity is in a loculation, a second injection must be done.

We then perform a thoracentesis immediately after the intraperitoneal dose of ^{99m}Tc MAA. If the pleural effusion is drained, the pressure in the thorax will be more negative with respect to the peritoneum, increasing the pressure gradient from peritoneum to pleural space. This facilitates the movement of ^{99m}Tc MAA across the diaphragm, increasing the sensitivity of the study for detecting diaphragmatic leaks.

CHAPTER 7

Hematologic

CASE 153

History.— 20-year-old patient with lymphoma.

Scan.—^{67}Ga citrate.

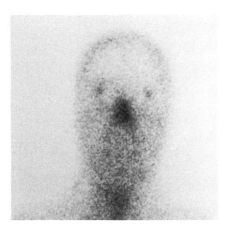
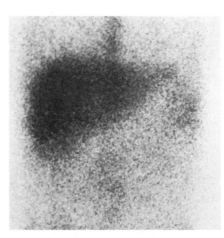
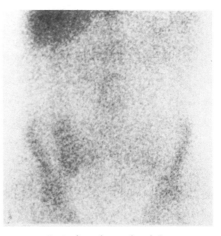

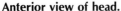

Anterior view of head.   **Anterior view of abdomen.**   **Anterior view of pelvis.**

Findings.— Uptake in lacrimal glands and GI tract. No abnormal areas of uptake.

Diagnosis.— Normal ^{67}Ga scan.

Gallium 67 is used to localize inflammatory lesions and some tumors. It has a half-life of 78 hours and decays by electron capture with photon energies of 93, 184, 296, and 388 keV.

After intravenous injection, ^{67}Ga binds to transferrin. This is the plasma protein responsible for iron transport in the blood. If a patient has hemochromatosis, which saturates the transferrin iron binding sites, a larger portion of the injected ^{67}Ga will be excreted through the kidneys, resulting in less soft tissue activity.

The main route of excretion of ^{67}Ga during the first 24 hours is the kidneys. Fifteen percent to 25% of the injected dose is excreted in the urine during this time. A small amount of activity may be seen in the kidneys on 48-hour images. After 48 hours, renal activity is abnormal. The colon becomes the main route of excretion after 24 hours. The colon is the critical organ, receiving 0.6 to 0.9 rad/mCi.

The biodistribution of ^{67}Ga is related to the concentration of lactoferrin in tissues. Lactoferrin is a protein with a high affinity for ^{67}Ga. It is found in high concentrations in lacrimal and salivary glands, the nasopharynx, bone marrow, and the spleen. Neutrophils have a high concentration of lactoferrin, which partly explains ^{67}Ga accumulation in abscesses. How-ever, ^{67}Ga accumulates even in sterile abscesses. The liver metabolizes both transferrin and lactoferrin, explaining ^{67}Ga activity seen there.

Tumor uptake of ^{67}Ga occurs because of specific transferrin receptors on certain tumor cell surfaces. The ^{67}Ga-transferrin complex is then taken up intact, with ^{67}Ga being deposited intracellularly.

In a normal patient, the ^{67}Ga scan shows prominent soft tissue activity on early images. Bowel activity should move and become less intense with time. Occasionally normal bowel activity will appear quite intense and mimic diffuse inflammatory bowel disease.

There is increased ^{67}Ga activity in the salivary glands and lacrimal glands. The breasts can accumulate ^{67}Ga, especially under the hormonal stimulation of pregnancy, menarche, or oral contraceptive use. The liver and spleen are commonly seen, as well as the thymus.

The lungs show prominent activity on early images, which normally fades with time. Prominent pulmonary activity may be seen if the patient has had a recent lymphangiogram.

^{67}Ga is a weak bone agent and will accumulate in the epiphyses of children. Uptake in the sternum of adults can mimic a mediastinal tumor.

CASE 154

History.— 29-year-old HIV-positive man with fever and productive cough.

Scan.— ^{67}Ga scan.

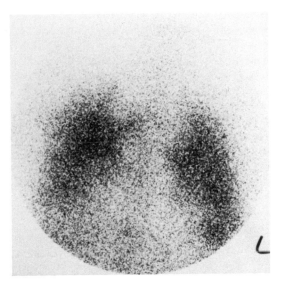

Anterior view of chest.

Findings.   Diffusely increased pulmonary uptake of ^{67}Ga.

Diagnosis.— AIDS, PCP.

The diagnosis of *Pneumocystis carinii* pneumonia (PCP) in a patient with acquired immunodeficiency syndrome (AIDS) can be difficult. The clinical findings of fever and respiratory symptoms are nonspecific. Appropriate therapy for PCP, when instituted early, can be of significant benefit to the patient.

PCP is a common infection in AIDS patients. Clinical symptoms are often out of proportion to the chest radiograph findings; up to one third of AIDS patients with documented PCP will have normal or equivocal chest radiographs. In such cases, a ^{67}Ga scan can be helpful. ^{67}Ga has the added benefit of accumulating in lymphoma, bacterial pneumonias, and other opportunistic infections.

^{67}Ga scan findings of PCP are increased heterogeneous or homogeneous diffuse pulmonary uptake. The likelihood of PCP increases if the chest radiograph is normal in the face of significant ^{67}Ga accumulation. Focal patterns of uptake are also seen in PCP, but a significant number of these patients will have bacterial pneumonia. If there is focal uptake in the hilar area, lymphadenopathy associated with lymphoma or mycobacterial disease should be considered.

The sensitivity of ^{67}Ga scanning for PCP when any intrapulmonary uptake is considered abnormal is greater than 90%; the specificity is about 75%. The positive predictive value of an abnormal finding representing PCP, however, is only about 60%. The negative predictive value for PCP in a patient with a normal ^{67}Ga scan is greater than 90%. Thus, a normal ^{67}Ga scan makes it very unlikely that a patient has PCP.

With pulmonary uptake of ^{67}Ga, further work-up with sputum examination, bronchoscopy, or both may be indicated. If lymphadenopathy is suspected, lymph node biopsy should be considered.

Kaposi's sarcoma can manifest with diffuse pulmonary abnormalities on chest radiograph. ^{67}Ga scans are normal in this disease.

CASE 155

History.—Postoperative patient with fever.

Scan.—^{67}Ga citrate scan.

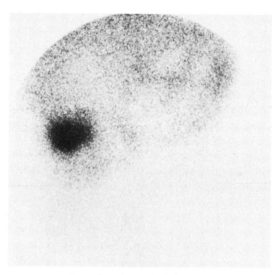

Anterior view of abdomen.

Findings.—Focal uptake right lower quadrant. No change over several days.

Diagnosis.—Intra-abdominal abscess.

In patients with localizing signs of an abscess, ultrasound or computed tomography (CT) should be performed. In true fever of unknown origin in which the site of infection is unknown, radionuclide imaging is useful because it evaluates the entire body. A recent study showed that even when the abdomen was the suspected site of infection, the actual site was outside the abdomen in 20% of cases.

Three different radiopharmaceuticals are available for imaging inflammatory lesions: ^{67}Ga citrate, leukocytes labeled with indium 111, or technetium 99m and radiolabeled antibodies. Each has advantages and disadvantages.

The ability of ^{67}Ga to accumulate in inflammatory lesions has been known for many years. ^{67}Ga has a high affinity for both transferrin and lactoferrin. After IV injection, ^{67}Ga is bound to circulating transferrin, the same protein responsible for transporting iron in the blood. The affinity of ^{67}Ga for lactoferrin explains its accumulation in abscesses because of high lactoferrin levels in neutrophils. ^{67}Ga can also accumulate in bacteria themselves, independent of the presence of neutrophils. In fact, neutropenic animals with abscesses will still accumulate ^{67}Ga.

The sensitivity of ^{67}Ga scans for abdominal abscesses is 80% to 90%, but with a significant number of false positive results. To improve specificity, one must have knowledge of the normal physiologic excretion of ^{67}Ga. Fifteen percent to 25% of the administered ^{67}Ga dose is excreted by the kidneys during the first 24 hours. Any renal activity after 48 hours in a patient with normal renal function is abnormal. After 24 hours, the colon becomes the major route of excretion. Activity excreted through the colon should decrease and move with time as opposed to an abscess that increases with time and remains stationary. Intense cecal activity is common and should not be mistaken for an abscess. The need for bowel preparation is debatable. Attempts at eliminating colonic activity using laxatives or enemas have been disappointing.

The liver accumulates ^{67}Ga because of the normal hepatic metabolism of transferrin and lactoferrin. A ^{99m}Tc sulfur colloid liver-spleen scan performed as part of this examination helps differentiate normal liver and spleen from an inflammatory focus, which frequently has uptake equal to the surrounding liver.

Because of the delay in physiologic excretion of ^{67}Ga from the gastrointestinal (GI) tract, localization of an abdominal abscess may take several days. This time delay is often unacceptable. The leukocyte scan is a better choice in most cases when an abdominal process is suspected. It has no normal gastrointestinal excretion to confuse interpretation. The leukocyte scan can be performed within 24 hours or less of injection and has sensitivity and specificity equal or superior to the ^{67}Ga scan.

CASE 156

History.— 62-year-old diabetic patient with right great toe swelling.

Scan.—^{67}Ga scan before and after therapy.

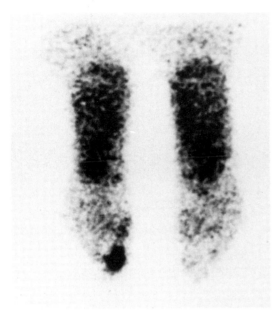

^{67}Ga scan of feet at onset of therapy.

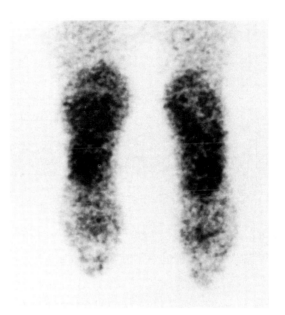

^{67}Ga scan of feet after 6 weeks of antibiotic therapy.

Findings.— Pretherapy scan: increased uptake right great toe.
Posttherapy scan: decreased activity.

Diagnosis.— Osteomyelitis responding to treatment.

^{67}Ga scanning is a valuable tool in the evaluation of patients with suspected osteomyelitis. It is often done in combination with a ^{99m}Tc methylene diphosphate (MDP) bone scan.

Plain films for osteomyelitis are normal early in the disease and become abnormal only after 10 to 14 days. The early diagnosis of osteomyelitis has become an important goal, because if appropriate antibiotic therapy is instituted early, the likelihood of chronic osteomyelitis is significantly decreased.

The diagnosis of osteomyelitis is complicated in the postorthopedic surgery patient. In these cases, bone scans are frequently not helpful. Bone scans normally show increased activity because of the increase in bony turnover after surgery. Even four-phase bone scans are abnormal whether or not the patient has osteomyelitis.

^{67}Ga has a sensitivity of nearly 100% in such postoperative cases, with a specificity, however, of only 25%. If the ^{67}Ga scan is normal, osteomyelitis can be effectively excluded. Also, if the degree of ^{67}Ga accumulation in the area of inter-est exceeds that of the bone scan or is in a different distribution from that of the bone scan, osteomyelitis is very likely. Leukocyte scans, by comparison, have a sensitivity of 60% to 100%, with a specificity of 97% for osteomyelitis in the postoperative patient. False positive leukocyte scans occur if there is an associated acute fracture or other noninfectious inflammatory process such as rheumatoid arthritis or heterotopic bone.

^{67}Ga scans can be used to follow patients with known bone infection. The degree of ^{67}Ga accumulation on serial scans of chronic osteomyelitis patients undergoing therapy have been shown to parallel the likelihood of recurrence of infection. If the ^{67}Ga scan returns to normal in such patients, it is likely that the patient has been adequately treated and the infection will not recur.

^{67}Ga scans appear to compete well with ^{111}In leukocytes scans in the evaluation of osteomyelitis of the spine. The sensitivity of leukocyte scans for chronic osteomyelitis of the central skeleton may be decreased.

CASE 157

History.—61-year-old man with lung cancer.

Scan.—^{67}Ga citrate scan.

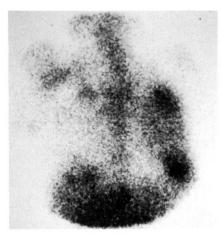

Anterior chest image of 72-hour ^{67}Ga scan.

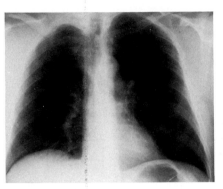

**Posteroanterior chest radiograph
6 months earlier.**

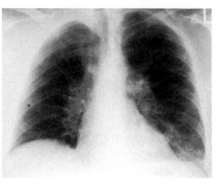

**Posteroanterior chest radiograph at time of
^{67}Ga scan.**

Findings.—Significant pulmonary uptake, left lung greater
than right.

Diagnosis.—Lung cancer with lymphangitic spread.

^{67}Ga uptake is seen in a variety of inflammatory and malignant conditions. In general, sarcoid and inflammatory lesions show greater ^{67}Ga uptake than carcinoma does.

Lung cancer accumulates ^{67}Ga. Because pulmonary background activity is low and tumor uptake of ^{67}Ga is high, ^{67}Ga scanning has been shown to be sensitive for detecting lung cancer. From 88% to 96% of primary lung cancers can be detected by ^{67}Ga scan. Most lesions that remain undetected are smaller than 2 cm. Although sensitivity for lung lesions is high, the specificity for malignant lung lesions is significantly less, approximately 50%, because of affinity of ^{67}Ga for nonmalignant, inflammatory lung lesions.

There is conflicting evidence regarding the efficacy of using ^{67}Ga scanning for the detection of distant metatases from a primary lung cancer. The use of ^{67}Ga for staging lung cancer is also controversial. Numerous studies have been performed and have given conflicting results. Single-photon emission computed tomography (SPECT) improves the accuracy of ^{67}Ga imaging for staging. At present, ^{67}Ga is not used frequently for preoperative staging.

CASE 158

History.— 22-year-old patient previously treated for lymphoma, who now has night sweats and fever.

Scan.—^{67}Ga citrate planar scan and ^{99m}Tc sulfur colloid scan.

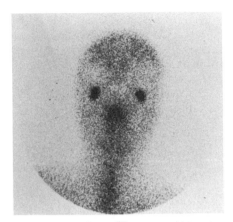

Anterior 72-hour ^{67}Ga scan of head.

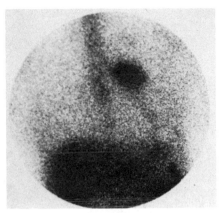

Anterior ^{67}Ga scan of chest.

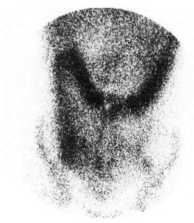

Anterior ^{67}Ga scan of abdomen.

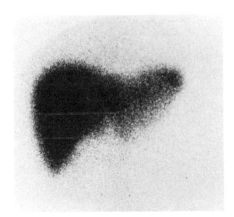

Anterior ^{99m}Tc sulfur colloid liver-spleen scan.

Findings.—^{67}Ga scan: focal uptake in left side of chest, with physiologic uptake in lacrimals and GI tract; ^{99m}Tc. Sulfur colloid scan: postsplenectomy.

Diagnosis.—Recurrent lymphoma.

^{67}Ga citrate is taken up by a number of malignant tumors, including lymphoma, hepatoma, lung cancer, melanoma, head and neck cancers (squamous cell and adenocarcinoma), sarcomas, leukemias (acute lymphocytic and myelogenous leukemia), and some GI cancers.

^{67}Ga is taken up by both Hodgkin's and non-Hodgkin's lymphomas. Overall sensitivity and specificity of ^{67}Ga scanning for lymphoma using high doses (7–10 mCi) and imaging on at least three photopeaks are approximately 90%. Accuracy by site of involvement is approximately 96%. ^{67}Ga is more sensitive in high-grade lymphomas and may be a useful adjunct to CT scanning in evaluating both the abdominal and mediastinal lymphatic chains.

Overall, ^{67}Ga's detection rate of non-Hodgkin's lymphoma is significantly lower than for Hodgkin's lymphoma. In non-Hodgkin's lymphoma, the sensitivity of the ^{67}Ga scan is highest in untreated histiocytic lymphoma and lowest in well-differentiated lymphocytic lymphoma. In both Hodgkin's and non-Hodgkin's lymphomas, the axillary, inguinal, abdominal, and pelvic nodes all are less accurately evaluated by ^{67}Ga than by lymphangiography.

^{67}Ga scanning can play a role in the follow-up of lymphoma patients. Although the sensitivity of ^{67}Ga is lower in posttherapy patients, an abnormal scan in those with nonspecific symptoms of recurrence (e.g., fever) can be helpful in directing further diagnostic or therapeutic measures.

CASE 159

History.— 49-year-old woman with fever and weight loss.

Scan.— ^{67}Ga citrate scan and chest x-ray.

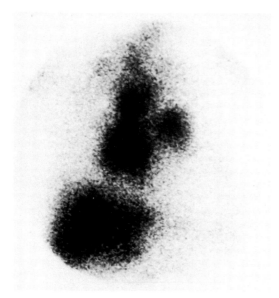

Anterior 72-hour Ga scan of chest.

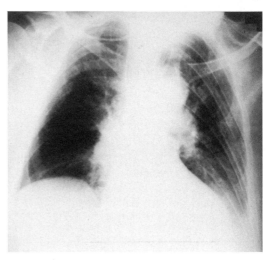

Posteroanterior chest radiograph.

Findings.— ^{67}Ga scan: increased mediastinal and left hilar uptake.
Chest x-ray: similar finding.

Diagnosis.— Sarcoidosis.

Sarcoidosis is characterized by noncaseating granulomas that can affect any organ system. The mediastinal lymph nodes and pulmonary parenchyma are frequently affected.

Sarcoidosis is caused by an amplified immune response to an inciting agent. The immune response involves primarily pulmonary macrophages and T lymphocytes, with a cytokine-mediated immune reaction. The result is the formation of a granuloma consisting of central macrophages, epithelioid and multinucleated giant cells, surrounded by lymphocytes, monocytes, and fibroblasts.

Chest radiograph changes of sarcoidosis involve both the parenchyma and lymph nodes. Bilateral hilar lymph node enlargement is the classic finding in sarcoid. Mediastinal lymph nodes may also be involved. Parenchymal disease usually manifests itself as small, irregular, nodular shadows, predominantly in the upper lobes.

In normal individuals, ^{67}Ga activity in the lungs is the same as that in the soft tissues of the neck and shoulders. With sarcoidosis, ^{67}Ga uptake may be seen in the mediastinal lymph nodes, producing the α sign, activity similar in appearance to the Greek letter α. The pulmonary parenchyma may also show ^{67}Ga activity in areas of radiographic abnormality. ^{67}Ga uptake is generally not evident in areas of normal radiographic appearance.

The response of sarcoid to therapy can be followed with ^{67}Ga scintigraphy. Uptake of ^{67}Ga either decreases or resolves with successful treatment. ^{67}Ga uptake does not correspond to the clinical picture, however. Both symptomatic and asymptomatic patients can show ^{67}Ga activity with no significant difference in the nature of uptake.

CASE 160

History.—52-year-old man with history of pulmonary fibrosis. We are asked to judge efficacy of corticosteroid therapy.

Scan.—Pretherapy and posttherapy ^{67}Ga citrate scans.

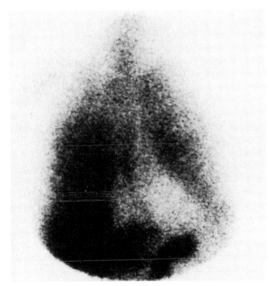

Anterior 72-hour ^{67}Ga image of chest.

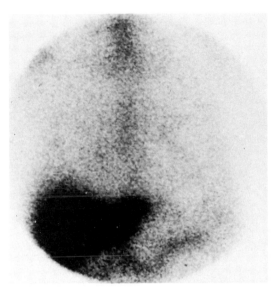

Anterior ^{67}Ga image of chest 2 months later.

Findings.—Pretherapy scan: diffuse pulmonary uptake equal to liver. Posttherapy scan: clearing of previous activity.

Diagnosis.—Interstitial lung disease improving with therapy.

Bilateral diffuse pulmonary uptake of ^{67}Ga occurs in a number of diseases and can be a normal variant. In the first 24 hours after injection, lung uptake of ^{67}Ga is common; it usually resolves on later images. The irritation of the contrast media of a lymphangiogram can also result in ^{67}Ga uptake. If ^{67}Ga imaging and lymphangiogram are used as part of the staging process in lymphoma, the ^{67}Ga scan should be done first. Drugs such as busulfan, cyclophosphamide, and amiodarone can also irritate the lung, resulting in ^{67}Ga accumulation.

Pneumocystis carinii infection in AIDS and other immunocompromised patients has become a common cause of ^{67}Ga pulmonary uptake. *P. carinii* pneumonia should be strongly suspected if significant ^{67}Ga accumulation is seen in the face of a normal chest radiograph.

Other causes of diffuse ^{67}Ga uptake in the lungs include bacterial pneumonia, tuberculosis, lymphangitic spread of tumor (lymphoma, lung, breast), pneumoconiosis, sarcoidosis, radiation therapy, and uremia.

Pulmonary fibrosis produces interstitial pulmonary parenchymal inflammation. ^{67}Ga accumulates in the lungs of patients with pulmonary fibrosis and is associated with the active inflammatory state. In these patients, ^{67}Ga uptake correlates with the percentage of neutrophils in the bronchoalveolar lavage.

Patients undergoing treatment of interstitial lung disease can be followed using serial ^{67}Ga scans. Rather than using the degree of uptake as judged visually, some type of index is usually calculated. This is done by drawing areas of interest over the lung and liver and calculating a ratio.

CASE 161

History.— 54-year-old alcoholic with abdominal pain and
increasing ascites.

Scan.—^{99m}Tc sulfur colloid and ^{67}Ga citrate scans.

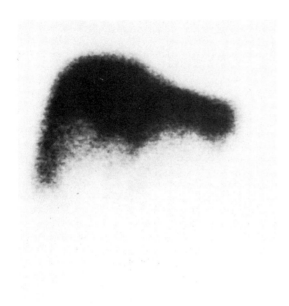

^{99m}Tc sulfur colloid liver scan.

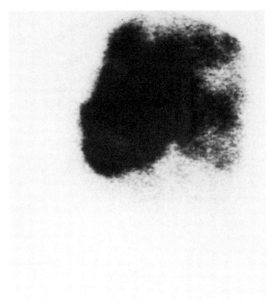

Anterior 72-hour ^{67}Ga scan of abdomen.

Findings.—^{99m}Tc sulfur colloid: cold defect in inferior portion of
right lobe. ^{67}Ga: uptake in region of cold defect.

Diagnosis.— Hepatoma.

Tumors known to show ^{67}Ga uptake include both Hodgkin's and non-Hodgkin's lymphomas, hepatoma, bronchogenic carcinoma, melanoma, leukemias (acute lymphocytic and myelogenous), and some tumors of the gastrointestinal tract.

Gallium, like indium and aluminum, is a group IIIA element. Because most of its salts are physiologically insoluble, soluble ^{67}Ga citrate is the compound of choice for human use. ^{67}Ga citrate is administered intravenously. It binds to plasma proteins, primarily lactoferrin and haptoglobin. At acid pH, ^{67}Ga shows high lactoferrin avidity. Consequently it is found in lactoferrin-rich tissues, which include the lacrimal glands and tears, salivary glands, nasopharynx, marrow, spleen, and gut. Hepatic uptake is also seen, probably because of hepatic lactoferrin and transferrin metabolism. The adrenal glands and lungs can also show ^{67}Ga uptake.

The mechanism of ^{67}Ga uptake by tumors and cause of variability of ^{67}Ga uptake between different tumor types is not known. Several factors may play a role, including transferrin receptor content, tumor viability, vascularity, permeability (either from neovascularity and inflammation or increased membrane pore size), histiocyte accumulation, tumor protein uptake of dissociated ^{67}Ga in a pH environment, and exchange of intracellular and extracellular ^{67}Ga pools. Elec-

tron microscopy shows prominent cytoplasmic ^{67}Ga uptake associated with lysozyme-like organelles. There is a correlation between the degree of ^{67}Ga uptake and the nuclear DNA content of tumors.

The usual adult dose of ^{67}Ga is 3 to 5 mCi; scanning is usually performed at 24 to 72 hours. For tumor imaging, this protocol is often modified to use a 10 mCi dose, with imaging at 2 to 7 days. Delayed imaging allows time for nonspecific GI tract activity to clear.

The association of alcoholic cirrhosis with hepatoma and their often similar clinical manifestations (abdominal mass, jaundice, ascites) make the clinical diagnosis of hepatoma difficult. The ^{67}Ga scan can help diagnose hepatoma when combined with ^{99m}Tc sulfur colloid liver scans. Hepatomas, because of the absence of Kupffer's cells, create cold defects on sulfur colloid liver scan. When these photopenic regions show ^{67}Ga uptake, hepatoma, as well as abscess and other causes, must be considered. If ^{67}Ga uptake is higher than surrounding hepatic uptake, hepatoma is likely. Conversely, if the lesion shows ^{67}Ga uptake less than the surrounding hepatic parenchyma, hepatoma is unlikely. Although ^{67}Ga scanning is not specific for hepatoma, it may be useful for directing biopsy in patients at high risk for hepatoma and for excluding biopsy in others.

CASE 162

History.— 23-year-old man with fever of unknown origin.

Scan.— ^{111}In leukocyte scan.

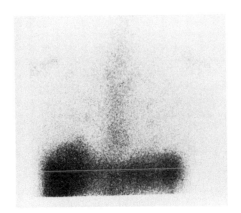 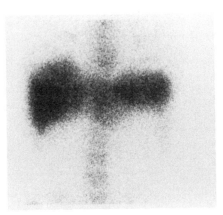 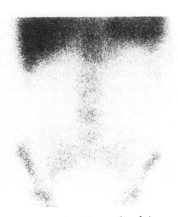

Anterior view of chest.　　　　Anterior view of abdomen.　　　　Anterior view of pelvis.

Findings.— Uptake in liver, spleen, and bone marrow.

Diagnosis.— Normal leukocyte scan.

Leukocytes are a heterogeneous group of cells that act as a group to protect their host from hazards such as infection and neoplasia and also aid in tissue repair. They spend only a fraction of their life in the peripheral circulation, using it mainly for transportation. The circulating leukocyte pool is composed of neutrophils (59%), lymphocytes (34%), monocytes (4%), eosinophils (3%), and basophils (0.5%).

Neutrophils have a life cycle of approximately 2 weeks. In the peripheral circulation, the neutrophils are in two pools, a circulating pool (44%) and a marginated pool (56%), in which neutrophils are either temporarily sequestered in capillaries or adhere to the endothelial surface of vessels. These two pools are normally in a dynamic equilibrium, although several factors can cause marginated neutrophils to move into the circulating pool. Demargination occurs with catecholamine release (stress, exercise, epinephrine administration) and with exposure to bacterial endotoxins.

Neutrophils have a circulating half-time of about 6 hours and normally migrate to the spleen, liver, lung, and, to a lesser extent, the gastrointestinal tract and oropharynx. Accumulation of neutrophils at sites of inflammation is stimulated by lactoferrin, neutrophil secretions, and other factors. Once at the site of inflammation, neutrophils reach the perivascular space by emigration and then migrate within the tissue via chemotaxis. Approximately 10% of circulating neutrophils will accumulate per day at sites of infection.

The primary radioisotope used for labeling leukocytes is ^{111}In. Because ^{111}In labels all cell types indiscriminately, leukocytes must be separated from the remainder of the blood before labeling. Although pure neutrophil populations are theoretically best, animal studies show there is no difference in concentrating ability between pure neutrophil populations and tagged cell preparations.

Oxine is the most commonly used agent for tagging leukocytes with ^{111}In. It is a lipophilic ligand that chelates bivalent and trivalent metallic ions such as ^{111}In. Plasma must be removed by centrifugation before labeling because ^{111}In has a higher affinity for the plasma protein transferrin than for oxine. The cells are then incubated with the ^{111}In oxine. Oxine allows the ^{111}In to enter the cell. Once inside the leukocyte, the ^{111}In oxine bond breaks. The ^{111}In then binds intracellularly, and the oxine leaves the cell. Before the labeled cells are reinjected into the patient, the cells are washed and recentrifuged to remove any excess oxine, unbound ^{111}In oxine, or both.

Neutrophils receive about 1,500 rad when labeled with 1 mCi of ^{111}In. These cells retain their normal metabolic and phagocyte function because they can withstand up to 50,000 rad. Radiation-induced oncogenesis is not a problem with these cells; neutrophils are postmitotic cells and relatively radioresistant. Radiation-induced oncogenesis is not a significant concern with lymphocytes in the mixed cell preparation either. The dose they receive (8,750 rad) is essentially a killing dose.

Normal variants or nonsignificant uptake on leukocyte scan may be seen with nasogastric tubes (nasopharyngeal uptake), swallowed leukocytes (anywhere in the GI tract), gastritis or low-grade GI bleeding, accessory or ectopic splenic tissue, intravenous catheters, colostomy sites, uninfected postsurgical wounds less than 10 days old, and hematomas. Delayed imaging to show movement with peristalsis is often helpful in cases of suspected benign GI tract activity.

CASE 163

History.— 39-year-old woman 2 weeks after hysterectomy, who now has increasing abdominal pain, chills, and fever.

Scan.—^{111}In leukocyte scan.

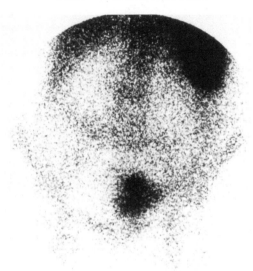

**Anterior leukocyte image of abdomen
and pelvis.**

Findings.— Focally increased uptake in pelvis.

Diagnosis.— Pelvic abscess.

Fever can be a perplexing problem in a patient without localizing signs. ^{111}Indium-labeled leukocytes are a valuable tool for localizing infection in patients with fever of unknown origin. In patients with localizing signs, CT or ultrasound is more appropriate.

Leukocytes are tagged by drawing 40 mL of blood into a tube containing anticoagulant and settling agent. The blood is then allowed to sediment by gravity. The leukocyte-rich plasma is drawn off and centrifuged to remove as much of the plasma and platelets as possible. ^{111}In will tag all cells indiscriminately, so separation from other cell types is important. ^{111}In has a higher affinity for transferrin in the plasma than oxine, the lipophilic chelating agent that allows ^{111}In to enter the cell.

Next, the leukocytes are resuspended in normal saline solution and incubated with ^{111}In oxine. The cells are then washed, resuspended in leukocyte-poor plasma, and reinjected into the patient. The radiolabeled leukocytes are given 24 hours to circulate and localize in sites of infection.

Normal sites of uptake vary with the imaging time. Early images 1 to 4 hours after injection show prominent pulmonary uptake. The cause of this is unknown. Delayed images at 24 hours show normal activity (from most to least intense) in the spleen, liver, and bone marrow. No renal or GI activity is normally seen with cells labeled with ^{111}In. ^{99m}Tc-labeled leukocytes frequently show gastrointestinal activity, however. Occasionally, blood pool is seen because of a small amount of red blood cell labeling. Other normal sites of uptake include IV catheters, colostomies, hematomas, accessory spleens, and uninfected surgical wounds 10 days old or less. Accumulation of leukocytes in other areas is abnormal and suspicious for infection.

The distribution and intensity of abnormal areas of activity is helpful in differentiating inflammation from true infection. Areas of activity more intense than the liver are more likely to represent infection, whereas those less intense than the liver are less likely to be infected. The pattern of abnormal activity is also useful. Diffuse pulmonary uptake represents infection only 10% of the time, whereas focal pulmonary uptake represents infection in 50% of cases.

The sensitivity and specificity of leukocyte scans for abdominal abscess are 90% and 95%, respectively. Abscesses of the liver or spleen may appear isointense with the rest of the liver or spleen and will be detected only when compared with a sulfur colloid liver-spleen scan. An abscess will appear as a cold area on colloid scan.

Activity that appears to be in the lumen of the bowel can be confusing. It represents the cause of fever only half of the time. True positive causes for gastrointestinal activity include pseudomembranous colitis, ischemic bowel, inflammatory bowel disease, and abscess communicating with bowel. False positive causes include swallowed leukocytes from sinusitis, nasogastric tubes, or pneumonia and gastrointestinal bleeding.

CASE 164

History.—48-year-old man with upper quadrant pain and fever.

Scan.—^{111}In leukocyte and ^{99m}Tc sulfur colloid scan.

Anterior leukocyte scan of abdomen.

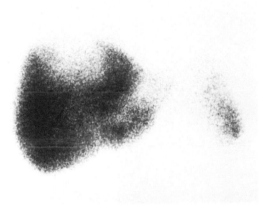

Anterior sulfur colloid scan of abdomen.

Findings.—^{111}In scan: homogeneous liver uptake. ^{99m}Tc sulfur colloid scan: cold defect in right lobe.

Diagnosis.—Hepatic abscess.

It is important to accurately diagnose abdominal abscesses. Untreated abscesses have an overall mortality of approximately 35%. Both ^{67}Ga citrate and ^{111}In leukocytes are sensitive for intra-abdominal abscess. ^{67}Ga, however, is primarily excreted by the bowel after the first 24 hours. The gastrointestinal uptake makes evaluating the abdomen difficult.

The sensitivity of the leukocyte scan for detecting abdominal abscess is 90%. Specificity has been reported as high as 95%. On leukocyte scan, abscesses appear as focal areas of increased uptake. There is no GI tract uptake.

Abscesses in the liver and spleen are difficult to detect solely on ^{111}In leukocyte images because the normal accumulation of activity in these organs may mask an adjacent in-

flammatory focus. This problem is overcome by comparing the leukocyte images with ^{99m}Tc sulfur colloid liver-spleen images. A hepatic abscess will show a cold defect on sulfur colloid images. This is because sulfur colloid uptake requires Kupffer's cell activity, which is not present in an abscess. This area "fills in" on ^{111}In leukocyte scan. Some studies indicate more than half of all upper quadrant abscesses will be missed if a combined ^{111}In leukocyte and ^{99m}Tc sulfur colloid scan is not done. Although computer-assisted subtraction of the ^{111}In leukocyte and ^{99m}Tc sulfur colloid images is possible, visual comparison of the two studies side by side on a viewbox is usually adequate.

CASE 165

History.— 30-year-old man with a history of IV drug abuse and fever.

Scan.—^{111}In leukocyte scan and ^{99m}Tc liver-spleen scan.

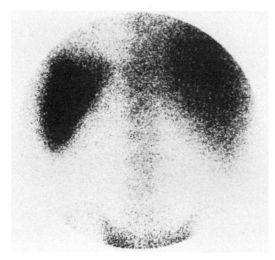

Posterior leukocyte scan of abdomen.

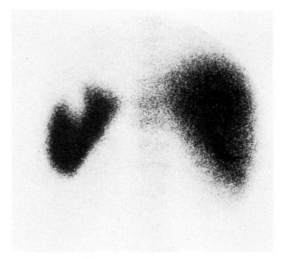

Posterior ^{99m}Tc colloid image of abdomen.

Findings.—^{111}In scan: homogeneous uptake in liver and spleen; ^{99m}Tc scan: defect in spleen.

Diagnosis.—Splenic abscess

Splenic abscess is an uncommon problem usually associated with sepsis. Hematogenous seeding of the spleen with bacteria occurs. Acute or subacute endocarditis is a common cause of splenic abscess. Other causes are intravenous drug use, direct extension of infection from an adjacent abscess, and secondary infection of a traumatic splenic hematoma.

Patients with splenic abscess often have abdominal pain, an enlarging spleen, and signs and symptoms of sepsis. In the majority of patients with splenic abscess, abscesses in other organs will also be present.

Imaging of the spleen can be performed with several methods, including computed tomography (CT), ultrasound, and radionuclide liver-spleen scan. A low-density area in the spleen on CT scanning can be confusing. Possible causes include splenic infarct, abscess, or hematoma. Metastatic disease involving the spleen, although rare, should also be considered. The liver-spleen scan shows cold defects in all these abnormalities as well.

Distinguishing splenic abscess from other causes of spleen abnormalities often requires a combination leukocyte and liver-spleen scan. A splenic infarct will appear as a cold defect on both studies. A splenic abscess, however, will appear warm or homogeneous on the leukocyte scan and cold on the liver-spleen scan.

The organ that receives the highest radiation dose from a leukocyte scan is the spleen. It receives 3 to 23 rad per dose. The splenic radiation dose may be even higher in children.

CASE 166

History.—57-year-old woman with productive cough and fever for 2 days.

Scan.—^{111}In leukocyte scan.

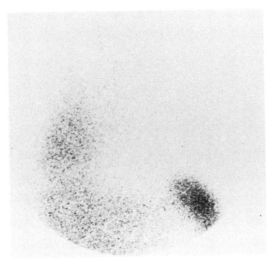

Anterior view of chest.

Findings.—Uptake in right lower lobe of lung.

Diagnosis.—Right lower lobe pneumonia.

A chest radiograph and sputum culture are the most appropriate tests for a patient suspected of having pneumonia. However, leukocyte scans in patients with fever of unknown origin will occasionally show pulmonary uptake. Studies of the clinical significance of pulmonary leukocyte accumulation have shown it is more difficult to distinguish infectious from noninfectious processes in the lung than in the abdomen.

Pulmonary uptake is routinely seen in the first hours following ^{111}In leukocyte reinjection. The significance of this is unknown, but it is thought that the leukocytes sustain some damage during the labeling process and, after reinjection, remain in the pulmonary vasculature for a short period to allow repair processes to occur. They are then released into the general circulation. An alternate explanation is that early uptake is simply physiologic margination.

One sixth of leukocyte scans will show pulmonary uptake. The pattern of activity is important in determining a cause.

Only 10% of patients with diffuse pulmonary activity will have a bacterial pneumonia. On the other hand, if the activity is focal, infection will be present in about 50%. Focal activity is seen with pneumonias, empyemas, and lung abscesses. The intensity of uptake can also be helpful. More intense uptake is more likely to represent infection.

Pulmonary uptake of leukocytes has a number of noninfectious causes, including:

1. Congestive heart failure
2. Adult respiratory distress syndrome
3. Atelectasis
4. Pulmonary emboli
5. Aspiration
6. Idiopathic

The mechanism of leukocyte accumulation for noninfectious processes appears related to complement activation.

CASE 167

History.— Patient 3 months after aortobifemoral bypass grafting who has a fever.

Scan.— ^{111}In leukocyte scan.

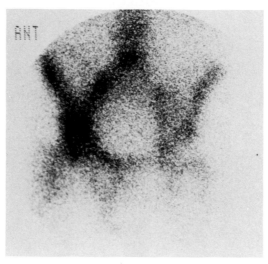

Anterior leukocyte scan of pelvis.

Findings.— Uptake in both limbs of the graft, right greater than left.

Diagnosis.— Aortic graft infection.

Infections of arterial grafts occur in up to 6% of grafted patients. This is a very serious complication, with mortality rates from 10% in femoropopliteal grafts to as high as 75% for aortofemoral grafts. About one-fourth of infected aortobifemoral bypass graft patients and one third of infected femoropopliteal graft patients require subsequent amputation.

Arterial graft infections are often quite indolent, and a high index of suspicion is required to diagnose them early. Several imaging modalities have been used to diagnose graft infections, including CT, ultrasound, ^{67}Ga scanning, and leukocyte scanning. The relative values of each of these studies is uncertain at this time.

^{111}In leukocyte studies are useful in detecting graft infections. The sensitivity and specificity of this study for graft infection in humans is not completely clear. In the first 2 to 3 months after graft placement, uptake can occur in noninfected grafts, presumably because of platelet adhesion to the graft. It is most remarkable in the early postoperative period and decreases over the next 10 to 12 weeks, possibly because of endothelialization of the graft.

Platelet activity can be seen in leukocyte scans because platelet tagging occurs during the leukocyte-labeling process. Indium oxine is an indiscriminate cell label. Before the addition of the indium oxine, cell separation is required. This is routinely done by gravity sedimentation enhanced by a settling agent (hydroxyethyl starch). The leukocyte-rich supernatant, which contains up to 70% of the neutrophils of the sample, is then drawn off, centrifuged, washed, and incubated with ^{111}In oxine. The cell mixture labeled by this method is about one-third platelets.

The other potential cause of vascular activity with leukocytes is excessive red blood cell labeling. This causes increased blood pool activity, which makes interpretation difficult.

Scans positive for graft infection generally show diffuse uptake along the infected portion of the graft. Often activity is increased at the anastamotic sites of the graft to the native vessel. Other vascular activity should be absent, assuming minimal red blood cell labeling. Correlation of leukocyte scan findings with CT or ultrasound will often reveal a fluid collection or gas formation in the area of the graft showing leukocyte uptake.

CASE 168

History.—52-year-old woman with fever and left upper quadrant
pain who has subacute bacterial endocarditis.

Scan.—^{111}In leukocyte and ^{99m}Tc sulfur colloid scans.

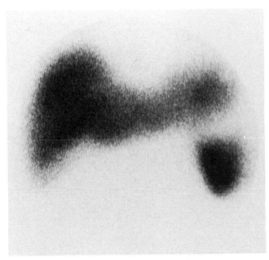

**Anterior ^{111}In leukocyte image of liver
and spleen.**

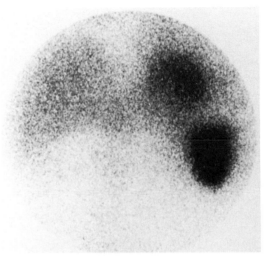

**^{99m}Tc sulfur colloid image of same area as
leukocyte scan (A).**

Findings.—Leukocyte scan: cold area in the spleen; ^{99m}Tc sulfur
colloid: matching defect.

Diagnosis.—Splenic infarct. No evidence of infection.

Splenic infarcts can become infected. Diagnosing an infected infarct is difficult with conventional imaging techniques. The combination of an Indium 111–labeled leukocyte scan and technetium 99m–sulfur colloid scan can be useful in such cases.

If the size of the defect on sulfur colloid is much larger than the cold area on leukocyte scan, the infarct is infected. If they are the same size, infection is unlikely.

As noted elsewhere, the combination of leukocyte and liver-spleen scan is imperative in making the diagnosis of upper quadrant abscesses in about one half of such cases. ^{99m}Tc sulfur colloid scans are helpful in evaluating the liver and spleen for abscess when using gallium 67 citrate as well.

CASE 169

History.— 55-year-old man with fever of unknown origin and bilateral pleural fluid collections on CT.

Scan.— ^{111}In leukocyte scan, followed by a ^{99m}Tc sulfur colloid liver-spleen scan.

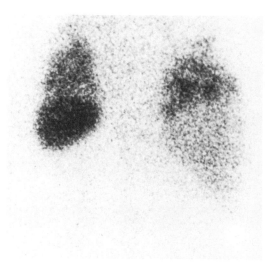

Posterior 24-hour leukocyte scan of chest and upper half of abdomen.

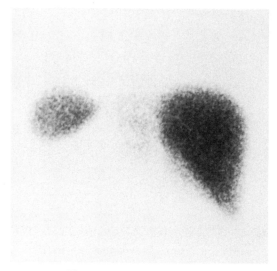

Posterior ^{99m}Tc sulfur colloid liver-spleen scan of chest and abdomen.

Findings.— There are bilateral dense collections of leukocytes. One is just superior to the spleen; the other is located posteriorly, just superior to the liver. These collections were believed to be in the posterior pleural space and corresponded to the fluid collections on CT scan.

Diagnosis.— Bilateral empyemas.

This is a case of focal leukocyte uptake in the chest, representing infection. A thoracentesis performed under ultrasound guidance documented purulent pleural fluid, and the patient was treated with bilateral thoracotomy tube drainage and antibiotic therapy.

Determining whether the infection is thoracic or abdominal is difficult in cases such as this where the abnormality is located above the liver and spleen. The liver-spleen scan is very helpful, but there still may be confusion. Correlation with other studies such as chest radiograph or CT will often answer the question. In this case, the chest CT showed bilateral pleural fluid that matched the leukocyte scan. For leukocyte collections above the liver, spleen, and diaphragm, pneumonia, pulmonary abscess, and empyema are the main considerations. The leukocyte scan alone cannot differentiate between these.

Leukocyte accumulations above the liver and spleen but below the diaphragm are most likely to be subphrenic abscesses. These can cause pleural effusions. This fluid is free flowing in distinction to empyemas, which usually are not.

CASE 170

History.— 55-year-old man 6 weeks after aortobifemoral grafting, now with intermittent GI bleeding, vague back pain, and fever.

Scan.—^{111}In leukocyte scan.

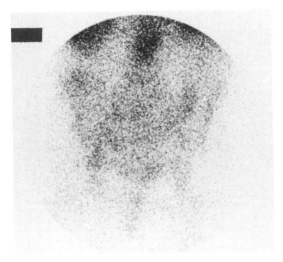

Anterior leukocyte scan of abdomen and pelvis.

Findings.— Uptake in graft in central portion of abdomen and bowel in lower quadrants.

Diagnosis.— Aortoenteric fistula.

Aortoenteric fistula is a disastrous complication of aortic graft placement. The most frequent cause is graft infection that erodes into the gastrointestinal tract. Usually there is intermittent GI bleeding; exsanguinating hemorrhage is the most feared complication. Other less specific symptoms include abdominal or back pain, anorexia, fever, and anemia.

Early diagnosis, as with any type of graft infection, is critical for lifesaving surgical intervention. Usually total graft removal with extraanatomic bypass for lower extremity limb salvage is required. Techniques used for diagnosis include endoscopy, arteriography, ultrasound, upper GI series, barium enema, computed tomography, gallium scan, leukocyte scan, and downstream blood cultures.

Indium-labeled leukocyte scanning has been shown to be useful in localizing sites of infection. If the bleeding rate is high, a GI bleeding study using technetium 99m—labeled red blood cells can be done. However, in the majority, the bleeding is intermittent. Graft infection is the more constant factor. This makes the leukocyte scan a good choice.

CASE 171

History.—45-year-old male alcoholic with abdominal pain.

Scan.—^{111}In leukocyte scan.

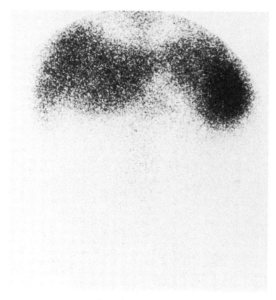

Anterior view of abdomen.

Findings.—Uptake in midabdomen, medial to left lobe of liver.

Diagnosis.—Pancreatitis.

Each day the pancreas secretes 1,500 to 3,000 mL of alkaline fluid containing about 20 enzymes and zymogens. These secretions contain the enzymes necessary for digestion and provide an optimal pH for their function.

Pancreatic inflammatory disease can be classified as either acute or chronic. In the United States, acute pancreatitis is most frequently caused by alcohol ingestion, although in middle-aged women cholelithiasis is the primary cause. Patients may have nonspecific symptoms, although abdominal pain is the most consistent finding.

Eleven factors have been identified that adversely affect survival in acute pancreatitis. These are known as Ranson's criteria and are advanced age, hyperglycemia, leukocytosis, significantly elevated lactic dehydrogenase and aspartate aminotransferase levels, fall in hematocrit, hypocalcemia, base deficit, rise in blood urea nitrogen level, hypoxemia, and significant fluid sequestration.

Computed tomography (CT) plays a role in the imaging of acute pancreatitis, with approximately 70% of patients showing abnormalities. CT findings include enlargement of the pancreas (diffuse more commonly than focal), calcifications (13%), pseudocyst (10%), and hemorrhage (5%). Gas or phlegmon, both associated with abscess, may also be seen occasionally.

The indium 111 leukocyte scan shows uptake in acute pancreatitis, which is often best appreciated on the posterior abdominal image. Uptake in mild cases of acute pancreatitis is generally absent. When correlated with prognostic criteria, leukocyte uptake is more common in patients with higher Ranson's scores and has been associated with the presence of significant pancreatic fat necrosis. The leukocyte scan may also be used in the evaluation of a pancreatic mass to distinguish pancreatic abscess from pseudocyst because both entities often have a similar clinical picture. As would be expected, a pancreatic abscess will show concentration of ^{111}In white blood cells, whereas an uninfected pseudocyst will not.

CASE 172

History.—49-year-old man with nasogastric tube after ulcer surgery.

Scan.—^{111}In leukocyte scan.

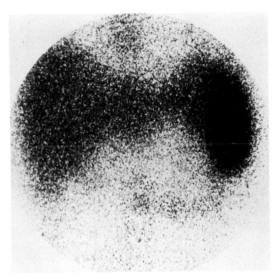

Anterior view of abdomen.

Findings.—Linear uptake in abdomen.

Diagnosis.—GI activity secondary to swallowed leukocytes.

Approximately 19% of patients with fever of unknown origin show leukocyte uptake in the GI tract; however, leukocyte uptake in the gastrointestinal tract correlates with the cause of fever in only about one half of these patients.

The most frequent cause of false positive findings in the GI tract are swallowed leukocytes and GI bleeding. Swallowed leukocytes occur in patients with indwelling endotracheal, nasogastric, and other tubes that cause significant inflamma-tion. Swallowed leukocytes may also be seen with pneumonia, empyema, and sinusitis. Common sources of GI bleeding include gastritis, ulcers, and diverticula. Bleeding tumors can also cause GI tract activity.

The most common causes of true positive GI leukocyte activity are intra-abdominal abscess that communicates with bowel, pseudomembranous colitis, inflammatory bowel disease, and necrotic bowel.

CASE 173

History.—39-year-old drug addict with recent removal of a bone spur from right heel, who developed swelling postoperatively.

Scan.—^{111}In leukocyte scan.

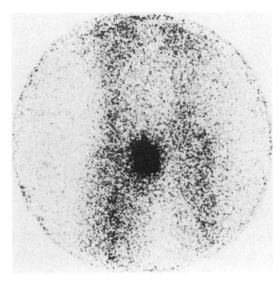

Leukocyte scan of feet.

Findings.—Intense uptake right heel.

Diagnosis.—Osteomyelitis of the right calcaneus.

The diagnosis of osteomyelitis can be difficult in patients with fractures, recent surgery, cellulitis, and diabetic osteoarthropathy. Bone scintigraphy is a valuable tool for the detection of osteomyelitis. But despite its sensitivity for osteomyelitis, lack of specificity for infection is a major limitation of the technique. Technetium phosphate bone scanning does not differentiate bone infection, fracture, postsurgical changes, heterotopic ossification, or arthritis. Gallium scanning has been found helpful in some patients. However, it is a weak bone agent and suffers from a similar lack of specificity.

Leukocyte scanning is useful in the evaluation of acute osteomyelitis. The sensitivity (true positives/all patients with disease), specificity (true negatives/all patients without disease), and accuracy (true positives and true negatives/all patients) of leukocyte scanning for bone infection have been reported as high as 97%, 82%, and 92%, respectively. Although the use of labeled leukocytes in chronic osteomyelitis is more controversial, recent studies indicate good sensitivities.

Osteomyelitis appears as an area of increased uptake on leukocyte scan. In patients with soft tissue ulcers or cellulitis, views in several projections with the skin markers can be helpful in differentiating osseous from soft tissue uptake. In about 12% of cases, osteomyelitis manifests as a cold defect on ^{111}In leukocyte scan. Because of the poor contrast with the small amount of activity normally in the marrow, these areas can easily be missed.

False positive ^{111}In leukocyte scans can occur in patients with prostheses, such as after total hip arthroplasty. The placement of hardware in the marrow cavity (e.g., rods) can push bone marrow forward and concentrate it at the tip of the prosthesis. Because ^{111}In leukocytes are normally concentrated in bone marrow, these focal collections can falsely be diagnosed as osteomyelitis. A ^{99m}Tc sulfur colloid scan can be done to outline the location of bone marrow. Uptake of ^{99m}Tc sulfur colloid in an area of leukocyte activity makes infection unlikely.

CASE 174

History.— 19-year-old black man with sickle cell anemia and complaint of deep bone pain in the distal right elbow.

Scan.—^{99m}Tc MDP bone scan.

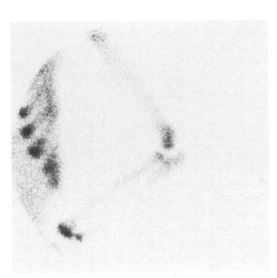

Left arm.

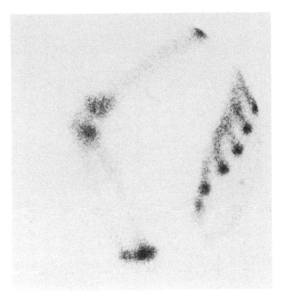

Right arm.

Findings.— Increased uptake in right distal humerus.

Diagnosis.— Bone infarct.

Bone marrow infarcts are a common complication of sickle cell disease. About half of patients with sickle cell anemia have a bone marrow infarct at some time during their disease because of sickling of the red blood cells in the small vessels and sinusoids of the bone marrow. This leads to ischemia and subsequent infarction of portions of the bone marrow. Predisposing factors for red blood cell sickling are slow blood flow and low oxygen saturation.

The clinical manifestation of a bone marrow infarct is characteristic with complaints of deep bone pain caused by swelling of the marrow after infarction. Joint pain and swelling are also characteristic and are thought to be caused by periarticular bone infarcts or microvascular occlusion in the synovium.

Plain films of acute bone marrow infarcts are almost always unremarkable. Even delayed films of bone marrow infarcts are abnormal only half of the time. Bone marrow imaging is a sensitive means of confirming bone marrow infarction.

^{99m}Tc sulfur colloid scans are frequently performed for marrow infarcts. These particles are rapidly cleared from circulating blood by the reticuloendothelial system (RES) of the liver, spleen, and bone marrow. In normal individuals, 86% of the injected colloid localizes in the liver, 6% in the spleen, and 8% in the bone marrow.

The normal marrow scanning dose is 12 to 15 mCi of ^{99m}Tc sulfur colloid. The increased dose is not to "saturate" the RES of the liver and spleen, allowing more activity to go to the bone marrow. Rather, it assures that 8% of the injected dose is sufficient to allow high-count images to be acquired within an acceptable time.

In normal individuals, and most disease states, the distribution of the RES and erythropoietic marrow elements are identical. Occasionally there is a discrepancy between the two, such as expansion of the RES without the presence of active erythropoietic elements.

Bone marrow infarcts appear as a cold area on sulfur colloid scans. Surrounding increased uptake in normally perfused marrow is sometimes seen. The cold defect is usually asymmetric and is most noticeable in areas of bone marrow expansion in the long bones. Because cold areas are present in up to half of asymptomatic patients with sickle cell anemia from previous infarcts that have subsequently fibrosed, false positive results are common.

If a bone infarct is present with a bone marrow infarct, the patient may develop extreme tenderness and swelling. The bone marrow scan is unable to differentiate between bone infarct and osteomyelitis. A bone scan also cannot distinguish these two diseases. Both can appear hot or cold on bone scan. A ^{67}Ga scan is the best test to differentiate the two.

The follow-up of patients with bone marrow infarcts shows these areas can repopulate with marrow elements or progress to fibrosis. Occasionally the necrotic marrow will become a nidus for infection or a site of pathologic fracture.

CASE 175

History.—47-year-old with an elevated hematocrit and headaches.

Scan.—After the intravenous administration of 12 mCi of ^{99m}Tc sulfur colloid, serial images of the entire skeleton were obtained.

Anterior view of skull.

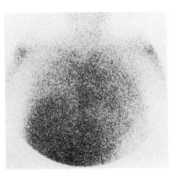

Anterior view of chest.

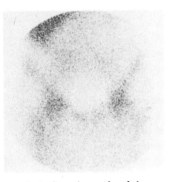

Anterior view of pelvis.

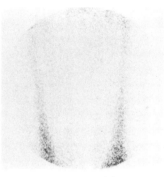

Anterior view of femurs.

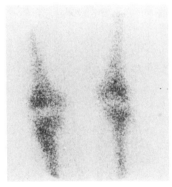

Anterior view of knees.

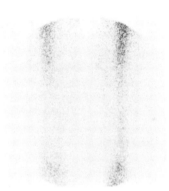

Anterior view of legs.

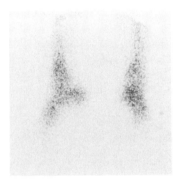

Anterior view of feet.

Findings.—Expansion of bone marrow into the long bones of the extremities is present. The central marrow is very active.

Diagnosis.—Polycythemia vera with marrow expansion.

Bone marrow expansion is a very nonspecific finding on bone marrow imaging. Possible causes include polycythemia vera, chronic iron deficiency anemia, hemolytic anemia, megaloblastic anemia, and leukemia. Clinical information and laboratory data are helpful in differentiating these diseases.

When increased red blood cell production is needed, the bone marrow expands its erythropoietic component. This occurs at the expense of fat in the marrow space. The distribution of this expanded marrow is similar to the normal bone marrow, so early in this process the bone marrow scan will be normal. As bone marrow expansion progresses, the active marrow extends more peripherally in the long bones of the extremities. In extreme cases, active marrow is found in the small bones of the hands. This expansion is normally symmetric, progressing centrally to peripherally. Any expansion of the active marrow past the junction of the proximal and middle third of the humerus or femur should be considered abnormal. Expansion of the bone marrow can also cause increased activity on a ^{99m}Tc MDP bone scan. The most characteristic finding is increased metaphyseal uptake, most apparent around the knees.

Early in polycythemia vera, normal or minimal expansion of bone marrow is seen. Later, more marked marrow expansion occurs. Ten percent to 20% of patients with polycythemia vera will progress to myelofibrosis. Myelofibrosis shows bone marrow expansion with decreased axial activity. These findings occur because of replacement of the central marrow by fibrosis. The presence of myelofibrosis is important in the consideration of phosphorus 32 therapy for polycythemia vera because ^{32}P can be toxic to the remaining bone marrow.

In more chronic hemolytic anemias and myeloproliferative disorders, erythropoietic marrow can be found in sites outside the bone marrow. This extramedullary hematopoiesis occurs most commonly in the liver and spleen but may be found in the adrenal glands, lymph nodes, retroperitoneal fat, breasts, pleura, lung, and falx cerebri. Both hematopoietic and reticuloendothelial system (RES) components are present in extramedullary hematopoiesis, allowing either ^{99m}Tc sulfur colloid, radioiron, or ^{111}In chloride to be used for imaging. These scans can be helpful in differentiating sites of extramedullary hematopoiesis from tumor in patients with a mass lesion.

In patients with symptomatic splenomegaly or hypersplenism secondary to extramedullary hematopoiesis in myeloid metaplasia, a bone marrow scan can determine the amount of active marrow outside the spleen when splenectomy is considered. This assures the patient is left with adequate marrow reserves.

Aplastic anemia is best evaluated with either ^{111}In chloride or radioiron because a total mismatch between RES and erythropoietic marrow occurs. A ^{99m}Tc sulfur colloid scan will overestimate marrow reserve.

The red, or erythropoietic, bone marrow is widely distributed in the body. It rivals the liver in size, weighing approximately 1,500 g. Marrow evaluation is usually done by bone marrow aspiration and biopsy. However, this technique samples only a small portion of the total bone marrow. Radionuclide bone marrow imaging allows evaluation of all of the body's marrow. It is also useful for detecting avascular necrosis of the femoral head, sites of extramedullary hematopoiesis, and areas of metastatic disease.

The distribution of marrow changes with age. At birth, active marrow extends the full length of the extremities. By age 10 years, the marrow has retracted to its adult distribution, with active marrow present in the axial skeleton (vertebral bodies, pelvis, sternum, ribs, scapulae, and skull) and extension into the proximal third of the femurs and humeri. Yellow marrow containing primarily fat replaces the active marrow as it retracts.

Bone marrow is comprised of two separate entities. Erythropoietic marrow contains the blood-forming elements. This portion of bone marrow is responsible for up to 90% of plasma iron turnover. The RES consists of phagocytic cells that remove foreign materials (e.g., bacteria, fungi, and senescent blood cells) from the blood. The RES also removes injected colloidal substances.

Radiopharmaceuticals for bone marrow imaging are divided into erythropoietic and RES agents. Radioisotopes of iron, such as ^{52}Fe and ^{59}Fe, label erythropoietic marrow. Radioiron is probably the most physiologic isotope available, but routine use is limited by characteristics of the isotopes. ^{52}Fe is a cyclotron-produced positron emitter. Cost and the availability of a PET scanner restrict widespread use. ^{59}Fe has a half-life of 45 days and has very high-energy photons (1.089 and 1.298 meV) that require heavy collimation and very low doses. Image quality is poor for these reasons.

RES bone marrow imaging is performed with ^{99m}Tc sulfur colloid. This material is taken up by the phagocytic cells lining the bone marrow sinusoids, as well as the RES of the liver and spleen. It is the most commonly used agent for bone marrow imaging because of its low radiation dose, ease of imaging, low cost, and ready availability. The RES and erythropoietic marrow nearly always show identical distribution.

Exceptions occur when RES cells proliferate in the absence of erythropoietic marrow. This is seen in pure red blood cell aplasia, DeGuglielmo's syndrome, hematologic malignancies, aplastic anemia, and myelofibrosis. In such cases, a ^{99m}Tc sulfur colloid scan may overestimate the amount of active bone marrow. Another disadvantage of sulfur colloid is that the vertebral bodies of the lower thoracic and upper lumbar spine are poorly seen because of normal uptake by the liver and spleen. Ninety-two percent of the injected dose localizes in these organs, with only 8% localizing in the marrow.

Another agent used for bone marrow imaging is ^{111}In chloride. Similar to iron, this agent binds to transferrin. In other ways it behaves like sulfur colloid, being phagocytized by the RES system. Good correlation is found between ^{111}In scans and the clinical status of patients with aplastic anemia, myelofibrosis, and other hematologic disorders. Some disparity exists in cases of pure red blood cell aplasia and other diseases, however.

The appearance of a normal bone marrow scan depends on the imaging agent used. Sulfur colloid scans show activity in the active bone marrow. This distribution is age related. The liver and spleen show intense activity. ^{111}In chloride scans show a distribution similar to sulfur colloid but with much less activity in the liver and spleen. Renal activity is also seen with ^{111}In. Radioiron scans show activity confined to the axial skeleton with little activity in the spleen.

CASE 176

History.—56-year-old woman with breast carcinoma who underwent radical mastectomy and was referred for radiation therapy. We were asked to determine the location and depth of the internal thoracic lymph node chain for radiation therapy planning.

Scan.—A subcostal injection of 500 μCi of ^{99m}Tc antimony sulfide colloid was followed by serial images of the chest. After visualization of the lymph node chain, the location and depth of each node were determined using skin markers and a rotating slant-hole collimator.

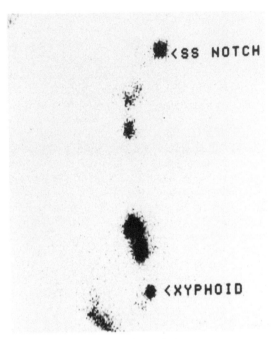

SS NOTCH

XYPHOID

Anterior view of chest.

Findings.—This study shows four lymph nodes of the right internal thoracic lymph node chain; the depths were noted. The location of each was marked on the patient's chest wall.

Diagnosis.—Localization of internal thoracic lymph nodes using lymphoscintigraphy in a patient with breast carcinoma. No evidence of macroscopic tumor involvement.

Internal thoracic lymph nodes can be accurately localized using parasternal lymphoscintigraphy. This information is important to assure adequate radiation treatment of all the lymph nodes draining the breast. As many as 40% of patients treated with standard tangential portals will have some internal thoracic lymph nodes outside the treatment field and will therefore be undertreated. Accurate localization of these nodes before radiation treatment allows modification of the standard port.

The technique involves the interstitial injection of 500 μCi of ^{99m}Tc antimony sulfide colloid about 3 cm lateral to the midsternal line and just below the costal margin of the affected side. The injection should be just anterior to the posterior rectus sheath.

Two to 3 hours later, images of the chest are obtained using a low-energy parallel-hole collimator. The location of each node visualized is determined using a radioactive marker on the skin. The skin overlying each node is then marked with an ink marker. The node's depth is determined using a rotating slant-hole collimator. With a radioactive source on the skin overlying each node, an image is obtained. Then, without the patient being moved, a second image is done after rotating the slant-hole collimator 180 degrees. Knowing the angle of the slant-hole collimator, one can determine the depth of each node using simple geometry. A second method determines depth using a lateral image and sternal skin markers.

An early image after injection should show the radioactivity to be confined to a point. If it is seen to spread out in the abdomen, the likelihood of an intraperitoneal injection should be considered. The visualization of at least one internal thoracic node ensures a technically satisfactory examination. Abnormal parasternal lymphatics have a variable appearance. They may show diminished activity in individual nodes or visualization of a few lower parasternal nodes because of obstruction of flow. Asymmetry may be demonstrable if both sides are injected. A gap in a chain is not considered abnormal.

In addition to draining the peritoneal cavity, the right internal thoracic chain also receives hepatic lymphatics, and an abnormality of this chain may be associated with metastatic tumor in the liver.

CASE 177

History.—28-year-old with newly diagnosed malignant melanoma on the scalp.

Scan.—^{99m}Tc lymphoscintigraphy.

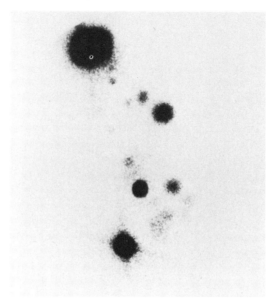

Left lateral view of head.

Findings.—Activity extending down the left side of the neck.

Diagnosis.—Drainage to the left side of the neck.

Malignant melanoma spreads early via lymphatics to the regional lymph nodes. Identifying the lymphatic drainage of the primary lesion and excising these nodes improves overall survival. Lymph node dissections are done not only to remove tumor already spread to regional lymphatics but also for staging. Lymphoscintigraphy is helpful in identifying the pattern of lymphatic drainage of melanoma lesions and in planning subsequent therapy.

There are some general rules for predicting the area of skin drained by each regional lymph node group. Sappey's line is a line from the level of the umbilicus extending around to the L-2 or L-3 vertebral body level in the back. The lymphatics above this line generally drain to the axillary lymphatics, whereas those below drain to the inguinal nodes. There is a similar demarcation line in the midline dividing drainage to the left or right side.

There is some overlap in lymph drainage near these lines, however, making prediction of drainage from these areas difficult. Lymph drainage of scalp lesions is also quite variable. Prediction of lymph drainage based only on the usual rules in these areas is wrong as often as half the time. In addition, many areas are drained by more than one regional lymph node group. This problem worsens when a lesion is located near the midline or Sappey's line. Lymphoscintigraphy involves the intradermal injection of 1 mCi of ^{99m}Tc antimony sulfide colloid circumferentially around the site of the original lesion. Because most melanomas have been excised before lymphoscintigraphy, these injections are placed circumferentially around the biopsy site. Two to 4 hours later, images of all regional node groups are obtained and examined for evidence of activity.

The results of lymphoscintigraphy are helpful if only one regional lymph node group drains the area of the lesion. In this case a lymph node dissection of this group is sufficient for therapy and staging. If more than one regional lymph node group drains the area of the lesion, the physician is left with the decision of whether to prophylactically resect more than one node group or not. The potential benefit of this treatment is under investigation.

Distal extremity lesions have a very predictable drainage pattern and lymphoscintigraphy is usually not necessary. If a lesion is located more proximally near the shoulder or buttocks, lymphoscintigraphy may be beneficial.

CASE 178

History.— 51-year-old man with anemia.

Scan.— Schilling's test parts 1 and 2.

Findings.— Part I: ^{57}Co B_{12} = 18% excreted; part II: ^{57}Co B_{12}-IF = 17%.

Diagnosis.— Normal Schilling's test results.

Schilling's test, parts 1 and 2, is useful in the evaluation of low vitamin B_{12} levels and in distinguishing between pernicious anemia and malabsorption.

Vitamin B_{12} is not synthesized by plants or animals but is produced by microorganisms found in soil and in the intestines and rumens of animals. Dietary vitamin B_{12}, therefore, comes from meat and dairy products.

Vitamin B_{12} is stored primarily in the liver. Total body stores are high, and daily excretion is low. Thus, it takes 3 to 5 years of dietary insufficiency (or malabsorption) to deplete the body's vitamin B_{12} stores. Vitamin B_{12} deficiency from diet alone is uncommon; it is seen almost exclusively in vegetarians.

Vitamin B_{12} must complex with intrinsic factor (IF), which is produced by the gastric parietal cells, before it can be absorbed in the terminal ileum. An alkaline pH and the presence of calcium are also required. In the terminal ileum, vitamin B_{12} dissociates from the intrinsic factor and is transported to the liver by binding to the carrier protein transcobalamin II. Over the next 8 to 12 hours, a portion of the vitamin B_{12} reenters the circulation and is bound to a larger transport protein, transcobalamin I. When the storage-transport capacity of transcobalamin is saturated, vitamin B_{12} is excreted into the urine by the kidneys. This is the basis for Schilling's test.

Vitamin B_{12} (cyanocobalamin) has cobalt as its central metal atom. Schilling's test substitutes radioactive isotopes of cobalt, producing a radiolabeled B_{12}. One isotope used is ^{57}Co, which has a physical half-life of 270 days and a photon energy of 122 keV. The other, ^{58}Co, has a physical half-life of 71 days and a photon energy of 810 keV.

For part 1 of Schilling's test, the patient swallows a capsule with 0.5 μCi of ^{57}Co B_{12} in 0.5 μg of B_{12}. One thousand micrograms of cold, or unlabeled vitamin B_{12} is then administered intramuscularly (or subcutaneously). The cold vitamin B_{12} saturates the transport proteins. Two consecutive 24-hour urine samples are then collected. Any ^{57}Co vitamin B_{12} absorbed across the ileum will not be able to bind to the transport proteins because they are saturated by cold vitamin B_{12}. Thus all absorbed ^{57}Co vitamin B_{12} will be excreted by the kidneys into the urine. After the volume of urine is measured and 2 mL aliquots of urine and dose standards are used, the percent of administered dose excreted over each 24-hour period is determined.

Schilling's examination part 2 is designed to determine if the cause of vitamin B_{12} deficiency is ileal malabsorption. The test is repeated just as in part 1 but with one difference: the 0.5 μCi of ^{57}Co vitamin B_{12} is complexed to human intrinsic factor.

CASE 179

History.—61-year-old woman with decreased serum vitamin B_{12} levels and anemia.

Scan.—Schilling's test parts 1 and 2.

Findings.—Part 1: 0.3%; part 2: 10.1%.

Diagnosis.—Pernicious anemia.

Pernicious anemia is an autoimmune disorder in which antibodies are directed against gastric parietal cells. Approximately 90% of patients with pernicious anemia have antiparietal cell antibodies; 60% have anti-intrinsic factor (IF) antibodies.

Pernicious anemia occurs most frequently in people of Northern European descent, affecting men and women equally. It is a disease of the elderly, rarely affecting patients younger than age 30 years. Gastric atrophy is the main feature of the disease. The antrum, which has no acid- or pepsin-secreting function, is spared. Among the consequences of gastric atrophy is the lack of production of IF, which is essential for vitamin B_{12} absorption by the ileum.

Without IF, there is no vitamin B_{12} absorption. Because of this, the urinary excretion of ^{57}Co B_{12} is low. Less than 6% excretion will be seen with pernicious anemia, although much lower uptakes, in the 3% or less range, are the rule. In pernicious anemia, vitamin B_{12} absorption corrects with Schilling's test, part 2, in which the ^{57}Co B_{12} is complexed to IF. The urinary excretion of ^{57}Co B_{12} complexed to IF will be greater than 10%.

CASE 180

History.—51-year-old man with sprue and anemia.

Scan.—Schilling's test, parts 1 and 2.

Findings.—Part 1: 4%; part 2: 5%.

Diagnosis.—Intestinal malabsorption of vitamin B_{12}.

Virtually any disorder that compromises the absorptive capability of the terminal ileum can result in vitamin B_{12} deficiency. Segmental involvement of the distal ileum by disease can cause megaloblastic anemia without any other manifestations of intestinal malabsorption. Specific entities include regional enteritis (Crohn's disease), Whipple's disease, and tuberculosis. Vitamin B_{12} malabsorption is also seen after ileal resection. Zollinger-Ellison syndrome (gastrinoma) can produce vitamin B_{12} malabsorption by acidifying the small intestine. An alkaline pH is necessary for vitamin B_{12} absorption.

The macrocytic anemia seen in association with intestinal strictures, diverticulae, anastomoses, and blind loops may be attributed to colonization of the small intestine by large masses of bacteria that divert vitamin B_{12} away from the host. For example, in Scandinavia, patients harboring the tapeworm *Diphyllobothrium latum* develop a megaloblastic anemia that corrects with destruction of the worm; competition for vitamin B_{12} by the worm has been attributed as the etiology.

Whatever the cause, with intestinal malabsorption the urinary excretion of ^{57}Co B_{12} (part 1) and ^{57}Co B_{12}–intrinsic factor (IF) (part 2) are both in the 6% or less range. Chronic cyanocobalamin deficiency from pernicious anemia can produce atrophy of the ileal mucosa, decreasing the ileal absorption of vitamin B_{12}. When malabsorption of vitamin B_{12} is from ileal mucosal atrophy, Schilling's test part 1 excretion (^{57}Co B_{12}) will be in the 1% to 3% range, with only minor correction with Schilling's test part 2 (^{57}Co B_{12}-IF). This is diagnosed by repeating Schilling's part 2 examination several weeks to months after vitamin B_{12} replacement therapy is instituted to allow mucosal regeneration. When repeated, part 2 excretion will be normal.

CASE 181

History.—60-year-old man with elevated hematocrit.

Scan.—Red blood cell and plasma volume determination.

Findings.—Red blood cell mass: 45 mL/kg (normal, 25–35 mL/kg); plasma volume: 38 mL/kg (normal, 30–45 mL/kg).

Diagnosis.—Polycythemia vera.

Red blood cell and plasma volume determinations are usually performed simultaneously. When combined, they yield the total blood volume. The most common reason for performing these studies is to differentiate polycythemia vera from stress erythrocytosis.

The tests are based on a dilution technique. A given amount of tracer is allowed to equilibrate with the space being measured; a sample is then obtained. Comparing the quantity of tracer given with the concentration of tracer in the obtained sample gives a volume. This volume may be expressed as :

$$Vp \; (mL) = \frac{VdCd \; (cpm)}{Cp \; (cpm/mL)}$$

where Vd = volume of dose given, Cd = concentration of dose given S, Cp = concentration of tracer in pool being measured, and Vp = volume of pool being measured.

As with other in vitro hematologic studies, the technique has been standardized. The following technique is used for determining RBC volume:

1. Draw 10 mL of blood; place 6 mL in a tube containing 2 mL of acid-citrate-dextrose (ACD) solution; place the remaining 4 mL in a tube containing ethylenediamine tetraacetic acid (EDTA); remove a 2 mL aliquot and perform a background count.
2. Incubate 35 μCi of chromium 51 chromate with the blood-ACD solution for 45 minutes.
3. Centrifuge the labeled blood at 1,000 G for 10 minutes; discard the plasma.
4. Wash with saline solution; recentrifuge to remove any unbound ^{51}Cr.
5. Resuspend in saline solution to original volume.
6. Make a counting standard by diluting 1 mL of labeled cells in 1,000 mL of distilled water; remove two 2 mL aliquots.
7. Have patient rest in recumbent position for 30 minutes; inject 5 mL of labeled cells; from the opposite arm, draw 5 mL samples at 10 and 40 minutes using EDTA as an anticoagulant.
8. Take 2 mL from each sample and count; perform a microhematocrit using the other 3 mL.
9. Calculate the RBC volume (RCV) by:
$$RCV = \frac{cpm/mL \quad Standard}{cpm/mL \quad Blood \; sample} \times Hct(0.98)$$
$$\times 1,000 \times 5$$
10. Total blood volume is calculated by:
$$TBV = \frac{RCV}{Hct \times 0.98 \times 0.91}$$
11. Calculate plasma volume (PV) by:
$$PV = TBV - RCV$$

The 0.98 correction is for plasma trapped in the red blood cell fraction. The 0.91 correction is total-body hematocrit, which, because some organs contain fewer red blood cells than the peripheral blood vessels, is lower than the peripheral hematocrit.

Polycythemia vera is characterized by overproduction of red blood cells. Leukocyte and platelet counts are often elevated as well. As the red blood cell mass increases, blood viscosity increases. Ultimately, increased blood viscosity may cause stroke, myocardial infarction, venous thrombosis, and even hemorrhage. However, the plasma volume is significantly decreased. With stress erythrocytosis, the red blood cell mass is either normal or slightly decreased.

The technique for performing plasma volume is similar to that for red blood cell mass except that iodine 125 human serum albumin is used as the dilution marker of the plasma space. Because of its low energy (32 keV), it is generally performed before red blood cell mass determination. In polycythemia vera, the plasma volume is usually normal but may be either mildly increased or mildly decreased.

CASE 182

History.— 52-year-old with splenomegaly and anemia.

Scan.— Red blood cell survival and sequestration study.

Findings.— Red blood cell survival: 10 days; sequestration study: spleen/liver ratio of 2:1, increasing to 5:1 over the course of the examination.

Diagnosis.— Decreased red blood cell survival with splenic sequestration of red blood cells

To determine if a patient's anemia is the result of decreased red blood cell survival or pathologic splenic sequestration of red blood cells, both red blood cell survival and splenic sequestration studies can be performed. For a red blood cell survival study, blood is collected in acid-citrate-dextrose, centrifuged (plasma is discarded), and the remaining packed red blood cells tagged with 0.5 μCi/kg of chromium 51-chromate. The cells are then washed and recentrifuged to remove any unbound ^{51}Cr.

After the volume is restored with isotonic saline solution, the cells are reinjected into the patient. Samples are then withdrawn every other day, beginning at 24 hours, for 21 days. A microhematocrit is performed on each sample, and the samples are counted in the well counter. The blood counts are plotted on semilog paper. Dividing the whole blood cell counts by the sample hematocrit improves accuracy, correcting for daily fluctuations of hematocrit.

The normal red blood cell survival study half-time is 25 to 35 days, based on a normal red blood cell life span of 120 days with a daily 0.8% senescence rate, and an additional 1% daily elution of ^{51}Cr off the red blood cells. Red blood cell survival of less than 25 to 35 days is abnormally low. Hematologic steady state is essential for diagnostic accuracy, because recent hemorrhage or transfusion affects the accuracy of the study.

Splenic sequestration studies are performed to determine if destruction of red blood cells, which causes decreased red blood cell survival, is caused by splenic destruction of red blood cells. The study may be performed in conjunction with red blood cell survival studies; imaging can be performed on the same every-other-day schedule as a red blood cell survival study. Activity is measured over the precordium, anterior liver, and posterior spleen.

In a normal study, the spleen/liver ratio is 1:1 and remains 1:1 over time. When splenic sequestration of red blood cells occurs, there is increased splenic/hepatic ratio that increases over the course of the study. Splenomegaly itself, without pathologic sequestration, can yield spleen/liver ratios from 2:1 to 4:1. Because of this, a rising spleen/liver ratio is the best and most specific evidence for significant sequestration.

CHAPTER 8

Neurologic

CASE 183

History.—18-year-old with a new-onset seizure disorder. MRI and CT are both normal.

Scan.—^{99m}Tc HMPAO SPECT brain scan.

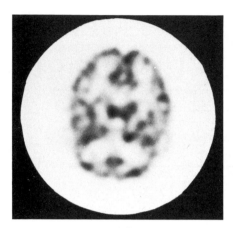

Transaxial view.

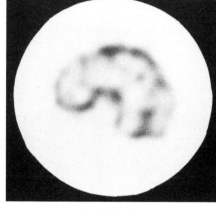

Sagittal view.

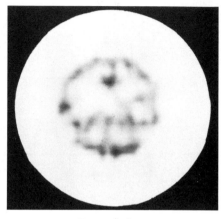

Coronal view.

Findings.—Symmetric, homogeneous uptake of ^{99m}TC HMPAO.

Diagnosis.—Normal ^{99m}Tc HMPAO brain scan.

Cerebral perfusion imaging is of significant importance in the evaluation of patients with cerebrovascular disease as well as a variety of disorders affecting cerebral blood flow, such as seizure disorders and dementia.

Isotopes used in evaluating these diseases are similar to thallium 201, with distribution proportional to blood flow. Radiopharmaceuticals with these properties include technetium 99m hexamethyl propylene amine oxime (HMPAO), and iodine 123 iodoamphetamine (IMP). They are fat soluble and cross the intact blood-brain barrier. Unlike pertechnetate, they are taken up by normal brain tissue. ^{99m}Tc HMPAO and ^{123}I IMP are highly extracted (about 80% during a single pass) from cerebral blood flow and reach equilibrium quickly. ^{99m}Tc HMPAO reaches equilibrium in about 5 minutes, with ^{123}I IMP reaching maximum extraction in about 20 minutes. ^{99m}Tc HMPAO does not undergo significant change in its distribution pattern with time. After crossing the blood-brain barrier, it binds intracellularly. ^{123}I IMP has been shown to redistribute or change its distribution pattern with time similar to ^{201}Tl in cardiac imaging. This allows evaluation of ischemic cerebrovascular disease with ^{123}I.

The identification of seizure foci is increased if the isotope is injected during a seizure rather than interictally. ^{123}I IMP is stable for about 12 hours. ^{99m}Tc HMPAO must be injected within about 45 minutes of being mixed because of gradual breakdown of the product into a more hydrophilic substance. Thus ^{123}I IMP has some advantages in imaging seizure foci; it can be kept at the bedside until a seizure occurs.

The study requires that the patient be placed in a subdued environment for about 30 minutes before injection. If there is excessive central nervous system stimulation at the time of injection, increased perfusion to the area of the brain involved with this stimulation (i.e., visual or auditory cortex) can be seen. Imaging can then be performed, in the case of ^{99m}Tc HMPAO, any time in the next 4 hours. Multiple-headed single-photon emission computed tomography (SPECT) cameras decrease the required imaging times. Sedation is occasionally required to keep the patient still during the acquisition period.

A normal ^{99m}Tc HMPAO brain scan shows increased activity in the gray matter and cerebellum, with a normal ratio of activity between these being about 1:1. The concentration of ^{99m}Tc HMPAO in white matter is normally about half that in gray matter. Symmetry is the hallmark of a normal study.

CASE 184

History.—73-year-old man with a 2-hour history of left hemiplegia.

Scan.—^{99m}Tc HMPAO SPECT brain scan.

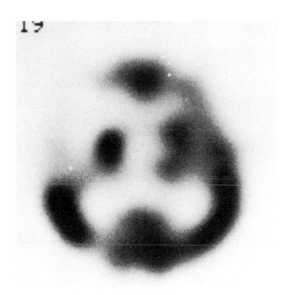

Transaxial SPECT reconstruction.

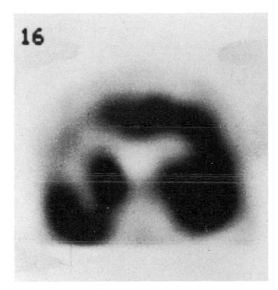

Coronal SPECT reconstruction.

Findings.—Defect in right frontoparietal region.

Diagnosis.—Cerebrovascular accident.

Cerebrovascular disease is the third most common cause of death in the United States. Cerebrovascular accidents (CVA), or strokes, are caused primarily by thrombosis, hemorrhage, and embolism. Three fourths of all thromboses involve the internal carotid or middle cerebral artery, usually at sites of branching, bifurcation, or curving. Radiopharmaceuticals initially used for imaging CVA were ^{99m}Tc pertechnetate, ^{99m}Tc diethylenetriaminepentaacetic acid (DTPA), and ^{99m}Tc glucoheptonate. These agents enter the brain if there is a breakdown in the blood-brain barrier. A major disadvantage of these agents is poor sensitivity for CVA in the first week (25%); the best sensitivity is 3 to 4 weeks after infarction.

Newer cerebral blood flow radiopharmaceuticals and single-photon emission computed tomography (SPECT) have made imaging of CVA much more clinically useful. ^{99m}Tc HMPAO and ^{123}I IMP have similar properties that make them useful for imaging stroke. Both are lipophilic and cross the in-

tact blood-brain barrier. They rapidly localize in the brain. Because of these properties, they act as regional cerebral blood flow markers.

A significant advantage of the newer agents is their sensitivity for acute CVA. Because regional cerebral blood flow is imaged, a SPECT image becomes abnormal earlier than anatomic modalities such as computed tomography (CT) and magnetic resonance imaging (MRI). Because of lower resolution, brain SPECT studies are not useful for suspected lacunar infarcts.

SPECT may be better than CT or MRI in defining the extent of an infarct. With ^{123}I IMP brain imaging, areas of infarct and ischemia can be differentiated by doing an initial image set and comparing these with delayed images. In cerebral ischemia, ^{123}I IMP will undergo "redistribution" with time just as ^{67}Tl does in the heart.

221

CASE 185

History.—72-year-old woman with the acute onset of right hemiparesis and aphasia.

Scan.—^{99m}Tc HMPAO SPECT brain scan.

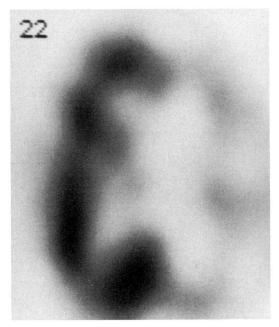

Transaxial SPECT image.

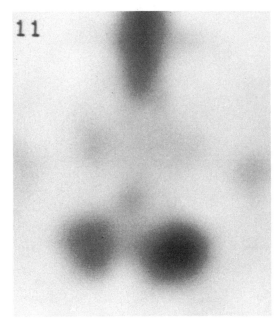

Lower transaxial view.

Findings.—Decreased activity in the left hemisphere and right cerebellum.

Diagnosis.—Left cerebrovascular accident, with crossed cerebellar diaschesis.

Cerebrovascular disease is manifested by symptoms of transient ischemic attacks (TIAs), reversible ischemic neurologic deficit, and cerebral infarction (CVA). The most common cause of cerebrovascular disease is atherosclerosis, with ulceration of the carotid artery bifurcation. Thrombus forms on the exposed ulcer and either lyses or detaches, with downstream embolization of the brain. The atheromatous plaque may also break loose and embolize the brain. In either case, if the embolism occludes a vessel with no collateral circulation, symptoms of cerebral ischemia result. The middle cerebral artery receives the largest share of blood flow of the three main intracranial vessels, and because of this, embolic events most commonly involve the middle cerebral artery distribution. When symptoms are present for less than 24 hours, it is referred to as a TIA. If the symptoms resolve after 24 hours, it is a reversible ischemic neurologic deficit. If the symptoms persist with incomplete recovery, a completed CVA has occurred.

The diagnosis of completed CVA usually is obvious by clinical examination. The cause of the symptoms is not always clear clinically, however. CT and MRI are successful in excluding hemorrhage as the cause, but definitive findings of cerebral infarction are often not seen for more than 24 hours. Radionuclide cerebral blood flow imaging has been shown to be abnormal earlier in stroke than either CT or MRI. The extent of the infarct is also better estimated with SPECT studies than with CT and MRI, which underestimate the size of the infarct.

SPECT cerebral blood flow imaging has been performed using several different isotopes, including xenon 133, ^{123}I IMP, ^{123}I HIPDM, and ^{99m}Tc HMPAO. Positron emission tomography (PET) also is useful in measuring regional cerebral blood flow. The study presented was performed using ^{99m}Tc HMPAO. This agent is a lipophilic agent that crosses the intact blood-brain barrier and has a high extraction on first pass through the brain. It provides a map of cerebral blood flow.

This study demonstrates the finding of crossed cerebellar diaschesis, a finding seen in CVA patients. A 15% to 20% decrease in regional blood flow to the cerebellar cortex contralateral to the infarction occurs. The proposed cause of this phenomenon, originally described on PET scans, is the interruption of the corticopontine or corticocerebellar neural interactions. It has been proposed that involvement of the motor cortex in the infarcted area is necessary for this to be seen.

Another cerebral blood flow characteristic seen occasionally in acute CVA is increased perfusion to the area immediately surrounding the infarction. This so-called luxury perfusion is thought to represent loss of autoregulation of cerebral blood flow in the peri-infarct region. This early hyperemia is transient and resolves on delayed scans performed 1 month later.

CASE 186

History.—66-year-old man with a history of transient left-sided weakness.

Scan.—^{123}I IMP SPECT brain scan.

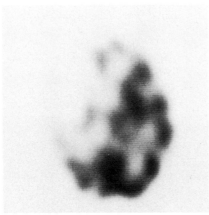

Immediate axial reconstruction.

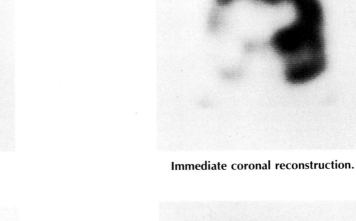

Immediate coronal reconstruction.

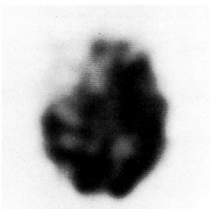

Four-hour axial reconstruction.

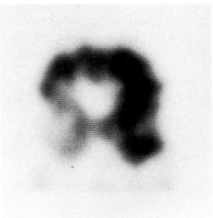

Four-hour coronal reconstruction.

Findings.— Decreased activity in right frontoparietal region, which fills in on delayed images.

Diagnosis.— Ischemia of the right middle cerebral artery.

The gold standard in the diagnosis of occlusive cerbrovascular disease has long been contrast angiography. It provides a reliable means of imaging arterial stenoses, ulcerations, and other cerebrovascular abnormalities. It is, however, not without risk. Complications occur in as many as 12% of patients and include embolic cerebrovascular accident (CVA), aortic dissection, and intravenous contrast reactions.

There are safer, noninvasive methods of evaluation for cerebrovascular disease. These include ophthalmodynamometry, oculoplethysmography, ultrasound Doppler examination of the carotid arteries, radionuclide angiography, and ^{123}I IMP brain scans.

At present, radionuclide angiography is rarely performed to diagnose cerebrovascular disease. The study is limited by low resolution and low count density and, because of this, is able to detect only major perfusion abnormalities. With an 80% or greater stenosis, 80% of lesions are detected. Fifty percent stenoses are detected only about half of the time. Lesser degrees of stenoses are identified in 10% or less of cases.

^{123}I IMP is a lipophilic agent that crosses the intact blood-brain barrier with a 74% to 92% extraction efficiency on first pass. Its uptake in the brain is dependent on regional cerebral blood flow, as well as binding to nonspecific, high-capacity binding sites for amines. Its distribution, and therefore the quality of the study, may be altered by sympathomimetic amines.

The initial uptake of ^{123}I IMP reflects regional cerebral blood flow. However, with time, the ^{123}I IMP undergoes "redistribution" similar to ^{201}Tl in the heart. The gray/white activity ratio changes with time from 2.4 immediately after injection to 0.6 at 24 hours. This redistribution phenomenon allows delayed imaging (e.g., as in cardiac imaging) to differentiate areas of infarction from ischemia. Cerebral infarction appears as a fixed photopenic area on both initial and delayed images, whereas ischemic areas fill in on later images.

The patient should be placed in a quiet room for 30 minutes before injection to prevent abnormal distribution as a result of sensory stimulation of cerebral cortex. The patient should also be pretreated with 3 drops of saturated solution of potassium iodide 30 minutes before the injection to minimize thyroid accumulation of the agent.

^{123}I is a cyclotron-produced isotope with a half-life of 13.2 hours. IMP needs to be specially ordered for each study at least 24 hours in advance. In addition to availability, disadvantages of ^{123}I IMP include its expense and poor photon flux for SPECT acquisitions.

CASE 187

History.—27-year-old woman with ataxia, decreased mental status, and the new onset of seizures. MRI of the brain with and without gadolinium was normal. She was in status epilepticus 7 hours before and during injection for this study, with a focal motor seizure involving her left shoulder and arm.

Scan.—Multiple SPECT images of the brain were obtained 2 hours after the ictal injection of 25 mCi of ^{99m}Tc HMPAO.

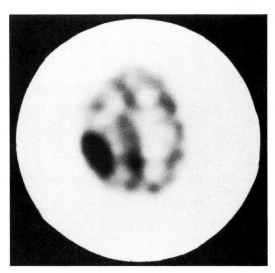

Transaxial SPECT reconstruction of brain.

Findings.—An area of markedly increased activity is seen in the high right parietal cortex.

Diagnosis.—Seizure focus in the right parietal cortex.

Brain SPECT studies are an important tool in the evaluation of epilepsy. They are most useful when used with magnetic resonance imaging (MRI), computed tomography (CT), and electroencephalographic (EEG) studies.

EEG is valuable in diagnosing seizure disorders but does not give detailed information about the location of the seizure focus. CT scanning demonstrates significant pathologic conditions in only about 10% to 40% of patients with partial seizures. MRI, CT, EEG, and SPECT combine to localize epileptic foci in 90% of cases.

The two most widely available agents for SPECT images are ^{99m}Tc HMPAO and ^{123}I IMP. Each has nearly equal sensitivities for brain pathologic conditions. HMPAO is a ^{99m}Tc agent and is readily available. It has superior counting statistics to ^{123}I IMP, reaches equilibrium in the brain quickly (about 2 minutes), and does not undergo redistribution with time. This allows injection during a seizure with delayed imaging when the patient is stable. ^{123}I IMP takes 15 to 20 minutes to reach equilibrium in the brain and must be ordered at least 24 hours in advance.

Another use of SPECT brain scanning is in differentiating epilepsy from pseudoseizures. Ictal injections of ^{99m}Tc HMPAO in epilepsy will show increased activity in the area of the seizure focus, with less marked uptake or normal uptake demonstrated with pseudoseizures.

CASE 188

History.— 55-year-old man with presenile dementia.

Scan.—^{99m}Tc HMPAO SPECT brain scan.

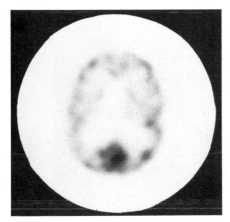

Transaxial view.

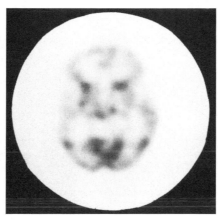

Lower transaxial view.

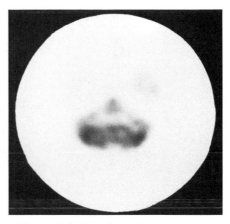

Transaxial view through cerebellum.

Findings.— The scan shows diminished activity involving the frontal and parietal cerebral cortical activity compared with the cerebellar hemispheres. The cortical/cerebellar uptake ratio was 0.75.

Diagnosis.— Alzheimer's disease.

Alzheimer's disease is a chronic, progressive, degenerative disease of the central nervous system that causes dementia. Memory, language, and cognitive abilities are affected. The disease is not uncommon; 2 million Americans older than 50 years of age are affected.

The diagnosis of Alzheimer's disease in its early stages can be difficult. Misdiagnoses occur in 10% to 30% of patients. Although standardized neurologic and neuropsychologic criteria for the diagnosis of Alzheimer's disease have been developed, it is often a diagnosis of exclusion.

SPECT has been shown to be an accurate technique for diagnosing Alzheimer's disease. It can solve the common clinical problem of differentiating Alzheimer's disease from multi-infarct dementia. In addition, SPECT scanning is used in some centers to follow progression or response to experimental therapy.

In demented patients the CT scan shows widened cortical sulci and enlarged ventricles. Brain SPECT scanning with either ^{123}I IMP or ^{99m}Tc HMPAO will show regionally de-creased blood flow in primarily the temporal and parietal lobes in Alzheimer's disease. Disseminated areas of decreased tracer uptake with no regional pattern are seen in multi-infarct dementia. Focal defects of perfusion in radiographically normal brain are seen more often in patients with Alzheimer's disease than in those with multi-infarct dementia.

Because of relative sparing of cerebellar perfusion in Alzheimer's patients, it has been shown that the cortical/cerebellar uptake ratio is reduced from a normal of about 1 to a value of less than 0.8. However, recent reports indicate the use of the cerebellum as an internal control may be unreliable when ^{123}I IMP is used. More study is needed in this area.

PET has documented abnormal patterns of cerebral blood flow and cerebral metabolism in patients with Alzheimer's disease. Areas of hypometabolism and corresponding hypoperfusion involving the posterior parietal and frontal lobes have been seen. The parallel relationship of metabolic activity and cerebral blood flow has also been demonstrated using PET imaging.

CASE 189

History.— 5-year-old girl being treated with radiation and chemotherapy for medulloblastoma, who now has recurrence vs. radiation necrosis on MRI.

Scan.— After intravenous administration of 3 mCi of ^{201}Tl, multiple SPECT images of the brain were obtained.

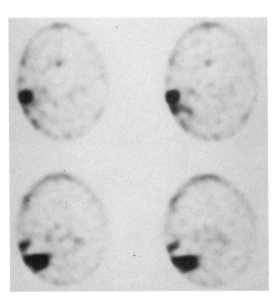

SPECT coronal image.

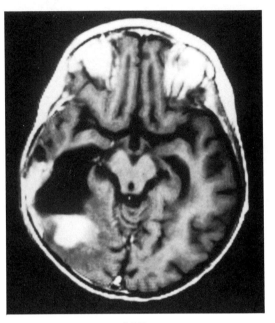

MRI.

Findings.— The MRI image shows gadolinium enhancement in the right parieto-occipital region. The ^{201}Tl scan shows increased activity corresponding to these areas of enhancement.

Diagnosis.— Medulloblastoma recurrence.

The initial evaluation of primary brain tumors is done with computed tomography (CT) and magnetic resonance imaging (MRI). Stereotactic or open biopsy provide the definitive diagnosis. These methods are all that is needed in the majority of patients.

The preoperative prediction of the glioma grade of a particular tumor is useful in light of the frequency of mixed tumor histology and sampling errors of stereotactic biopsy. Thus far positron emission tomography (PET) has been most reliable in predicting the metabolic activity of a particular tumor. The more metabolically active a tumor is, the more likely it is to behave as a higher-grade tumor. The availability of PET, however, is still limited.

Another problem with gliomas is differentiating recurrent tumor from necrotic tumor, radiation necrosis, or scar tissue in a patient already treated for a brain tumor. Contrast-enhanced CT and MRI have difficulty because enhancement occurs in any area where there is breakdown of the normal blood-brain barrier, whether the cause is recurrent tumor, necrotic tumor, or radiation necrosis.

Thallium 201 SPECT brain imaging has been proposed as a means of assisting in the previously mentioned clinical situations. The use of ^{201}Tl for imaging tumors is not new. It has been shown to accumulate in several tumors, including thyroid, lung, liver, and esophageal cancers. The mechanism of uptake of ^{201}Tl in tumors is not known for certain but likely is similar to the uptake of potassium via the sodium-potassium pump. ^{201}Tl accumulation is related to the growth rate; increased uptake occurs in rapidly growing tissue, and little uptake is seen in slowly growing tissues.

Normal brain tissue demonstrates very little accumulation of ^{201}Tl. Primary brain tumors have been found to show increased accumulation of ^{201}Tl, with the intensity of uptake related to histologic grade of the tumor. When normal brain contralateral to the tumor is used as a baseline, if the degree of tumor uptake is greater than 1.5 times that in normal brain, the tumor behaves as a high-grade lesion. If the uptake is less than 1.5 times normal, it is more likely to act as a low-grade lesion.

A similar principle can be used in following patients treated for brain tumors. In cases where there is contrast enhancement on CT or MRI at the site of the previously treated primary tumor, a ^{201}Tl brain scan can help differentiate recurrent tumor from necrotic tissue. This is because ^{201}Tl uptake is not dependent on blood-brain barrier breakdown but is an active process that is increased in malignant tissues. Significant uptake indicates tumor recurrence.

CASE 190

History.—50-year-old woman with headaches.

Scan.—After intravenous administration of 20 mCi of ^{99m}Tc pertechnetate, serial angiographic images of the brain were obtained in the anterior view at 2-second intervals for 60 seconds with immediate blood pool images and 3-hour delayed images in multiple projections of the brain.

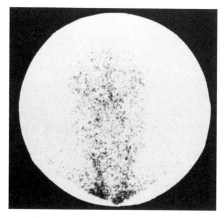

Anterior flow study arterial phase.

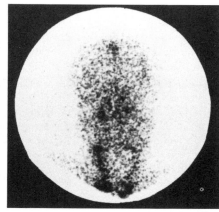

Flow study venous phase.

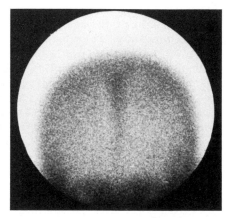

Anterior delayed image.

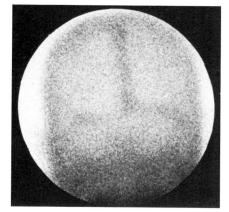

Right lateral view.

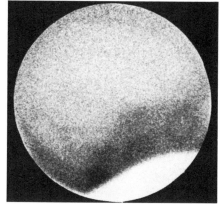

Posterior delayed image.

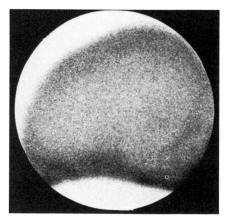

Left lateral view.

Findings.— No abnormal areas of uptake.

Diagnosis.— Normal conventional brain scan.

Imaging of the brain before computed tomography (CT) and magnetic resonance imaging (MRI) was performed by either cerebral angiography or conventional radionuclide brain scan. The indications for conventional radionuclide brain scans are quite limited now because of the much higher-resolution CT and MRI; however, there are occasions when conventional brain scans are still of significant clinical use, as in brain death and inflammatory disease.

The blood-brain barrier acts to prevent most bloodborne materials from entering the brain. Anatomically, brain capillaries are unique in that they have a continuous basement membrane and closed endothelial clefts, preventing exit of large molecular-weight proteins. Passive diffusion, pore filtration, and pinocytosis normally do not occur in the brain. Rather, substances enter the brain by way of active transport across the capillary walls. The blood-brain barrier normally prevents entry into the brain of radiopharmaceuticals such as ^{99m}Tc pertechnetate, ^{99m}Tc glucoheptonate, or ^{99m}Tc diethylenetriaminepentaacetic acid (DTPA). Abnormal accumulations of these radiopharmaceuticals are primarily the result of breakdown of the blood-brain barrier.

Tumors cause increased accumulation of conventional radiopharmaceuticals because of increased vascularity, abnormal permeability, pinocytosis, direct cellular uptake, and accompanying cerebral edema, in addition to blood-brain barrier breakdown.

Each of the radiopharmaceuticals used for conventional brain scans has advantages and disadvantages. ^{99m}Tc pertechnetate is most commonly used because of its availability and low cost. It is loosely bound to albumin, which causes slow blood clearance. Because of this, a delay of 3 to 4 hours is required before scanning. ^{99m}Tc pertechnetate is normally concentrated by the choroid plexus, which can con-

fuse interpretation. This uptake can be blocked by pretreating the patient with oral potassium perchlorate.

^{99m}Tc DTPA and ^{99m}Tc glucoheptonate are two other agents used in conventional brain imaging. They have an advantage over ^{99m}Tc pertechnetate because of their enhanced washout by the kidneys. This increases the target/background ratio and allows earlier imaging (delays of only 1–3 hours) and, theoretically, increased sensitivity. These agents are also not normally concentrated in the choroid plexus, and therefore pretreatment with perchlorate is not required.

The sensitivity of ^{99m}Tc DTPA and ^{99m}Tc glucoheptonate is increased over ^{99m}Tc pertechnetate in acute infarcts, well-differentiated gliomas, and tumors near the base of the brain. ^{99m}Tc glucoheptonate is slightly more sensitive than ^{99m}Tc DTPA for brain disease. Its cost, however, is also much greater.

A normal brain scan includes an angiographic phase performed in the anterior projection, with blood pool images done in multiple projections. Delayed images are then obtained.

The flow on angiographic images should show symmetric activity in the common carotids, middle cerebral arteries, and midline anterior cerebral arteries. The anterior cerebral arteries appear as a single midline structure, with the two middle cerebral arteries and the carotid arteries forming a five-pointed star. The capillary phase of the study shows symmetric activity in the region of both cerebral hemispheres. The venous images show activity in the superior sagittal and transverse sinuses and in the jugular veins.

Delayed static images should show symmetric activity in the scalp and venous sinuses, with normal brain being devoid of significant tracer accumulation.

CASE 191

History.— 26-year-old man with a history of a recent intracranial arteriovenous malformation rupture. The patient was clinically brain dead but was being considered as a potential transplant donor. We were asked to confirm brain death.

Scan.—Twenty-five millicuries of ^{99m}Tc TcO$_4$ was administered intravenously. Serial images were obtained at 2-second intervals for 30 seconds, with delayed images in multiple projections.

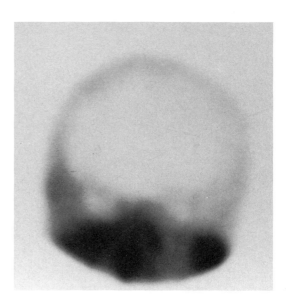

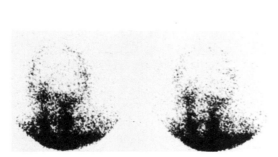

Cerebral flow study.

Immediate anterior static image.

Findings.— No arterial flow above the circle of Willis and no activity in the superior sagittal sinus or the transverse sinuses.

Diagnosis.— Brain death.

The radionuclide cerebral perfusion study is a noninvasive indicator of cerebral viability. In critically ill patients it can be performed at the bedside.

In patients with cerebral death, increased intracranial pressure causes diminished or absent intracranial blood flow, eventually resulting in total cerebral infarction. A radionuclide brain scan is performed in two stages to determine if arterial blood flow to the brain is present. Angiographic images are obtained in the anterior projection, followed by blood pool images in the anterior and both lateral projections. A good bolus injection is important. A tourniquet around the scalp may be used to prevent flow to the scalp through the external carotid system.

A normal study shows flow in the carotid arteries bilaterally that enters the anterior cerebral arteries (which overlap on this study) and both middle cerebral arteries. If a tourniquet is not used, external carotid system flow is seen. Blood pool images show visualization of the superior sagittal and transverse sinuses.

In brain death there is no flow above the circle of Willis during the angiogram. Because of shunting of blood from the internal carotid system to the external carotid system, increased activity in the face often causes the "hot nose" sign. Blood pool images classically show no uptake in the superior sagittal sinus or transverse sinuses.

Occasionally, slight activity in the superior sagittal sinus is seen. This is caused by perforating veins from the scalp and does not preclude the diagnosis of brain death in a patient with no evidence of intracranial flow during the arterial phase. In children, visualization of cranial sutures is also considered a sign of brain death because of diminished background activity without cerebral perfusion.

CASE 192

History.— 62-year-old woman with sudden onset of right hemiplegia.

Scan.—^{99m}Tc pertechnetate planar brain scan.

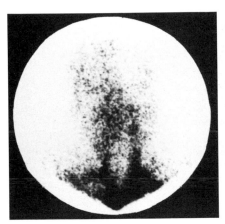

Anterior angiographic image of head.

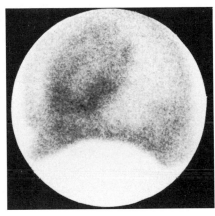

Left lateral view of head.

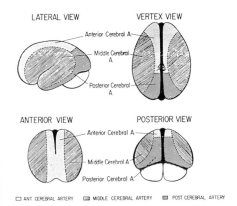

Vascular territories of each of three main cerebral arteries.

Findings.— The angiographic images demonstrate diminished activity in the left middle cerebral arterial distribution. The delayed static image in the left lateral projection shows a flame-shaped area of increased activity in the distribution of the left middle cerebral artery.

Diagnosis.— Left middle cerebral CVA on conventional brain scan.

The pathogenesis of cerebrovascular accident (CVA) as an embolic occlusion of a cerebral vessel, which usually originates at the carotid artery bifurcation, is discussed in detail in another case. Other mechanisms for CVA include thrombosis of an artery compromised by atherosclerotic disease, intracranial hemorrhage, or hemorrhagic stroke.

The evaluation of suspected cerebral infarction is normally done using computed tomography (CT) or magnetic resonance imaging (MRI). However, brain death studies are sometimes done in CVA patients; therefore, knowledge of the findings of stroke on conventional brain imaging can be useful.

All of the radiopharmaceuticals normally used for conventional brain imaging are labeled with ^{99m}Tc and include pertechnetate, glucoheptonate, and DTPA. They require breakdown of the blood-brain barrier for lesion visualization. In CVA the abnormal activity accumulates in the distribution of a cerebral blood vessel. The diagram illustrates the distribution of the three main cerebral vessels.

With strokes, the radionuclide cerebral angiogram shows asymmetric decreased flow. A "hot nose" may be present because of shunting of blood from the internal to the external carotid systems. A "flip-flop" sign is another indication of stroke. In the early arterial phase of the study, diminished perfusion to the involved side is seen, with normal flow on the contralateral side. Later in the arterial phase, activity is increased on the involved side, with decreased activity on the normal side because of slower collateral circulation to the infarcted area. Occasionally the cerebral angiogram will demonstrate increased flow to the involved side because of "luxury perfusion" or reactive hyperemia in the peri-infarct zone seen in the early weeks after CVA.

The static image shows a characteristic flame-shaped area of increased activity. The sensitivity of static images depends on the time since the initial event. Early, the images may be normal in both an ischemic and hemorrhagic stroke. After this time, some, but not all, will demonstrate diminishing uptake on subsequent studies. Static images of a hemorrhagic CVA will be abnormal only about 25% of the time in the first week. The scan findings then fade by about 6 to 8 weeks. The sensitivity of static images for detection of an ischemic CVA in the first week is even poorer.

CASE 193

History.—60-year-old woman with headache.

Scan.—After intravenous administration of 20 mCi of ^{99m}Tc pertechnetate, multiple images of the brain were obtained.

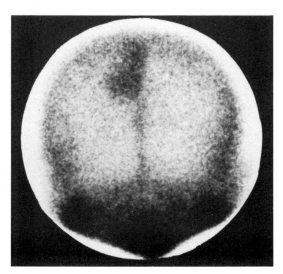

Anterior view of head.

Findings.—Delayed anterior image shows intense uptake just to the right of midline overlying the frontal lobe. Angiographic images (not shown) demonstrated hyperemia to this area.

Diagnosis.—Meningioma.

Meningiomas are slow-growing benign tumors that arise from cells of the pia-arachnoid and comprise 20% of all primary brain tumors. They occur commonly in the midline along the falx cerebri and along the sphenoid ridge. Other sites of occurrence include the lateral cerebral convexities, the olfactory groove, the tentorium of the cerebellum, and near the foramen magnum. Women are affected more than men. Meningiomas are very vascular tumors and have a tendency to calcify (10%). About half of meningiomas have associated hyperostosis of the overlying bone.

The sensitivity of the conventional radionuclide brain scan for detection of a meningioma is greater than 90%. The meningioma on brain scan is hypervascular throughout the arterial and venous phase. Delayed images show significantly increased uptake, which becomes more intense with time as further delayed images are obtained.

This appearance, although typical of meningiomas, is not specific for meningiomas alone. Other primary or metastatic brain tumors may also share this appearance. The appearance of a meningioma is quite distinct on contrast-enhanced computed tomography (CT). The lesion displays variable calcification but enhances intensely with sharp rounded borders.

Radionuclide brain scanning has largely been replaced by CT and magnetic resonance imaging (MRI). These have much higher resolution and have tomographic capabilities that nuclear medicine has subsequently borrowed in the development of SPECT imaging. Studies by the National Cancer Institute indicate that essentially no tumors missed on CT will be seen on radionuclide studies. Therefore, patients with normal CT or MRI scans in whom clinicians have a strong suspicion of tumor should not undergo radionuclide brain scanning.

Current radionuclide brain imaging, however, continues to expand into areas of SPECT and PET as new radiopharmaceuticals become available. These agents focus on diagnosing physiologic disorders of the brain rather than anatomic lesions.

CASE 194

History.— 12-year-old boy with the acute onset of fever, confusion, and headache. He also complained of olfactory hallucinations.

Scan.— ^{99m}Tc pertechnetate planar brain scan was performed.

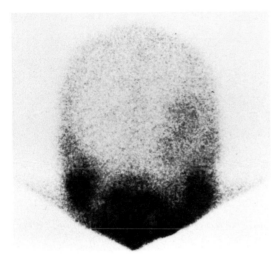

Anterior view of head.

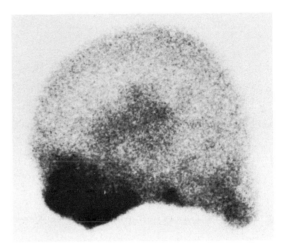

Left lateral view of head.

Findings.— Angiographic images are not shown. The 3-hour delay scan shows increased activity in the region of the left medial temporal lobe.

Diagnosis.— Herpes simplex encephalitis.

A subsequent work-up, including a brain biopsy, confirmed the diagnosis of type I herpes simplex encephalitis. Encephalitis caused by the type I herpes simplex virus is the most common sporadic form of necrotizing viral encephalitis. Herpes is a severe, rapidly progressive, central nervous system infection that often results in significant neurologic sequelae or death. Early detection of this infection is important so that appropriate antiviral therapy can be instituted to minimize long-term effects. Therapeutic trials found that if a definitive diagnosis can be established before the fourth day of symptoms and appropriate antiviral therapy instituted, morbidity and mortality will be minimized.

Common symptoms of herpes simplex encephalitis include the acute onset of fever and focal neurologic symptoms. Symptoms related to temporal lobe dysfunction are more common because the temporal lobes are the most consistently involved parts of the brain in herpes simplex encephalitis. Early symptoms may be more insidious, including malaise, lethargy, headache, and confusion. Seizures, coma, and death can result.

Computed tomography (CT) has reduced sensitivity for this disorder until later in the course of the disease. When abnormal, the CT shows a low-density lesion in the medial portion of the temporal lobe. Mass effect with streaky linear enhancement of this lesion is also seen. Magnetic resonance imaging (MRI) is the imaging procedure of choice. Temporal lobe edema can be detected earlier with MRI than CT. The overall sensitivity for detection of herpes simplex encephalitis by radionuclide imaging ranges from 50% to 85%. If CT or MRI is normal and the clinicians have a strong clinical suspicion of herpes, a radionuclide brain scan can be performed. The radionuclide scan relies on breakdown of the blood-brain barrier for lesion detection.

The most specific radionuclide brain scan findings of herpes simplex encephalitis are bilateral hyperperfusion, with delayed images showing bilateral temporal increased activity. A less specific but common pattern is unilateral hyperperfusion, with unilateral temporofrontal uptake on delayed images. If scans are performed late in the course of disease, decreased flow may be seen because of necrosis. Differential diagnoses of these findings include cerebritis, abscess, cerebral infarction with luxury perfusion, and a vascular tumor.

CASE 195

History.— 42-year-old man with a seizure disorder.

Scan.— After intravenous administration of 20 mCi of ^{99m}Tc pertechnetate, serial angiographic images of the brain were obtained in the anterior view at 2-second intervals for 60 seconds, with immediate blood pool images and 3-hour delayed images in multiple projections.

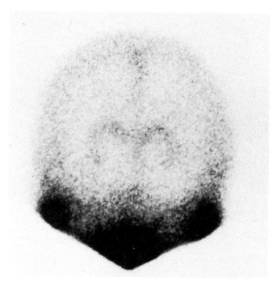

Anterior view of head.

Findings.— The angiographic images are not shown but were normal. The 3-hour delayed images show significant activity in the roof and lateral walls of the lateral ventricles. The scan is otherwise normal.

Diagnosis.— Choroid plexus visualization of ^{99m}Tc pertechnetate.

The most commonly used agent for conventional brain scans is ^{99m}Tc pertechnetate. It is readily available without special preparation. It is obtained simply by "milking" a molybdenum generator. It is inexpensive, and its 140-keV photon is ideal for imaging with the Anger camera. Its 6-hour half-life results in a low-delivered radiation dose to the patient.

In about 20% of patients, ^{99m}Tc pertechnetate is concentrated by the choroid plexus to a degree that interferes with interpretation of the study. The choroid plexes are specialized areas of the brain located primarily in the walls of the lateral ventricles but also located on the roof of the third and fourth ventricles, which are very vascular and are involved in the production of cerebrospinal fluid (CSF). CSF is often thought of as an ultrafiltrate of serum; however, it is evident that active transport of certain materials by the choroid plexus also occurs.

^{99m}Tc pertechnetate accumulation in the choroid plexus can be competitively inhibited by pretreatment with perchlorate. This is similar to the use of perchlorate to wash out ^{99m}Tc pertechnetate in the thyroid gland.

The oral dosage of perchlorate as the potassium salt is 200 mg for an adult, 100 mg for children 2 to 12 years old, and 50 mg for children up to age 2 years. For maximal blocking effect, ^{99m}Tc perchlorate should be administered 30 to 60 minutes before ^{99m}Tc pertechnetate injection.

^{99m}Tc perchlorate administration does not significantly alter uptake of ^{99m}Tc pertechnetate in the salivary glands. This can be a significant problem in detecting lesions located near the base of the brain.

Choroid plexus visualization can also result from choroid plexus papilloma, intrathecal methotrexate, intraventricular hemorrhage, and infection.

CASE 196

History.—53-year-old woman with breast carcinoma and suspected metastases. She had undergone a bone scan 3 days earlier, which was normal.

Scan.—The patient was pretreated with 200 mg of ^{99m}Tc perchlorate orally. ^{99m}Tc pertechnetate planar brain scan was performed.

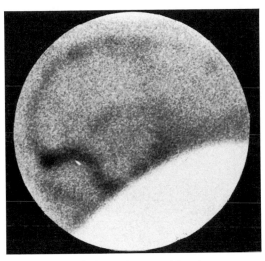

Right lateral view of head.

Findings.—Angiographic images are not shown. Prominent venous sinus activity in the superior sagittal sinus, the transverse sinus, and the choroid plexus is seen. No other significant intracranial pathologic condition was identified.

Diagnosis.—Brain scan with red blood cell labeling secondary to previous tin administration.

This case demonstrates an important technical error that can dramatically alter the biodistribution of ^{99m}Tc pertechnetate. ^{99m}Tc pertechnetate scans (e.g., brain, Meckel's, thyroid) performed after the previous administration of tin can result in the in vivo labeling of red blood cells.

In vivo labeling of red blood cells is widely done. The in vivo technique involves the intravenous administration of 0.5 to 1.0 mg of stannous (tin) ion in the form of cold stannous pyrophosphate. Ten to 20 minutes is allowed for equilibration of the stannous ion. Fifteen to 30 mCi of ^{99m}Tc pertechnetate is then injected intravenously. The intracellular stannous ion acts as a reducing agent for the ^{99m}Tc pertechnetate, allowing it to bind to the hemoglobin molecule in red blood cells. This results in about 60% to 90% binding to the red blood cells. The remaining activity concentrates in the stomach, thyroid gland, and salivary glands or is excreted through the kidneys in the urine.

The excretion of tin from the body is very slow. Any test such as a bone scan that has tin as the reducing agent will result in high levels of circulating tin for an extended period. Subsequent administration of ^{99m}Tc pertechnetate for further diagnostic studies can result in significant red blood cell la-

beling. This effect is most marked in the first few days after tin administration but has been seen out as late as 8 weeks. A common cause of this problem in the past was a ^{99m}Tc pertechnetate brain scan being performed after a ^{99m}Tc pyrophosphate (PYP) bone scan. A more common problem today occurs when Meckel's scan is performed after in vivo tagging of red blood cells for a gastrointestinal bleeding study. Thyroid scans may show diminished thyroid activity as well if performed after significant tin administration.

The other commonly used brain scanning agents, ^{99m}Tc DTPA and ^{99m}Tc glucoheptanate, do not share this problem with ^{99m}Tc pertechnetate. They are prepared using tin; their biodistribution is not altered by previously administered tin. Other radiopharmaceuticals prepared using tin as a reducing agent (and therefore may cause red blood cell labeling with subsequently administered ^{99m}Tc pertechnetate) include methylene diphosphonate, DTPA, PYP, HMPAO, mertiatide, glucoheptanate, human serum albumin, macroaggregated albumin (MAA), and diisopropyliminodiacetic acid. An exception to the use of tin in ^{99m}Tc radiopharmaceutical preparation is sulfur colloid.

CASE 197

History.— 62-year-old woman with dementia.

Scan.—^{111}In DTPA cisternogram.

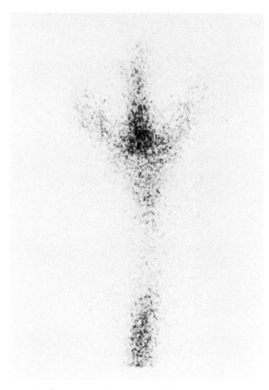

Six-hour anterior view of head and neck.

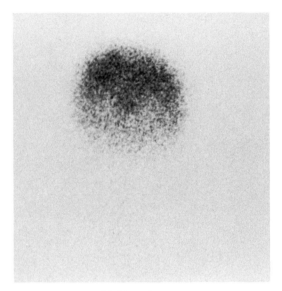

24-Hour image.

Findings.— Visualization of activity in the basal cisterns by 4 hours and ascent of activity over the convexities of the brain by 24 hours. No evidence of ventricular reflux.

Diagnosis.— Normal cisternogram.

Cerebrospinal fluid (CSF) imaging is useful in the diagnosis of communicating and obstructive hydrocephalus CSF leaks and in the evaluation of CSF shunt function.

CSF is formed in the choroid plexus located in the lateral ventricles of the brain. It flows from the lateral ventricles into the midline third ventricle through the foramen of Monroe. It then flows through the aqueduct of Sylvius to the fourth ventricle and exits the ventricular system through the foramen of the fourth ventricle (foramen of Luschka and Magendie).

The total volume of CSF is about 120 mL in a normal adult, with about one third of this located in the ventricular system of the brain. The other two thirds bathe the brain and spinal cord. CSF circulates and is reabsorbed into the vascular system through the arachnoid granulations located near the superior sagittal sinus. A small amount of CSF absorption also occurs across the ependymal lining of the ventricular system and the meninges.

CSF imaging is performed using primarily Indium 111 DTPA. This agent is diffusable in the CSF. It remains in the CSF space until absorbed through the arachnoid granulations, similar to CSF. ^{111}In DTPA distributed in the extracellular space is cleared by the kidneys via glomerular filtration.

^{111}In's 67-hour half-life allows imaging over several days. ^{111}In DTPA cisternography delivers 0.1 rad/mCi total-body radiation, 2.3 rad/mCi to the brain, and 1.3 rad/mCi to the spinal cord.

CSF imaging requires the subarachnoid administration of the radiopharmaceutical. This is performed through a lumbar puncture using a 21- or 22-gauge spinal needle. The dose is injected after the establishment of free CSF flow. An early image is usually obtained to ensure an adequate injection. This normally appears as a smooth column of activity. Serial delayed images are then obtained in anterior, posterior, vertex, and both lateral views at 1, 3 to 6, 24, 48, and 72 hours after injection.

About 15% of the time, an extradural injection occurs. The activity remains stationary, with no basal cistern activity by 3 hours. In this case, the injection needs to be repeated.

The normal scan shows activity ascending in the spinal canal, with activity visible in the basal cisterns by 3 to 4 hours. As activity fills the interhemispheric and sylvian fissures, a three-pronged Neptune's trident appearance is seen. By 24 hours, the activity ascends over the convexities of the brain. Normally no reflux of activity is seen into the lateral ventricles, although a small amount of transient ventricular activity seen before 24 hours is not considered abnormal.

Flow of the CSF from the puncture site to the basal cisterns can be speeded by mixing the ^{111}In DTPA with 2 to 3 mL of 10% dextrose solution to make the injectant hyperbaric. The patient can also be placed in the Trendelenburg position.

CASE 198

History.—61-year-old man with dementia and incontinence.

Scan.—^{111}In DTPA cisternogram.

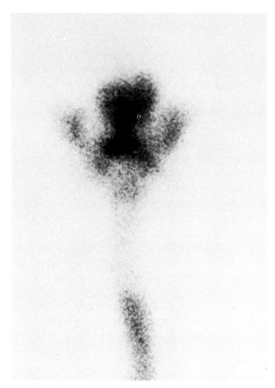

Six-hour anterior view of head and neck.

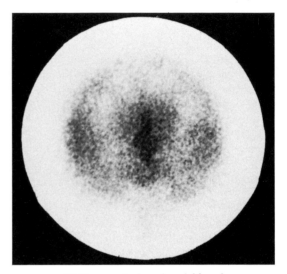

48-Hour anterior view of head.

Findings.—Reflux into ventricles at 6 hours, which persists at 48 hours. Delayed flow over the convexities.

Diagnosis.—Normal-pressure hydrocephalus.

Normal-pressure hydrocephalus can be difficult to diagnose. It is characterized by the triad of dementia, gait disorder, and urinary incontinence. Some patients respond dramatically to ventricular shunting. Because this disease is one of the few causes of presenile dementia that is treatable, tests like the cisternogram that can make the diagnosis of normal-pressure hydrocephalus are important.

The cause of normal-pressure hydrocephalus is unknown. It is thought to begin with an obstruction to CSF flow in the ventricles or basal meninges, with resulting dilatation of the ventricles. The CSF pressure then gradually returns to normal levels. The enlarged ventricles damage the adjacent brain parenchyma and decrease blood flow, causing dementia. The pattern of CSF flow is abnormal in NPH and can be assessed by following intrathecally injected ^{111}In DTPA.

Normally, after the lumbar injection of ^{111}In DTPA, activity appears in the basal cisterns by 3 hours. This activity then enters the inner hemispheric and sylvian fissures, forming Neptune's trident. CSF flows over the convexities by 24 hours. Usually there is no reflux into the lateral ventricles, although transient reflux at 12 to 24 hours is not considered significant.

In normal-pressure hydrocephalus, there is reflux into the lateral ventricles that persists on the 24-, 48- or even 72-hour images. The flow over the convexities of the brain is delayed or absent.

It is important to realize that the relationship between the CSF flow pattern on cisternography and the patient's response to shunting is variable. If the patient has had long-standing disease, chances are low that shunting will help. The ultimate decision whether to shunt should be based on clinical data.

CASE 199

History.—6-month-old boy with a history of meningitis and increasing head size. CT demonstrated dilated ventricles without an obstructing mass.

Scan.—^{111}In DTPA cisternogram.

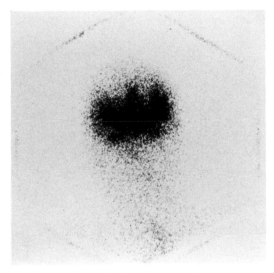

Anterior 48-hour image of head.

Findings.—Activity in the cisterns, with delayed flow over the convexities.

Diagnosis.—Obstructive (communicating) hydrocephalus.

Hydrocephalus indicates an excess of cerebrospinal fluid (CSF) in the brain. The pathophysiology includes cerebral atrophy, overproduction of CSF, poor absorption of CSF, or a blockage of CSF flow.

Obstructive hydrocephalus is caused by obstruction to CSF flow. It can be further subclassified as communicating or noncommunicating. Obstructive communicating hydrocephalus indicates an extraventricular block of CSF flow. There is free passage of CSF from the fourth ventricle to the cisterna magna. Obstructive noncommunicating hydrocephalus occurs when there is a block of CSF flow within the ventricular system. This usually occurs when tumors, other mass lesions, or developmental abnormalities block the flow of CSF from its site of production in the choroid plexus (in the third and fourth ventricles) to the site of exit of CSF from the brain near the fourth ventricle.

Attempting to discover the exact etiology of obstructive communicating hydrocephalus is often frustrating. Some are caused by arachnoid adhesions after meningitis or subarachnoid hemorrhage.

The scintigraphic pattern of CSF flow in obstructive communicating hydrocephalus shows slow transit of activity. There is reflux of activity into the lateral ventricles that persists beyond 24 hours. It may persist without clearing on delayed images. The other main finding is a delay in ascent of activity over the convexities of the cerebral cortex. Normal individuals usually have flow over the convexities by 24 hours. In obstructive communicating hydrocephalus, this is prolonged.

Cisternography is often performed for investigation of obstructive communicating in children. The normal and abnormal patterns of CSF flow are similar to those of an adult; however, normal CSF flow is more rapid in children. Intrathecal tracer injections are usually visible over the convexities of the brain by 12 hours.

CASE 200

History.—38-year-old woman with headaches. She had a ventriculoperitoneal shunt for obstructive communicating hydrocephalus.

Scan.—A needle was inserted into the shunt port and a small amount of CSF withdrawn to check for proximal limb patency. Three millicuries of ^{99m}Tc DTPA were then injected into the port, with serial delayed images being obtained over the entire length of the shunt.

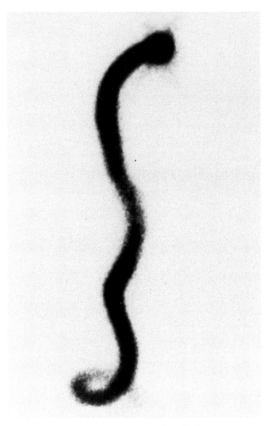

Anterior view of head and chest.

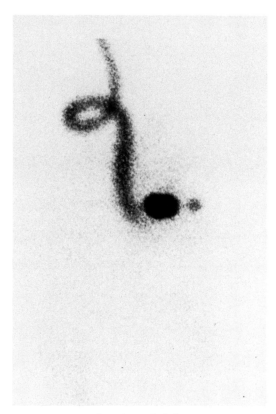

Anterior view of abdomen.

Findings.—This scan shows activity visible from the site of injection down the length of the shunt tubing into the coiled portion in the abdomen. The delayed image over the distal portion of the shunt demonstrates diffusion of activity into the peritoneum.

Diagnosis.—Ventriculoperitoneal shunt patency.

Hydrocephalus is caused by excess production, underabsorption, or blockage of cerebrospinal fluid (CSF). This results in enlargement of the ventricular system of the brain. The patient's symptoms may include headache, vomiting, incontinence, seizures, increasing head circumference or bulging fontinelles (in pediatric patients), and decreased consciousness. These patients require shunting of CSF flow to minimize permanent pressure-induced CNS damage.

The most common types of shunts redirect CSF flow from a lateral ventricle of the brain to the peritoneal cavity (ventriculoperitoneal, or VP, shunt) or to the right atrium (ventriculoatrial, or VA, shunt). These shunts have one or more one-way valves to assure unidirectional flow from the dilated ventricle to the peritoneum or right atrium. Also, they often have a port, or "pump," that can be used by the patient or physician to manually pump CSF simply by repeatedly depressing it.

The radionuclide evaluation of VP or VA shunt function involves the injection of a small amount of radioactive tracer into the port. If a one-way valve is located proximal to the port, no reflux of activity will be seen into the ventricular system of the brain. Patency of the proximal portion of the shunt is evaluated by attempting to aspirate 2 to 3 mL of CSF before injecting the radionuclide. If this is easily accomplished and a one-way valve is located distal to the port, patency of the proximal portion of the shunt can be assumed.

Serial delayed images over the distal portion of the shunt should be acquired to assure activity is seen diffusing freely into the peritoneum. If a VA shunt is being evaluated, demonstration of activity elsewhere is required to prove distal limb patency. In the case of DTPA, a delayed image over the kidneys should show excretion of the tracer if the distal limb is patent. A superior radiopharmaceutical for evaluation of VA shunts is ^{99m}Tc MAA, which demonstrates distal limb patency by embolizing the lung.

Another means of evaluating for VP and VA shunt dysfunction is CT scanning. Shunt malfunction is suspected in patients with enlarging ventricular size. There are occasional false negatives (shunt malfunction with normal ventricular size) and false positives (dilated ventricles with normal shunt function) with this more indirect method of determining shunt patency.

CASE 201

History.— 18-year-old man with a basilar skull fracture and persistent rhinorrhea from a motorcycle accident.

Scan.—Multiple 1 cm square cotton pledgets attached to a string were placed in the nasal cavity. After the subarachnoid injection of 500 μCi of ^{111}In DTPA via a lumbar puncture, multiple images of the head in various projections were obtained at 60-minute intervals for 6 hours. The pledgets were removed at 6 hours (after arrival of the radioactive bolus to the basal cisterns) and counted in a well counter. A simultaneous 0.5 mL serum sample was obtained and also counted.

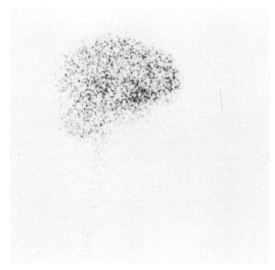

24-Hour right lateral view of head.

Findings.—Images: no evidence of a leak. Pledget/serum counts: left: high 1.0, middle 4.8, low 4.1; right: high 0.9, middle 0.8, low 1.0.

Diagnosis.—CSF rhinorrhea.

Rhinorrhea after head trauma may indicate the presence of a CSF leak or fistulous connection between the subarachnoid space and nasal cavity. The most common sites of a CSF leak after basilar skull fracture are the cribiform plate and ethmoid-sphenoid sinus areas. CSF otorrhea may occur if the fracture involves the temporal bone. CSF leaks can be difficult to diagnose because of their intermittent nature.

The radionuclide evaluation of CSF rhinorrhea is performed after injecting a radionuclide into the CSF space as in cisternography. Pledgets are placed high in each nostril (or in the external ear in cases of suspected CSF otorrhea) before radioisotope injection. At our institution this is usually done by otolaryngology, with three to four pledgets being placed on each side of the nasal cavity. The pledgets are numbered according to their location. ^{111}In DTPA is injected by lumbar puncture into the dural sac. The pledgets are removed 4 to 6 hours after isotope injection and counted in a well counter. Blood samples obtained at the same time are allowed to clot, and 0.5 mL samples of serum are also counted. This is done because as the ^{111}In DTPA is reabsorbed by the arachnoid granulations, it is distributed in the extracellular space. (It is excreted via glomerular filtration by the kidney.) Because of this, some radioactivity is expected in normal nasal secretions. In most patients with a CSF leak the pledget/serum ratio is greater than 1. It is also considered abnormal if there is marked asymmetry in the pledget counts from side to side.

Index

A

Abdomen, abscess in, 188
Abscess
  abdominal, 188
  hepatic, 197
  pelvic, 196
  splenic, 198
Achalasia, 133
Acquired immunodeficiency syndrome,
    Pneumocystis carinii pneumonia
    in, 187
Adenoma
  parathyroid, 18
    simulated, 19
  thyroid, 6, 8
Adriamycin cardiotoxicity, 78
AIDS, *Pneumocystis carinii* pneumonia
    in, 187
Alzheimer's disease, 227
Anemia, pernicious, 214
Aneurysm
  apical, 71
  of left ventricle, 80
  true vs. false, 80
Angina, unstable, 88
Angiography, radionuclide, in
    cerebrovascular studies, 225,
    230–231
Ankle cellulitis, 43
α_1-Antitrypsin deficiency, 177
Aortic graft infection, 200
Aortic regurgitation, with diminished
    left ventricular
    function, 77
Aortoenteric fistula, 203
Arterial graft infection, 200

Artifact
  on liver-spleen scan, 104
  on lung scan, 179
Asplenia, functional, 110
Asthma, bronchial, 171
Avascular necrosis, of hip, 39

B

Biello criteria, for V/Q scan
    interpretation, 169, 175
Bile duct obstruction, 117–118
  simulated, 119
Bilirubin, 111
Bleeding studies, gastrointestinal,
    122–125
Blood-brain barrier, 231
Blood pool imaging, 73
Bone disease, metabolic (*see* Metabolic
    bone disease)
Bone lesion, solitary, 25
Bone marrow, 208–209
  infarct, 207
Bone metastases
  compression fracture vs., 27
  of lumbar spine, 29
  from lung cancer, 34
  from prostate cancer, 26
  from renal cell carcinoma, 24–25,
    57
  of spine and ribs, 28
Bone scan
  hot and cold defects, 28
  for metastases, 29
  normal, 22–23
  phosphate agents, 23
  simulated lesions, 23

Bone tumors
  enchondroma, 41
  osteoid osteoma, 40–41
  osteosarcoma, 56
Brain death, 232
Brain scan, normal conventional,
    230–231
Brain SPECT studies, for epilepsy, 226
Brain tumors
  medulloblastoma, 228–229
  meningioma, 234
Breast carcinoma, lymph node
    localization after mastectomy,
    210–211
Breast-feeding, radioiodine uptake and,
    17
Bronchial asthma, 171
Bronchitis, chronic, 170–171
Bronchogenic carcinoma, 180
  soft tissue uptake of ^{99m}Tc in, 52
Budd-Chiari syndrome, 101

C

Captopril, renal scans and, 146–147
Cardiomyopathy, idiopathic, 79
Cardiotoxicity, 78
Cardiovascular system, 60–89
  apical thinning, normal, 61
  stress scan, normal, 60
Cardioversion injury, 86–87
Catheter placement, for liver cancer
    chemotherapy, 128
Causalgia, 36–37
Cellulitis, of ankle, 43
Cerebral artery ischemia, 224–225
Cerebral infarction, 223